Ventricular
Function

Edited by
David C. Warltier, MD, PhD

Professor of Anesthesiology, Cardiology and Pharmacology
Vice Chairman for Research, Department of Anesthesiology
Medical College of Wisconsin
Milwaukee, Wisconsin

With 16 contributors

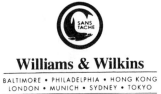

Williams & Wilkins

BALTIMORE • PHILADELPHIA • HONG KONG
LONDON • MUNICH • SYDNEY • TOKYO

A WAVERLY COMPANY

Ventricular Function

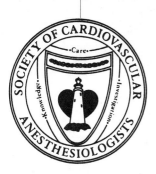

A Society of
Cardiovascular Anesthesiologists
Monograph

Copyright © 1995
SOCIETY OF CARDIOVASCULAR ANESTHESIOLOGISTS

Accurate indications, adverse reactions, and dosage schedules for drugs are provided in this
book, but it is possible that they may change. The reader is urged to review the package
information data of the manufacturers of the medications mentioned.

Printed in the United States of America
(ISBN 0-683-08794-0)

95 96 97 98
1 2 3 4 5 6 7 8 9 10

Contributors

Matthew J. A. Benson, MB, BS, FANZCA
Visiting Assistant Professor of Anesthesia
University of California, San Francisco
San Francisco, California

Michael K. Cahalan, MD
Professor of Anesthesia
University of California, San Francisco
San Francisco, California

Che-Ping Cheng, MD, PhD
Assistant Professor of Cardiology
Bowman Gray School of Medicine
Wake Forest University
Winston-Salem, North Carolina

Stefan G. De Hert, MD, PhD
Head of the Division of Cardiac Anesthesia
Department of Anesthesiology
University Hospital Antwerp
Edegem, Belgium

Douglas A. Hettrick, MS
Biomedical Engineer
Department of Anesthesiology
Medical College of Wisconsin
Milwaukee, Wisconsin

David A. Kass, MD
Associate Professor of Medicine and Biomedical Engineering
Division of Cardiology
Department of Internal Medicine
Johns Hopkins Medical Institutions
Baltimore, Maryland

William C. Little, MD
Professor of Medicine
Chief, Cardiology Section
Bowman Gray School of Medicine
Wake Forest University
Winston-Salem, North Carolina

Carl Lynch III, MD, PhD
Professor of Anesthesiology
University of Virginia Health Sciences Center
Charlottesville, Virginia

Dennis T. Mangano, PhD, MD
Professor of Anesthesia
Vice Chairman, Department of Anesthesia
University of California, San Francisco
San Francisco, California

Robert G. Merin, MD
Professor of Anesthesiology
Medical College of Georgia
Augusta, Georgia

Paul S. Pagel, MD, PhD
Assistant Professor of
 Anesthesiology
Medical College of Wisconsin
Milwaukee, Wisconsin

Kathryn Rouine-Rapp, MD
Assistant Professor of Anesthesia
University of California, San
 Francisco
San Francisco, California

Manfred D. Seeberger, MD
Visiting Assistant Professor of
 Anesthesia
University of California,
 San Francisco
San Francisco, California

Damon C. Sutton, MB, BS,
 FANZCA
Visiting Assistant Professor of
 Anesthesia
University of California,
 San Francisco
San Francisco, California

Arthur W. Wallace, MD, PhD
Assistant Professor of
 Anesthesiology
University of California,
 San Francisco
San Francisco, California

David C. Warltier, MD, PhD
Professor of Anesthesiology,
 Cardiology & Pharmacology
Vice Chairman for Research,
 Department of Anesthesiology
Medical College of Wisconsin
Milwaukee, Wisconsin

Contents

Preface

The objective of the 1995 Society of Cardiovascular Anesthesiologists Monograph is to provide the cardiac anesthesiologist with a primer on ventricular function covering a broad series of topics which extend from the biochemical and cellular biology of the myocyte to perioperative assessment of cardiac function. Over the last ten to fifteen years, a considerable number of discoveries have occurred on the molecular and cellular level revealing basic mechanisms of normal cardiac function and dysfunction coincident with a variety of cardiovascular diseases. Certainly, the role of the sarcoplasmic reticulum as a pivotal point in the regulation of contraction and relaxation has continued to evolve. New pharmacological agents for the treatment of heart failure are presently being developed as greater information about the mechanism of myocardial contraction and relaxation has become available. These agents possess different mechanisms of action as compared to presently available drugs and may offer important alternatives in the armamentarium of drugs for congestive heart failure. A greater awareness of the importance of diastole in overall ventricular performance has occurred. Cardiac function cannot be optimal without adequate diastolic filling, and, in fact, manifestations of many cardiac diseases can be related to abnormalities that occur only in diastole. Development of pharmacological agents used to improve cardiac performance must not only focus on increasing contractile function during systole but now must also consider effects occuring during diastole. New information concerning the molecular basis of remodeling of ventricular myocardium during disease states and the influence of neural and hormonal factors on the pathophysiology of ventricular function has grown exponentially. Even investigation of the anatomical ultrastructure of the cardiac muscle cell and cytoarchitecture of ventricular myocardium has brought forth a multitude of novel findings. A rather recent development has been the discovery that the endothelial lining of the cardiac chambers may significantly contribute to alterations in left ventricular function in both the normal and diseased heart.

The study of ventricular function in systole and diastole continues in experimental animals *in vitro* and *in vivo* by the use of pressure-dimension relations. Initially popularized by Professors Kiichi Sagawa and Hiroyuki Suga, these investigators led a group of physiologists in the reexploration of an old relationship initially studied by Otto Frank almost a century ago. The relationship of pressure and volume during the cardiac cycle allows for the precise determination of ventricular systolic and diastolic function, ventriculo-arterial interactions, myocardial efficiency and energetics, and alterations produced by drugs in the presence of regional or global cardiac disease. Techniques for the diagnosis of cardiovascular injury and subsequent therapeutic management have been extended to patient care from these initial experimental observations. The goal immediately on the horizon is to apply those methodologies that have been developed in the physiology laboratory over the last ten years to the study of ventricular function in humans. There is a major problem inherent in this jump from animal to human. Relatively invasive, instantaneous measurements of chamber pressure and dimension are required in order to provide accurate data regarding ventricular function. The information that can be acquired by determination of ventricular pressure and volume is substantial, but these methods of approach remain highly experimental and are, at present, confined to a few centers using the "conductance catheter" technique in the cardiac catheterization laboratory or in the operating room. New techniques such as on-line automated border detection or acoustic quantification *via* transesophageal echocardiography may offer a means whereby such procedures can be performed considerably less invasively in patients. Such approaches are increasing our understanding of not only the pathophysiology, progression, and chronic treatment of cardiac disease but also the acute effects of inotropic drugs and anesthetic agents. The purpose of this Monograph is to present this new knowledge in a concise format and, hopefully, to act as a stimulus to fill a void in our knowledge of the effects of anesthetic agents in patients with cardiac disease through the conduct of more definitive research.

I gratefully acknowledge the help of all the participating authors who have devoted their time and energies to the construction of a well-needed overview on ventricular function for anesthesiologists. The summary this work provides is up-to-date but only for an instant in time in the continuum of the study of ventricular function. It is important to realize that this area is still in evolution and information acquired today, including the advocation of certain technologies used to assess cardiac performance, will undoubtedly change over the next few years. Nevertheless, previously defined relationships between ventricular pressure and dimension will continue to form a basis for measurement of the effects of alterations occurring at the molecular and cellular level on the whole organism.

DAVID C. WARLTIER, MD, PHD
MEDICAL COLLEGE OF WISCONSIN

Ventricular Function

Carl Lynch III

The Biochemical and Cellular Basis of
1 Myocardial Contractility

Excitation-contraction (EC) coupling is the mechanism by which depolarization of the cell membrane activates contraction. The essence of the process involves regulation of the intracellular concentration of Ca^{2+} ($[Ca^{2+}]_i$) and its consequent modulation of the interaction of the contractile proteins (actin and myosin) which causes myocyte shortening and force development. The control of $[Ca^{2+}]_i$ is achieved via an intracellular compartment, the sarcoplasmic reticulum (SR), from which Ca^{2+} can be rapidly released and reaccumulated. The entry and efflux of extracellular Ca^{2+} across the surface membrane is responsible for triggering the release of Ca^{2+} as well as maintaining the quantity of Ca^{2+} in the SR. The Ca^{2+} fluxes are mediated via a variety of channels, exchangers, and pumps which are distributed in a highly regimented manner within the external and intracellular membranes, which are likewise exquisitely structured around the contractile proteins.

In contrast to skeletal muscle, in which the strength of contraction is controlled by the number of fibers activated by motor neurons, cardiac muscle is an electrical syncytium in which *all* cells are stimulated to contract under normal conditions. The strength of the cardiac contraction is instead controlled by the degree of activation of the myocytes, which is determined by the amount of activator Ca^{2+} and the length of the initial degree of sarcomere overlap. The entry of Ca^{2+} and Na^+ and their interaction via the Na-Ca exchange also mean that elec-

Ventricular Function, edited by David C. Warltier. Williams & Wilkins, Baltimore © 1995.

trophysiological behavior and EC coupling are highly integrated, interdependent functions. The varied tension generation that is observed with changes in cardiac volume (Starling's Law of the Heart[1]) or rate of beating (positive frequency staircase) results from two intrinsic characteristics of the myocardium: 1) variation in the myofibril Ca^{2+} sensitivity; and 2) alteration in the amount of activator Ca^{2+}. A variety of extrinsic factors, such as inotropic stimulation or ischemia, exert their effects by alterations in these intrinsic determinants of cardiac contractility. In addition to functional constraints determined by the fine subcellular structure, the Ca^{2+} fluxes, as well as the response by actin and myosin, are tightly modulated by regulation of the activity of various enzymes and transport proteins.

BASIC STRUCTURE OF THE CARDIAC MYOCYTE

Unlike skeletal muscle, which is composed of long, multinucleated fibers, atrial and ventricular muscle in mammals is composed of individual myocytes (mono- or binucleate). These cells are typically 80 to 150 μm in length with elliptical cross-sections of 5 to 15 × 20 to 30 μm (Fig. 1–1).[2] The myocytes are connected longitudinally end-to-end and also end-to-side, resulting in interconnected strands in which an average cardiac myocyte is electrically and mechanically connected to ~seven other myocytes.[3] Myocytes are coupled at intercalated discs, a complex interdigitation of membrane structures which maintain mechanical integrity via cytoskeletal membrane proteins such as vinculin and permit electrical continuity via transmembrane ion channels called connexons (or gap junctions).[4–6] Connexons in the heart are formed from six monomers of connexon 42 (molecular weight: 42 kilodalton (kD)), a member of a large family of gap junction-forming proteins. Two of the large homohexameric connexon hemichannels present in the membrane of adjacent cells become juxtaposed end-to-end to form a highly conductive channel between the cells. Previous work employing isolated myocytes has suggested that one effect of volatile anesthetics is to depress coupling between myocytes, particularly at higher anesthetic concentrations.[7,8] If individual myocytes become electrically isolated, they will not shorten and contribute to cardiac contraction; however, it is not known whether such cell uncoupling occurs either in intact tissue or is clinically significant.

The sarcomere is the basic functional unit of contraction in striated muscle and is remarkably similar in both skeletal and cardiac muscle. This subunit is a 2.0 to 2.5-μm segment in which an array of myosin filaments (1.55-μm long) is centered between the interdigitates with two arrays of actin filaments (1.15-μm long). At the Z-line, the ends of the actin filaments from adjacent sarcomeres meet and combine with a va-

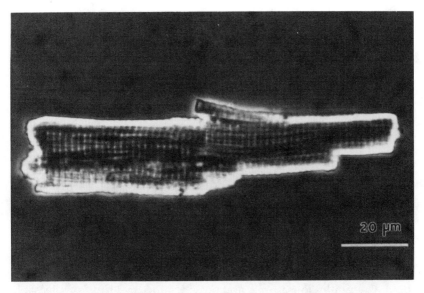

FIGURE 1-1. Phase contrast light micrograph of enzymatically isolated rat ventricular myocardial cell. Periodic banding pattern of myofibrils is evident secondary to the sarcomeric striations of the myofibrils (Fig. 1–2). The uneven contour of the cell is the result of myofibrils of different overall lengths and the formation of junctions with other myocytes along the length of the cell. *(Courtesy of Michael S. Forbes)*

riety of cytoskeletal proteins (α-actinin, talin, integrin) and anchor fibers. The surface membrane is linked to the Z-line by the structural protein vinculin. In addition, stretching between the Z-lines and running parallel to the actin and myosin filaments are long protein strands, which are composed of a very high molecular weight polypeptide called titin.[9] The actin and myosin filaments are also separated into bundles 0.5 to 1-μm in diameter (myofibrils), each containing 300 to 1000 filaments of each type. In addition, microtubules (tubulin) and longitudinally oriented intermediate filaments (primarily desmin) are also present in myocytes, partitioning them into quasi-compartments to prevent disruption of the complex intracellular architecture. These structural cellular components also increase the passive stiffness of the cardiac myocytes, at least in comparison with skeletal muscle.[10]

The surface membrane (plasmalemma) of the myocytes is a typical lipid bilayer containing the various receptors, transport proteins, and structural components. A cylindrical sheath enclosing the cell contents and structural proteins, it may be removed (chemically or mechanically) without disturbing the organized structure of sarcomeres, which can continue to function as long as they are bathed in solutions appropriate for the intracellular milieu. However, the plasmalemma and the closely adherent extracellular mucopolysaccharide basement membrane have a complex structure. At each Z-line, the sarcolemma forms tubular invaginations (0.1-μm diameter) called transverse tubules, or T-tubules, which create a network across the ventricular myocyte. T-tubules are critical for carrying the surface depolarization and providing Ca^{2+} entry to activate the myofibrils in the interior of the myocyte. Such structures are frequently not seen in small diameter atrial myocytes.

Each of the 10 to 70 myofibrils observed in a cross-section of a myocyte is surrounded by a membranous network, the sarcoplasmic reticulum (SR), the lumen of which contains a high concentration of Ca^{2+} (Fig. 1–2). The network of SR is juxtaposed to the T-tubules at the Z-line. The SR membrane which faces the T-tubules contains an array of highly specialized, very large homotetrameric protein complexes, the Ca release channels. These are responsible for controlling the release of Ca^{2+}, which activates tension development. This junctional SR is also characterized by a larger lumen which contains calsequestrin, a protein which binds Ca^{2+} with a low affinity and provides an extra "sink" of releasable Ca^{2+}. In addition to couplings with the T-tubules, the SR occasionally forms junctions with the surface membrane, another location where Ca^{2+} release may be activated. The functional structure here is similar to that usually found in smooth muscle. Free SR vesicles, or corbular SR, may also be found in mammalian myocytes.[2]

Myocytes require a large number of mitochondria because of the continuous high rate of energy consumption by the myocardium. A very high density of ATP-producing organelles is obviously critical in a continuously active tissue like the heart, in contrast with most types of skeletal muscle. Myocardial mitochondria frequently occupy 30 to 40% of the cell-volume, depending upon the species, and are organized in rows between the separate myofibrils. While this architecture provides a short diffusion distance between the sites of ATP production and utilization by the SR and myofibrils, it may present a partial diffusion barrier to other intracellular substances.[11]

The interconnected strands of myocytes are enmeshed in a thin network of collagen fibers and gathered into small interconnecting bundles which are also sheathed in connective tissue. While mechanical continuity within the myocytes is generated by the cytoskeletal proteins (talin, α-actinin, integrin, dystrophin, and titin), tissue-level structural organization and generation of macroscopic force by the heart is due to the microfibrils and extracellular lamina which connect the plasmalemma to the collagen matrix surrounding cell bundles. The connective tissue and collagen present in the extracellular space is 2 to 6% of muscle dry weight, far greater than that in skeletal muscle. While there do not appear to be any passive, noncontractile elements in series with the myocytes,[12] this extracellular matrix provides an important elastic component parallel to

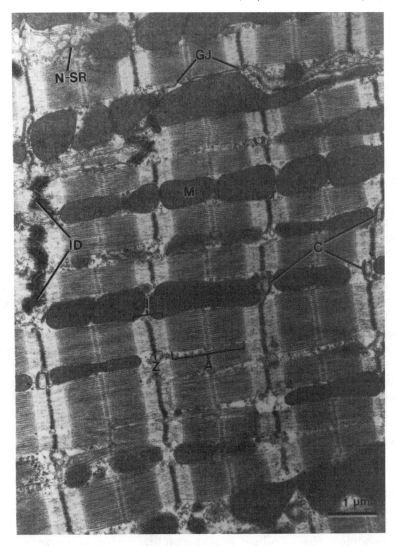

FIGURE 1-2. Transmission electron micrograph of a longitudinal thin section through rat ventricular myocardial cells. The bulk of each cell is occupied by the myofibrils, oriented along the long axis of each cell and exhibiting the characteristic banding pattern formed by the A-bands (where actin and myosin filaments overlap). I-bands (consisting primarily of actin filaments), and Z-lines (composed in large part of α-actinin) which bisect each I-band. At the end of myofibrils, specialized junctions (the intercalated discs (*ID*)) connect adjacent cells at the position Z-lines would occupy. Mitochondria (M) are arranged either in rows among the myofibrils or in clusters beneath the cell membrane, where they are frequently closely apposed to gap junctions (*GJ*). The membrane systems of myocardial cells include the sarcoplasmic reticulum (*SR*), most of which is in the form of tubular retes (network SR (N-SR)) on the surfaces of myofibrils. Continuous with the network SR are specialized flattened saccules of junctional SR (Fig. 1–6), which are apposed either to the surface sarcolemma or its tubular extensions, the transverse tubules, to form couplings (C), which frequently are located at the levels of the Z-lines. (*Courtesy of Michael S. Forbes*)

the contractile cellular elements, which can generate considerable passive tension when myocardium is stretched. In addition, the collagen fibers, endomysial mesh and struts which attach to the sarcolemma at the Z-line of myocytes, protect them from being overstretched and maintain the unloaded geometry of the left ventricle (LV).[13]

REGULATION OF INTRACELLULAR Ca^{2+}

The major determinant of myocardial contractility is the regulation of the amount of Ca^{2+} made available to activate during each beat of the heart. More myofilaments within a myocyte will be activated to generate tension when more Ca^{2+} is released. The amount and source of activator Ca^{2+} in the myoplasm surrounding the myofibrils in mammalian hearts are determined by an intermixture of Ca^{2+} entering from the extracellular milieu and Ca^{2+} released from the intracellular SR pool. Upon depolarization, Ca^{2+} enters the cell through the surface membrane, which triggers release of a far greater amount of Ca^{2+} from the SR store into the myoplasm. Since the extracellular and SR lumen have a free Ca^{2+} concentration of ~1 mM, versus a myoplasmic [Ca^{2+}] surrounding the myofibrils of 0.1 μM, Ca^{2+} flows passively down an enormous concentration (and electrical) gradient. Intracellular Ca^{2+} binds to the myofibrils to activate contraction, and relaxation ensues as Ca^{2+} is removed from the myoplasm. The majority of Ca^{2+} is taken up into the SR; however, an amount equal to that which entered the cells is transported outside the cell through the sarcolemma. In either case Ca^{2+} must be moved against a large concentration gradient, which requires the consumption of energy. The mixture of activator Ca^{2+} from the extracellular space and SR lumen varies according to such factors as age, species, heart rate, and temperature, all of which frequently differ in experimental studies.

In order to rapidly conduct an ion such as Ca^{2+} through the hydrophobic milieu of a lipid bilayer membrane, channel proteins, exchangers, and pumps must span the membrane. Recent molecular biological studies have permitted amino acid sequencing of a large number of the membrane proteins responsible for transporting Ca^{2+} through the membrane. These proteins either permit Ca^{2+} to flow down its electrochemical gradient (channels) or use an energy source to transport Ca^{2+} against the gradient (pumps and exchangers).

Cardiac Surface Membrane Calcium Channels

The voltage-gated surface membrane channel proteins are large, complex molecules which possess a similar structure among the major ion channel types.[14–26] Although they are typically composed of three or four different subunits, the central conducting region of both sodium (Na) and calcium (Ca) channels are similar large proteins composed of 2000 to 2500 amino acids, termed the α_1 subunit. A proposed structure for these channels is now generally accepted in which there are four major domains (I to IV), each formed from six hydrophobic transmembrane α-helical segments (Fig. 1–3.)[27–29] This similarity in structure may explain in part the fact that a number of drugs show only partial specificity for a particular channel. For example, both the phenylalkylamines (the verapamil family of drugs) and the dihydropyridines (nifedipine, nicardipine, etc.) can also block Na channels as well as Ca channels, al-

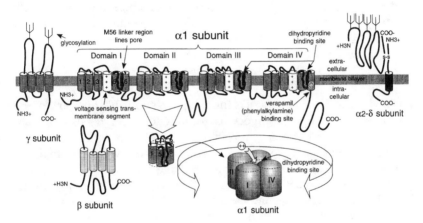

FIGURE 1-3. Structural model of the L-type Ca channel based upon amino acid sequence analysis. The $\alpha1$ subunit is composed of a sequence of 2171 amino acids in which 24 hydrophobic regions are hypothesized to form alphahelical transmembrane segments (indicated by the small cylinders).[16] As shown for domain II, the six transmembrane segments (S1 to S6) coalesce to form four domains (*I* to *IV*). The four domains gather as indicated to form a tetrameric structure with a central pore through which the ions pass. The pore itself appears to be lined by the extracellular linking segment between helix spans 5 and 6, which is thought to fold back into the pore so that the polar or negatively charged sites become available for binding by ions as they pass through the channel. The fourth transmembrane segment (S4) of each domain contains a number of positively charged amino acids (typically arginine) which can respond to the membrane voltage field, acting as a "voltage sensor" and inducing a conformational change which will permit ions to flow through the central pore.[28] It is at the junction between this region and S6 of domains III and IV that the dihydropyridines such as nifedipine appear to bind, while the diphenylalkylamines (e.g., verapamil) bind at the intracellular aspect of the α_1 subunit. Also shown in the figure are the other subunits which occur with the α_1 subunit. The β subunit, which appears to adjoin an intracellular aspect of the $\alpha1$ subunit, enhances channel opening and activation. The α_2-δ subunit also appears to modulate channel voltage responses, while the role of the γ subunit is unclear.

though not necessarily at clinical concentrations.[30–32] Likewise, local anesthetics as well as phenytoin can block Ca as well as Na channels.[33–35] Three additional subunits are typically present in Ca channels in addition to the major pore-forming α_1 subunit. Furthermore, the selective conductance of Ca^{2+} can be conferred on the Na channel by specific point mutations in the 5 to 6 linker region, which also determines how the ions bind as they pass through the center of the protein.[36]

Based on biophysical and pharmacological characteristics as well as cloning of channels, at least seven types of Ca channels are present in mammalian cells (three dihydropyridine-sensitive forms (cardiac, skeletal, and endocrine L-types), as well as T-, N-, R-, and P-types (? Q-type). Two forms of Ca channels have been described in cardiac myocytes; the distinction is based on the depolarization required to cause opening, the rate at which ions pass through (conductance), and their pharmacological sensitivity (Table 1–1).[37–39]

L-Type Ca Channel

The major cardiac Ca channel is the L-type, responsible for ≥90% of the Ca current in ventricular myocytes. Initially termed L for its long-lasting single channel opening, this channel requires a depolarization of the membrane potential more positive than -40 mV to activate opening, so they are also designated high-voltage activated (HVA). The L-type channels are also highly sensitive to dihydropyridine drugs (nifedipine, nicardipine, Bay k 8644). In addition to the cardiac L-type channel which is also present in vascular smooth muscle, distinct dihydropyridine-sensitive L-type channels are also present in endocrine tissue and in skeletal muscle. These channels serve as voltage sensors to activate Ca^{2+} release from the SR in skeletal muscle.[19] The L-type channel is the best characterized of all Ca channels. The primary amino acid structure of the various subtypes and subunits is clearly defined, providing the postulated secondary and tertiary structure shown in Figure 1–3.[19,40] The cloning of the genes for the various subunits has permitted the expression of each of the protein subunits alone or in combination, typically in *Xenopus* oocytes which normally possess no such channels. These additional peptides are usually smaller than the α_1 subunit; however, in certain instances their presence is required for the α_1 subunit to act as a channel. In the case of the Ca channel, the β and $\alpha_2\delta$ subunit make the channel behave in a more physiological fashion.[41]

Ionic Effects

Ca^{2+} normally binds quite tightly within the pore when passing through the L-type Ca channel actually preventing other ions from en-

TABLE 1–1. CHARACTERISTICS OF L- AND T-TYPE CA CHANNELS IN CARDIAC TISSUE

Characteristic	L-type Channel	T-type Channel
Voltage dependence (threshold)	< -40 mV (high-voltage activated, HVA)	< -70 mV (low-voltage activated, LVA)
Kinetics	Slow, voltage-dependent inactivation in the absence of Ca^{2+}, more rapid Ca^{2+} dependent inactivation	Rapid inactivation, Ca^{2+}-independent Persisting inactivation leading to increased inhibition at high-stimulation frequencies
Conductance (in 10 mM Ba^{2+}	25 pS (~9,000 ions/msec at 0 mV)	8 pS (~3,000 ions/msec at 0 mV)
Ion selectivity	$Ba^{2+} > Ca^{2+}$ (2X) Blocked by $Cd^{2+} > Ni^{2+}$	$Ba^{2+} = Ca^{2+}$ Blocked by $Ni^{2+} = Cd^{2+}$
Pharmacological sensitivity	Dihydropyridines inhibit or potentiate (e.g., Bay k 8644) Frequency-dependent blockade by phenyl-alkylamine (e.g., vera-pamil) and benzothiaze-pines (e.g., diltiazem)	?Blocked by amilo-ride (also blocks Na^+/H^+ antiport) ?Tetramethrin
Density and distribution	1–5 channels/μm^2 >90% of Ca current in ventricular myocytes	0.1–0.3 channels/μm^2 Absent in calf and rabbit myocardium, rat ventricle Possibly >50% of Ca current in pacemaking tissues
Modulation	Highly sensitive to phos-phorylation by cAMP- and Ca-calmodulin-dependent protein kin-ase, and possibly protein kinase C.	?Modest effect of β-adrenergic stimulation Minimal Ca^{2+} potentiat-ing effect

(Adapted from McDonald TF et al. Physiol Rev 74:365–507, 1994)

tering. When Ca^{2+} is reduced to very low levels (<1 μM) in the medium, L-type channels will actually pass Na^+ at a very high rate, generating a far greater current than observed when Ca^{2+} is present. Ba^{2+} does not bind in the channel as tightly. When substituted in an equal concentration for Ca^{2+}, channel conductance (rate of ion passage) with Ba^{2+} is approximately twice as great, a fact that also separates L-type from certain other Ca channel. Mixtures of Ca^{2+} and Ba^{2+} lead to surprisingly small currents (the "anomalous mole fraction effect"), which has led to specific models of binding within the channel pore. Although Mg^{2+} is frequently described as a Ca channel blocker, it actually has very little blocking action. Its ability to decrease Ca^{2+} entry into cells via Ca channels is probably related to its action to reduce the Ca^{2+} concentration electrostatically attracted to the membrane surface, providing fewer Ca^{2+} in the vicinity of the channel mouth. Transition metal ions bind even more tightly than Ca^{2+} and block the Ca channel: Mn^{2+} passes very slowly, partially blocking the channel[42]; La^{3+} or Cd^{2+} block the channel at 1 to 100 μM.[43] Ni^{2+}, like Mn^{2+}, passes slowly through the L-type channel while having a far greater blocking action on T-type channels.

Channel Gating and Modulation

Single L-type channels exhibit a complex pattern of opening and closing, which is responsible for the time-dependent changes (kinetics) observed in the Ca^{2+} currents of whole myocytes (Fig. 1–4). There is a variable delay before channels open following membrane depolarization, and most models of the molecular behavior suggest that the channel molecule undergoes a number of molecular rearrangements before finally assuming an open configuration. While the open state typically lasts for only 0.6 msec, the channel can close and then reopen a number of times before inactivating. The sum of individual currents through a large number of such channels in a myocyte can generate the long-lasting inward current. Some channels may not open at all in response to depolarization, while other channels remain open for a far more sustained period.[44] While such channels are clearly L-type, their gating appears to be governed by somewhat different operational rules. These non-opening, short-opening and long-opening behaviors have been termed modes 0, 1, and 2, respectively. The intrinsic behavior of the Ca channels is in large part controlled by the phosphorylation of the amino acids, primarily on the α_1 subunit. Such phosphorylation by cAMP-dependent protein kinase, activated by β-adrenoceptor stimulation, leads to distinct behavioral changes, as if the L-type channel shifted from mode 0 and 1 to mode 2, with far longer open times, and consequently far greater Ca^{2+} current.[45]

In addition to its binding within the Ca channel pore, the Ca^{2+} ion itself plays a complex role in modulating L-type channel function, causing both inactivation as well as facilitation. In many studies in which Ba^{2+} is used as the charge-carrying ion or in which intracellular Ca^{2+} is heavily buffered, the Ca^{2+} currents observed may not reflect the inactivation of the channel more likely to occur in physiological settings (Fig. 1–4B). In these studies, facilitation is also not observed.[46,47] Chemically caged Ca^{2+} was freed at the intracellular surface by a photolytic light flash to explore these opposing mechanisms.[48] The results were consistent with a model in which a fraction of Ca^{2+} binds to a site (separate from those in the pore) on the open channel to inactivate it.[48] A component of Ca^{2+}-mediated potentiation is also present which seems to re-

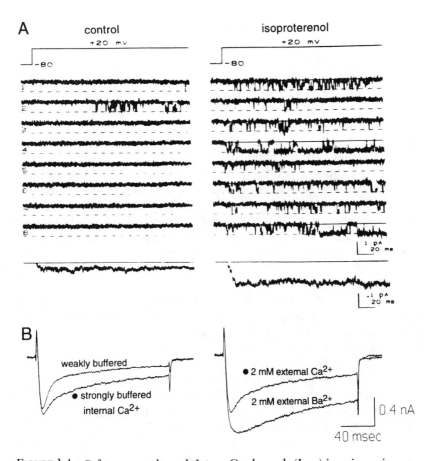

FIGURE 1-4. Ca^{2+} currents through L-type Ca channels ($I_{Ca,L}$) in guinea pig ventricular myocytes, demonstrating short- or long-opening modes of gating (A) and
Ca^{2+} dependent inactivation (B). Inward current is a downward deflection. (A)
Single channel recordings of single L-type channels from a patch of myocyte
membrane containing two channels which was depolarized from -80 to $^+20$ mV
(*dashed line* represents single open-channel current). The lowest tracing in each
panel shows the average response from 200 to 300 sweeps. (*Left*) Normal brief
openings (mode 1) or absent responses (mode 0). (*Right*) longer sustained channel openings typical of mode 2 gating observed with β-adrenergic stimulation.
(*Reproduced with permission from, Yue DT et al. Proc Natl Acad Sci USA*
87:753–757, 1990) (B) Whole cell Ca^{2+} currents observed in response to a depolarization from -80 to 0 mV (corrected for capacitance and leakage currents).
Na^+ currents were blocked by 10 μM tetrodotoxin, and K^+ currents were blocked
by 20 mM TEA$^+$ and 120 mM Cs$^+$. (*Left*) More rapid rate of inactivation of $I_{Ca,L}$
when myoplasmic Ca^{2+} is weakly buffered with 0.5 mM EGTA in the pipette vs
more strongly buffered with 10 mM EGTA (●). (*Right*) Currents observed in 2
mM external Ca^{2+} (●, same cell as in A), and subsequently with substitution of 2
mM Ba^{2+} for Ca^{2+} in the same cell. In spite of strongly buffering intracellular
Ca^{2+} with 10 mM EGTA ([Ca^{2+}]$_i$<0.05 μM), the $I_{Ca,L}$ showed some inactivation
when carried by Ca^{2+} compared with Ba^{2+} current. (*Courtesy of Pancrazio JJ and
Lynch C, unpublished results.*)

quire ATP or a nonhydrolyzable analog, suggesting a direct modulation by the Ca-nucleotide complex. A similar mechanism has also been described with Mg^{2+}-nucleotide chelates.[49] There may also be a component due to Ca-calmodulin-dependent protein kinase (CaMK II), which may have an important role in Ca^{2+}-dependent potentiation of $I_{Ca,L}$.[50] An important feature contributing to Ca^{2+} regulation may be the clustering of Ca channels, since the entering Ca^{2+} can achieve higher local concentrations when a number of channels are aggregated,[51] thereby enhancing potentiation and/or inactivation. Increased Ca^{2+} accumulation appears to activate a greater degree of channel opening with the clustering of channels.[51] While the Ca^{2+}-dependent inactivation is an important process, there is also an inherent voltage-dependent inactivation of Ca channels, which also causes channel time-dependent turnoff of current.[52] Both processes probably contribute to normal inactivation under physiological conditions.

Pharmacology

Gene cloning has also permitted selective modification of the amino acid sequence to actually determine which parts of the protein bind to certain drugs. Catterall and coworkers using this technique have demonstrated in an elegant series of modifications of the channel that the binding site for dihydropyridine calcium antagonists is in domain III at the external pore mouth.[29,53] Binding can either inhibit channel opening or cause channels to remain open longer depending upon the structure of the particular dihydropyridine. For example, the dihydropyridine compound Bay k 8644 is closely related to the structure of nifedipine but is a calcium agonist. This agent causes the channel to assume mode 2 gating, in which the channel stays open for a longer time. This results in larger Ca^{2+} currents and entry into the cell[54] and a positive inotropic action in intact myocardium. Such results suggest that dihydropyridines do not directly block the channel but rather modulate the channel's conformational change in response to the voltage change. This molecular evidence fits with results demonstrating that dihydropyridines act from an extracellular location.[55] In contrast, the phenylalkylamines act intracellularly,[56] and the binding site for verapamil is at the internal Ca channel pore mouth on the pore lining S5-S6 linker. Verapamil shows a clear frequency-dependent blockade of Ca channels and appears to more clearly occlude the pore, behaving as a local anesthetic for Ca channels.

T-Type Ca Channel

The T-type, in contrast to the L-type channel is activated by a smaller depolarization to less positive membrane potentials (hence low-voltage activated, or LVA). It also has a lower conductance and generates a more transient current (hence the T designation).[37–39,57] T-type channel inactivation occurs even with heavy Ca^{2+} buffering, suggesting that Ca^{2+} does not contribute prominently to this process. Little is known regarding details of T-type channel structure and function. The channel has not yet been isolated or cloned, nor has a highly specific blocking agent or toxin been delineated. In ventricular myocytes, T-type channels are responsible for a modicum of I_{Ca}, probably less than 10%. Although Ca^{2+} entry through this channel may be sufficient to activate release of Ca^{2+} from the SR, its seems unlikely that it contributes significantly to normal activation. T-type channels constitute a greater proportion of channels in Purkinje fibers and may play a role in diastolic depolarization, as postulated in sinoatrial and atrioventricular nodes.

The SR

As in skeletal muscle, in mammalian myocardium the Ca^{2+} that activates myofibrils is primarily derived from the SR that envelops each myofibril. An important feature in each type of muscle is the very large tetrameric channel located at the couplings between the T-tubules and the SR. The high affinity of the plant alkaloid (and insecticide) ryanodine has permitted isolation of these channels, also termed ryanodine receptors, and the cloning of the genetic substrate for three different forms. The regulation of these channels has also been widely investigated using ryanodine, which binds to the channels when they assume an open configuration.

The Ca Release Channel

Each Ca release channel (CaRC) is a homotetramer, composed of four monomers arranged with a rosette or quatrefoil symmetry.[58–60] Each monomer is thought to have transmembrane domains which extend to the SR lumen and a very prominent cytoplasmic domain on the N-terminus (Fig. 1–5A). The cytoplasmic domains occupy space between the SR membrane and the T-tubular membrane and are sufficiently large that they are seen in micrographs as the electron-dense "foot" structures which bridge between the adjacent membranes (Fig. 1–6A). This cytoplasmic domain may contain an internal channel, as well as the various binding sites for Ca^{2+}, ATP, anthraquinones, and other drugs which regulate the opening of this channel. Of the three CaRC isoforms isolated by molecular genetic techniques,[59–65] the cardiac isoform is designated RYR2 (for ryanodine receptor) and

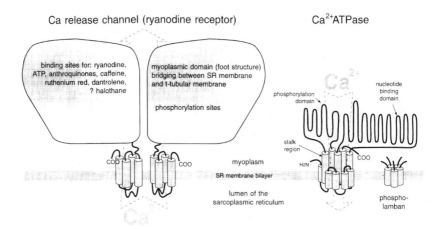

FIGURE 1-5. Proposed structure of the cardiac Ca release channels (CaRC, ryanodine receptor) and of the Ca^{2+}-ATPase of cardiac SR. (*Left*) Two of the four monomers (each containing ~5000 amino acids) which compose the CaRC are shown, the four subunits being arranged in a radially symmetrical pattern around a central axis (?pore). Based on the hydrophobic nature of the amino acids, four transmembrane helices have been proposed,[347] although other investigators have suggested 10 or 12 such helical regions.[62] (*Right*) The SR Ca^{2+}-ATPase (SERCA) composed of ~1000 amino acids has five extended transmembrane helical domains, which form a stalk region to two large cytoplasmic domains.[90] Phosphorylation by ATP and subsequent dephosphorylation generates changes in the configuration of the protein so that two Ca^{2+} which bind from the myoplasm in the transmembrane region are released into the SR lumen. Phospholamban is a small pentameric transmembrane protein which in its dephosphorylated form inhibits the activity of the SERCA. It may also behave as a Ca^{2+}-conducting channel, although its physiological role is unclear.

is also present in the brain. RYR1, the first described,[62,63] is present in skeletal muscle, while RYR3 is present in brain and smooth muscle.[65] The cardiac CaRC isoform is structurally very similar to RYR1 but has 63 fewer amino acids and has 66% amino acid identity.[64] Each of the monomers is composed of ~5000 amino acids, over twice the size of the entire α_1-subunit of the L-type plasmalemmal Ca channel. The total weight of the tetrameric CaRC complex is over 2,000 kD. These channels have been incorporated into artificial bilayers and have a very single high-channel conductance, capable of permitting a high rate of Ca^{2+} efflux from the SR lumen. However, like the L-type Ca channel, Ca^{2+} selectivity arises from a tighter binding of the ion as it passes through the channel. Monovalent ions pass through more rapidly, and the pore is of sufficient magnitude to permit small sugar molecules to pass.[60]

After opening, ryanodine binds tightly, which causes the channel to remain open but with a conductance less than half of the control value. By blocking the CaRCs open, ryanodine causes loss of Ca^{2+} from the SR, resulting in marked depression of cardiac contractions. Using single-channel studies or ryanodine binding to define open channels, the gating and conductance states of both skeletal and cardiac muscle CaRC have been extensively investigated.

Ca^{2+}-Induced Ca^{2+} Release

In skeletal muscle entry of Ca^{2+} is not the physiological activator of CaRC opening, but rather a specialized and truncated L-type Ca channel (class S) located in the T-tubules appears to be directly coupled to CaRCs. The voltage-induced conformational change in the L-type Ca channel is transmitted via an intracellular loop to the CaRC, which then opens to permit Ca^{2+} efflux from the SR into the myoplasm. Although the skeletal muscle CaRC (RYR1) can be activated by Ca^{2+}, no entry of extracellular Ca^{2+} is actually required. In cardiac tissue, the CaRC (RYR2) requires entry of Ca^{2+} to be activated. The cardiac L-type channel does not undergo structural change to activate CaRCs.[66,67] The cardiac CaRC does not appear to be inactivated by high $[Ca^{2+}]$, at least at the single-channel level incorporated into artificial bilayers.[68]

Some fraction of entering Ca^{2+} may bind to troponin C to activate contractions, but, in large, the Ca^{2+} which enters by the plasmalemmal L-type Ca^{2+} channels is insufficient by itself to activate the myofibrils directly. Its primary function is to bind to receptors on the CaRC to activate opening and release of SR Ca^{2+}, a process termed Ca^{2+}-induced Ca^{2+} release (CICR).[69] Because the CaRC has a very high single-channel conductance (about 10 times greater than the L-type Ca channel) the stored Ca^{2+} rapidly enters the myoplasm to bind to troponin C. Since each myofibril is typically less than 1 μm in diameter, and each half sarcomere is less than 1.2 μm long, the distance over which Ca^{2+} must diffuse from the junctional SR during activation is very short, so that the time dependence of this process is minimal. The activated Ca^{2+} release is detectable as a transient increase in intracellular Ca^{2+} which precedes tension development, representing a transient excess in myoplasm until the Ca^{2+} binds to troponin on the actin filament.

While CICR from the SR now seems well established,[70,71] the question remains as to its exact control. A positive feedback loop would be anticipated because the Ca^{2+} entry stimulates Ca^{2+} release. That is, once Ca^{2+} flux from a CaRC was initiated, all CaRCs in the vicinity would be activated.[70,72] This would result in a release of all of the SR Ca^{2+} store.

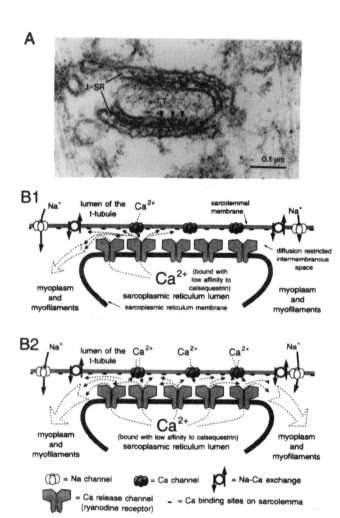

FIGURE 1-6. Coupling between the T-tubule and SR of a cardiac myocyte. (A)
High-magnification electron micrograph of a myocardial coupling in a rat ventricular cell. The internal membrane component is the junctional SR (*J–SR*),
characteristically flattened and containing dense granular material within the lumen (in part calsequestrin). In the cleft between junctional SR and a transverse
tubule (*TT*) there appear periodically spaced opaque structures known as "SR
feet" or "junctional processes" (*arrowheads*), which are the Ca^{2+} release channels
(CaRC, ryanodine receptors) that open to release sequestered Ca^{2+} from the SR
lumen. (*Courtesy of Michael S. Forbes*) (B) Cardiac tissue demonstrates a graded
release of Ca^{2+} from the SR store, in spite of the fact that the Ca release channels
(Ca RC) are Ca^{2+} activated. This effect may in part be explained by the diffusion-
restricted space created by the junctional cleft between the cytoplasmic faces of
the T-tubule and JSR membranes, indicated schematically. (*B1*) With small de-
polarizations or partial Ca^{2+} channel blockade, some CaRCs are activated. How-

However, there instead appears to be a finely graded release, with the quantity of Ca^{2+} released dependent upon the amount of entering Ca^{2+}. Between the T-tubule, where Ca^{2+} enters, and the opposed SR membrane containing CaRC there is restricted diffusion or "fuzzy" space.[70,73,74] This region may be of critical importance in regulation of CICR and the graded release which appears to occur with Ca^{2+} entry. An appropriately graded response can be provided by local control models which depend upon Ca^{2+} gradients in the neighborhood of a channel: a "calcium synapse" in which Ca^{2+} entry through an L-type channel activates a single CaRC and a "cluster bomb" model in which a small group of CaRC can be activated together. There currently is no definitive answer, but these models can at least demonstrate the graded behavior observed experimentally when local domains of Ca^{2+} are permitted, as shown in Figure 1–6B. Low affinity sites on the sarcolemmal membrane and Na-Ca exchange may also contribute to buffering of Ca^{2+} release[75,76] and muting the response of nearby CaRCs. A purely descriptive model has also been proposed by Callewaert.[77] While massive activation of release occurs during each beat, in quiescent cells the spontaneous opening of a single CaRC may result in a localized "spark" of Ca^{2+},[78] which does not go on to cause a regenerative release of a large quantity of Ca^{2+}.

Channel Modulation and Drug Effects
The cardiac CaRC also appears to be more readily phosphorylated than the skeletal muscle isoform by protein kinase A (cyclic AMP-dependent) and Ca^{2+}-calmodulin-dependent kinases.[79] Such phosphorylation provides an additional modulatory mechanism which is associated with increased channel opening.[80] It may also explain how perfusion of hearts with decreased or increased extracellular Ca^{2+} (0.2 to 5.6 mM) caused a subsequent down- or up-regulation of CaRC Ca^{2+} flux, respectively, which was maintained when SR was subsequently isolated.[81]

A variety of drugs also may play modulatory roles. The best example is the effect of caffeine, which in pharmacological concentrations (1 to 25 mM) is widely used to "empty" Ca^{2+} stores from various tissues, a process mediated by opening of the CaRC.[82] More clinically rel-

---

ever, because of the low-affinity binding sites on the sarcolemma or prolonged exposure to Ca^{2+}, the Ca^{2+} released from the CaRC is not sufficient to activate all surrounding CaRCs. (B2) With more profound Ca^{2+} entry into the intermembranous space, most or all of the CaRCs will be activated, resulting in complete release of SR Ca^{2+}. Calculations suggest that in this space $[Ca^{2+}]$ may rise to 100 to 500 μM.[76,348]

evant are the anthroquinone antineoplastic drugs that induce CaRC opening,[83,84] a process which may contribute to the cardiomyopathy associated with these agents. The immunosuppressant drug FK506 binds to a specific protein which is closely associated with the CaRC, although its physiological function is unclear.[85]

The Sarcoplasmic/Endoplasmic Reticulum Ca^{2+}-ATPase (SERCA)

Critical to relaxation within mammalian heart is the ability to decrease the Ca^{2+} concentration well below the threshold (near 0.10 μM) at which it activates contraction. In the normally working heart, the bulk of this role is usually carried out by the SR Ca pump, which is responsible for reaccumulating all of the released Ca^{2+} back into the SR lumen. The cardiac SR Ca^{2+}-ATPase is one of three isoforms of intracellular Ca pumps or SERCAs which are expressed on the intracellular membranes of a wide variety of cells.[86] The cardiac Ca^{2+}-ATPase (SERCA2) is a 105-kD protein composed of 997 amino acids and is also the isoform expressed in slow skeletal muscle.[87,88] As typical of membrane transport proteins, this protein has hydrophobic regions representing probably intramembranous helices (Fig. 1–5B), and it is within these structures that ions are thought to bind and translocate. The bulk of the protein is not present in the 10 membrane domains but is instead located in the myoplasmic domains. These include an ATP-binding region, as well as regions which modulate function.

The cycle by which Ca^{2+} is translocated involves an initial binding of two Ca^{2+} from the myoplasmic side to a site within the transmembrane region when the protein is in its high-affinity state (E_1) ($K_M \sim 0.2$ μM, which is the [Ca^{2+}] for 50% binding). ATP then phosphorylates an aspartate residue in the myoplasmic domain ($2Ca \bullet E_1P$). The protein subsequently undergoes a conformational change ($2Ca \bullet E_2P$) in which Ca^{2+} affinity is decreased while the binding site becomes exposed to the luminal side. The protein (E_2P) dephosphorylates and resumes the conformation in which the low-affinity site is exposed on the myoplasmic side after Ca^{2+} diffuses off of the protein into the lumen. As a consequence, 1 ATP is hydrolyzed to transfer 2 Ca^{2+} into the SR lumen (coupling ratio of 2).[89,90]

The primary means by which cardiac Ca^{2+}-ATPase activity is modulated occurs by regulation of the number of active ATPase molecules. Phospholamban is a homopentameric protein[91] (each monomer having 52 amino acids[92]) which in its unphosphorylated state binds to and inhibits SERCA2, thereby reducing the rate of Ca^{2+} accumulation into the

SR. When the protein kinases become activated and phosphorylate phospholamban, its inhibitory action on Ca^{2+}-ATPase ceases.[93]

After its initial release from the SR, Ca^{2+} binds to the regulatory troponin-tropomyosin complex which actually regulates myosin-actin interaction. Ca^{2+} will dissociate from troponin and can either rebind, continuing to activate the myosin-actin interaction, or bind to the higher affinity Ca^{2+} binding sites on the SERCA. Ca^{2+} binds to the ATPase because of the dense distribution of the ATPase on the longitudinal (or network) SR which surrounds the length of the myofibrils, and because it has a higher affinity for Ca^{2+} than the Ca^{2+} binding troponin subunit (TnC, $K_M = 0.5$ μM Ca^{2+}).[94] Ca^{2+} is translocated into the SR lumen after binding to the ATPase and is unavailable for the rest of that contraction. From its location in the longitudinal SR, it diffuses to the junctional SR which contains the CaRCs.

The SERCAs are specifically inhibited by the terpenoid drug thapsigargin,[95] which completely eliminates the twitch response in isolated myocytes by preventing uptake of Ca^{2+} into SR, ultimately resulting in its depletion.[96,97] Curiously, the effect of thapsigargin or cyclopiazonic acid, another SERCA inhibitor, is far more limited in intact muscle.[98]

Calsequestrin

Another important constituent of the SR is the 45-kD protein calsequestrin, which binds up to 40 Ca^{2+} per molecule and is about half-saturated at ~500 μM Ca^{2+}.[99,100] Of the 391 amino acids which compose the cardiac isoform of this protein, 109 are negatively charged to provide the multiple binding sites for Ca^{2+}.[100] Such low-affinity binding reduces the effective [Ca^{2+}] within the SR lumen from 1 to 5 mM down to 0.1 to 0.5 μM, so that the gradient against which the SR Ca^{2+} ATPase has to pump is considerably reduced, yet at the same time permits rapid mobilization and efflux from the SR when the CaRCs open. In addition to calsequestrin, a protein called triadin has been identified in skeletal junctional SR which may coordinate release between the CaRC and calsequestrin.[101–103] Its possible role in cardiac muscle activity remains undefined.

Removal of Ca^{2+} from the Myocyte

Although Ca^{2+} entry via Ca channels is insufficient by itself to activate a normal contraction, a substantial influx of Ca^{2+} does enter with each depolarization, which must be eliminated from the myocyte during steady-state beating to prevent overloading of Ca^{2+}. The system primarily responsible is the Na-Ca exchanger,[104,105] which employs an entry of 3 Na$^+$ to eliminate a Ca^{2+}, although supplemental elimination of Ca^{2+} does occur via a sarcolemmal Ca^{2+} pump.

The Na-Ca Exchanger

The Na-Ca exchanger of the myocardium is a 108-kD, 970 amino acid protein present in the plasmalemma.[106] The Na-Ca exchanger has a number of hydrophobic regions previously described for other ion transport proteins. Twelve helical transmembrane domains have been proposed, with a large cytoplasmic domain located between the sixth and seventh transmembrane domains.[106] The exchanger does not consume ATP as do the ion ATPases ("pumps") but rather employs the potential energy in the Na$^+$ gradient to translocate Ca^{2+} against its gradient in a process which is reversible.[107,108]

Critical to its behavior is the fact that the exchanger is electrogenic, that is, 3 Na$^+$ exchange for 1 Ca^{2+}. Thus there is a net transfer of 1 charge *into* the cell for 1 Ca^{2+} moved *out* of the cell (or vice versa). The Ca^{2+} flux is measurable as a current (I_{NaCa}) in the opposite direction.[109] Furthermore, the membrane potential can greatly alter the amplitude of the Ca^{2+} flux, as well as its direction. The membrane potential at which the Ca^{2+} flux reverses ($E_{rev,Na-Ca}$) is given by: $E_{rev,Na-Ca} = 3 \bullet E_{Na} - 2 \bullet E_{Ca}$, where E_{Na} and E_{Ca} are the Na$^+$ and Ca^{2+} equilibrium potentials defined by the Nerst equation.[110] For example, 3 Na$^+$ enter the cell down their 10-fold gradient (E_{Na} ~+60 mV) through the exchanger and are able to move 1 Ca^{2+} against its 10,000-fold gradient (E_{Ca} ~+120 mV) when the membrane potential is negative to −60 mV. This can occur during rest since the normal resting potential is < −80 mV. During the peak of an action potential when the potential increases to +40 mV, the exchanger reverses direction and mediates Ca^{2+} entry (and an outward I_{NaCa}), augmenting entry via the L-type Ca channel. Such entry declines sharply after Ca^{2+} release and the entry has raised [Ca^{2+}] to ~1 μM and made $E_{rev,Na-Ca}>0$ mV.[111] Ca^{2+} entry via the exchanger is clearly sufficient to activate Ca^{2+} release from the SR[112,113] and may also serve to load the SR stores.[114] While a large Na$^+$ gradient is required to eliminate Ca^{2+} during diastole, too large a gradient may prevent Ca^{2+} entry by this pathway during the peak of the action potential.[115] Calculations suggest that the exchanger may contribute as much as 65% of the entering Ca^{2+} which triggers release from the SR,[115] but there is disagreement as to whether such reversed Ca^{2+} flow into the myocyte has physiological relevance.[71,113] It is unclear whether Na$^+$ enters and accumulates in a "fuzzy" subsarcolemmal space, decreasing its gradient and thereby inducing greater exchanger-mediated Ca^{2+} entry.[116,117]

Nevertheless, an accepted corollary to exchanger function is that when Ca^{2+} is released from internal stores during rest, there is a net inward I_{NaCa} as 3 Na^+ enter to remove each Ca^{2+} released. Such release from the SR may be induced by caffeine,[118] or it can be spontaneous in situations of Ca^{2+} overload.[119] The resulting transient inward current can reach the action potential threshold and may account for triggered dysrhythmias under a variety of settings.[120] When Ca^{2+} is released during an action potential and active Ca^{2+} release, the action potential plateau and $E_{rev,Na-Ca}$ are closer in value, with a smaller resulting I_{NaCa}.

Obviously, the Na+ gradient that is maintained by the Na^+, $K^+ - ATPase$ ("Na pump") is critical to eliminating Ca^{2+}. The Na pump is also electrogenic, normally pumping 3 Na^+ out and 2 K^+ into the cell, employing energy derived from ATP hydrolysis.[121] Although not directly coupled, between the exchanger and the Na pump, 1 ATP is consumed to "pump" 1 Ca^{2+} out (and 2 K^+ in). The Na pump is also required to eliminate the Na^+ which enters via Na channels as well as that which enters by the exchanger.

The Plasma Membrane Ca²⁺-ATPase (PMCA)

Ca^{2+} can also be eliminated from the myocyte via a Ca^{2+} ATPase (Ca pump) located in the surface plasma membrane (PMCA). Four distinct isoforms of PMCAs have been described with at least one form present in most cell types, and these are particularly important in tissues such as erythrocytes which contain no Na-Ca exchanger. These proteins are vanadate-inhibited and are similar in basic conformational structure to the SERCAs. Distinct differences from SERCAs include a lower apparent coupling ratio (1 Ca: 1 ATP) and distinctly different modulatory pathways. PMCAs contain a specific binding site for Ca^{2+}-calmodulin, which is a prominent regulatory mechanism.[122] In addition, acidic phospholipids can enhance the turnover rate of the pump, as can phosphorylation by protein kinases.[122] The PMCA has a low capacity and does not contribute substantially to myoplasmic Ca^{2+} removal under normal settings.[74,123] It is likely that <1% of activator Ca^{2+} is eliminated by this pathway because on any cardiac beat <10% of the Ca^{2+} increase is due to Ca^{2+} influx and >90% (and possibly all) of entering Ca^{2+} is eliminated by the Na-Ca exchanger.[104,109]

Continuous Ca²⁺ Circulation and Rate Dependence

There is little change in the ability of skeletal muscle (which remains inactive) to generate tension with a depolarization, since the internal store of Ca^{2+} which binds to the myofibrils to activate contraction is readily available after long periods of rest. This behavior is in sharp contrast to the contractility of myocardium of most mammalian species, which shows an exponential decline with rest (rat myocardium is an important exception). Unlike skeletal muscle in which the SR tightly retains Ca^{2+}, the Ca^{2+} activating cardiac myofibrils undergoes active exchange across the sarcolemma. Fetal and neonatal mammalian myocardium is similar to frog heart in having a far less developed SR structure and function. Thus, immature myocardium relies far more on extracellular Ca^{2+} entry, by both the Ca channel and Na-Ca exchanger, for contraction.[124] Adult myocardium relies primarily on the SR to supply the activator Ca^{2+}, although that store can be rapidly depleted.

Effects of Rest

During inactivity, Ca^{2+} is eliminated from cardiac SR Ca^{2+} stores, a process that occurs without any apparent increase in resting myoplasmic $[Ca^{2+}]$ or tension development. Perhaps mediated by such events as the incrementally "sparks" of Ca^{2+} release from the SR in the absence of depolarization,[78] the incrementally released Ca^{2+} is gradually eliminated by the Na-Ca exchanger. With sustained (>5 min) rest, Ca^{2+} is eliminated from the SR so that the resulting "rested state" contraction is minuscule compared to those at normal rates, and the SR is depleted of Ca^{2+}.[125] It may require 20 to 100 beats for the myocyte SR store to be replenished with Ca^{2+} and show an unchanging contraction at any given rate after prolonged rest. The importance of the exchanger is evidenced by the fact that in low external Na^+, the rest contraction is not depressed but enhanced and the SR store remains replete with Ca^{2+}. The importance of the Na^+ gradient is also exemplified by the study of rat heart, in which contractions after rest are sustained or increased in amplitude. Rat heart has a higher intracellular $[Na^+]$ of ~13 mM (vs 7 mM in rabbit), and the smaller Na^+ gradient favors Ca^{2+} entry rather than elimination during rest.[126] Therefore, the SR pool stays filled with Ca^{2+}, an effect seen with low extracellular Na^+ in other species.[127] The observation that rat heart relies more on sarcolemmal Ca^{2+}-ATPase for Ca^{2+} elimination is not surprising in view of the increased intracellular $[Na^+]$.[128]

Relevant to such discussion is the distribution of the Na-Ca exchanger, which is located throughout the sarcolemma,[129] although a somewhat higher density appears to be present in the T-tubules when tested with monoclonal antibodies.[130] As such it may be located strategically to eliminate Ca^{2+} as it is slowly lost from junctional SR, particularly since the junctional cleft represents a diffusion-restricted space (Fig. 1–5).[74] In fact, the cytoplasmic Ca^{2+} binding (K_D) of the Na-Ca exchanger is only 0.6 μM,[131] which would be inadequate to rapidly reduce myoplasmic Ca^{2+} to the typical resting levels of 0.1 μM. The presence of release at a diffusion-restricted site such as the junctional cleft and other subsarcolemmal sites would permit a locally elevated Ca^{2+} concentration at which the exchanger could work.

Rate Effects
An obvious example of intrinsic variation of Ca^{2+} stores occurs with variation in heart rate. At physiological rates, the bulk (90 to 95%) of activator Ca^{2+} is derived from loaded SR stores, although the small amount entering from outside is responsible for inducing Ca^{2+} release and contributing to 5 to 10% of Ca^{2+} for myofibrillar activation. As indicated in Figure 1–7, these two sources of Ca^{2+} are apparently intermingled. Relaxation occurs as 90 to 95% of Ca^{2+} is reaccumulated in the SR, and 5 to 10% of the Ca^{2+} (equal to the amount that entered) is eliminated from the cell by the Na-Ca exchanger before depolariza-

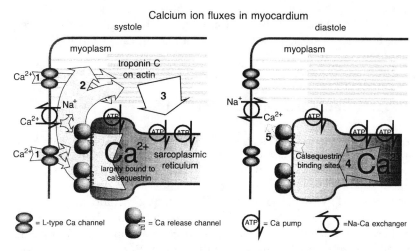

FIGURE 1-7. Ca^{2+} cycling by myocardial SR. (*Left*) Upon depolarization, Ca^{2+} enters via L-type Ca channels and also via the Na-Ca exchanger to initiate systole (step 1). While a small fraction of entering Ca^{2+} may reach the myofibrils, the major role of Ca^{2+} entry is to bind to the Ca release channels of the JSR to activate release of Ca^{2+} (step 2), which represents the bulk of the activator Ca^{2+} that binds to troponin C to permit actin-myosin interaction. Following tension development, Ca^{2+} diffuses off of troponin C and binds to the higher affinity binding sites of the Ca-ATPase ("Ca pump") located on the longitudinal (or network) SR which then transports it to the SR lumen (step 3). (*Right*) During diastole, Ca^{2+} moves toward the J-SR lumen (step 4), and the Ca^{2+} which "leaks" from the SR is slowly eliminated from the myocyte by the Na-Ca exchange (step 5). If diastole is not prolonged, the bulk of the Ca^{2+} is still present in the JSR lumen and available for release with the subsequent depolarization. With prolonged rest (>30 sec) the SR gradually is depleted of its Ca^{2+} store.

tion stimulates the next beat. At lower rates with more time for the SR to lose Ca^{2+} the contractions are smaller and the entering Ca^{2+} now represents a higher fraction (perhaps 10 to 20%) of activator Ca^{2+}. As heart rate is increased, a well-described "positive frequency staircase" or increased contraction at higher heart rates results. This phenomenon has been demonstrated in human hearts. As the diastolic rest interval is decreased, there is less time for Ca^{2+} to "leak" from the SR and be removed by the Na-Ca exchanger, so a greater SR Ca^{2+} store is available for release. There is evidence that a very small fraction of time (50 to 200 msec) may be required to transfer Ca^{2+} from the longitudinal to the junctioned SR, so that at very high heart rates with short diastolic intervals, not all of the SR pool of Ca^{2+} is at a release site. When a premature beat occurs, the contraction may be reduced because Ca^{2+} is not yet in a releasable junctional SR location. However, during the subsequent pause there is time for accumulation in the junctional SR release site of an enhanced Ca^{2+}, including that from the extra beat. There is a marked potentiation of the next beat (postextrasystolic potentiation).[132] The continued Ca^{2+} entry at very high heart rates with reduced time between contractions for Ca^{2+} elimination can result in SR Ca^{2+} overload.

OTHER EFFECTS ON Ca^{2+} STORES

As noted previously, $E_{rev,NaCa}$ becomes much more positive after Ca^{2+} release, with calculated values of +10 to +40 mV,[111,133] which are in the range of the action potential plateau. When the voltage is clamped near these potentials, there is no longer a decline in measured Ca^{2+} transients caused by Na-Ca exchange.[109,134] Both $[Ca^{2+}]_i$ (and consequently $E_{rev,NaCa}$) and the plateau of the action potential also decline together.[111,133] Consequently, modest change in action potential plateau amplitude and duration may alter the time during which Ca^{2+} enters through the exchanger, before Ca^{2+} elimination begins. The period of exchanger Ca^{2+} influx may be extended with a very positive plateau of extended duration (as when repolarizing K+ currents are inhibited.) Conversely, when the plateau is short and more negative, more Ca^{2+} can be eliminated by the exchanger. Since the exchanger competes to a small extent with the SR Ca^{2+}-ATPase for ions, when Ca^{2+} removal begins later (as in the former case) more Ca^{2+} will accumulate in the SR and contractility will be greater. Contractility will be reduced in the latter case when the exchanger eliminates more Ca^{2+}.

Pharmacological blockade of Ca^{2+} channels can also decrease cardiac contractility. This effect is both direct and indirect. By decreasing the amount of triggering Ca^{2+}, the activation of Ca^{2+} release may be reduced. It is unknown whether there may be a substantial excess of Ca^{2+} normally entering to activate release of the much greater SR store. Initially with Ca^{2+} channel blockade and decreased Ca^{2+} entry, Ca^{2+} elimination via the surface membrane will exceed Ca^{2+} entry, resulting in a gradual reduction in the SR Ca^{2+} store and reduced contractility.

The Role of the Mitochondria

Mitochondria carefully regulate Ca^{2+} via a Ca^{2+}-H^+ exchanger and Ca^{2+} uniport pathways in addition to synthesizing ATP by employing a proton gradient across the inner and outer membranes. While the rate of Ca^{2+} uptake has been shown to be too slow to contribute to Ca^{2+} regulation within a contractile cycle,[135] over a time course of seconds increased myoplasmic Ca^{2+} can be assimilated by the mitochondria.[136] The loss of the proton gradient during hypoxia or ischemia may also result in Ca^{2+} loading of mitochondria. Sustained Ca^{2+} overload leads to mitochondrial swelling and ultimately to disruption. However, in contrast to pathological conditions, the increased "average" myoplasmic $[Ca^{2+}]$ which occurs with increased heart rates during β-adrenergic activation may be reflected by a more modest increase in mitochondrial $[Ca^{2+}]$. This may in turn enhance the activity of intramitochondrial dehydrogenases, leading to an appropriate increase in ATP synthesis.[136]

MYOFILAMENT RESPONSE TO Ca^{2+}

Control of contractility is determined by the quantity of Ca^{2+} released to the myofibrils. The myofibrils themselves also have a variable Ca^{2+} sensitivity which depends upon the length of and tension generated within the myocyte sarcomeres.

The Myofilaments

Actin Filaments

The thin filaments of striated muscle are composed of F-actin, a helical polymer composed of two intertwined strands of single actin molecules. Each actin monomer is composed of two side-by-side peanut-shaped domains. These monomers are held together in a strand by strong noncovalent interactions, in which a divalent cation (Ca^{2+}, Mg^{2+}) and an adenosine nucleotide (ATP or ADP) are critical cofactors.[137] Each F-actin filament has two helical grooves formed by the intertwined actin strands. An elongated molecule of tropomyosin overlapping seven actin monomers lies in

each of the grooves. Each tropomyosin has an associated complex of troponin comprised of an inhibitory (TnI), Ca^{2+}-binding (TnC), and
tropomyosin-binding (TnT) subunit. The position of the tropomyosin
molecule within the actin filament groove determines whether sites on the
actin monomers are accessible to interact with myosin. The myoplasmic
$[Ca^{2+}]$ at rest (during diastole) is approximately 80 to 100 nM ($\sim$0.1μM),
and no Ca^{2+} is bound to the regulatory Ca^{2+} site on troponin C (TnC). The
troponin complex stabilizes the position of the tropomyosin molecule so
that the sites on actin for myosin attachment are occluded. When $[Ca^{2+}]_i$
surrounding the myofibrils rises to the 0.5 to 2 μM range, Ca^{2+} binding to
TnC appears to couple TnI to TnC[138] and uncouple TnI from actin.[139,140]
This results in a conformational shift of tropomyosin in the actin filament
groove and reveals the active sites on actin to which the myosin head
groups can bind (Fig. 1–8). Activator Ca^{2+} acts like a switch to turn on
actin-myosin interaction by binding to TnC.

Myosin

Myosin is comprised of two heavy chains (MHC), each containing globular head domains (subfragment 1 (S1)), a tightly coiled rod section (S2),
and a light meromyosin, as well as two pair of light chains. Myosin
(thick) filaments are formed by the aggregation of the individual
myosins with the head groups facing outward to bind to actin. It is the
flexion or rotation of the 19-nm-long head group after binding to an actin
monomer which generates the tension on the myosin filament, and the

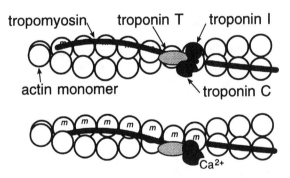

tropomyosin   troponin T   troponin I

actin monomer   troponin C

Ca^{2+} binding reveals myosin binding sites (m)

FIGURE 1-8. Schematic of the Ca^{2+} activated "switch" of the troponin-
tropomyosin complex on actin. When Ca^{2+} binds to troponin C (TnC), the at-
traction for the inhibitory subunit troponin I (TnI) is increased. When TnT is
moved into closer aposition with TnC, the tropomyosin strand rotates further
into the tropomyosin groove, revealing the myosin binding site (m) on actin. Recent molecular models suggest that myosin may actually bind to sites on two adjacent monomers.[141]

total tension generated within the muscle is proportional to the total number of head groups actively cycling. A schematic of this contractile apparatus is indicated in Figure 1–9.[141] After head group rotation, ADP is released, and the myosin and actin remain attached (a rigor complex) unit ATP can combine to uncouple the proteins, freeing myosin to combine again with actin. If other myosin head groups are generating tension and shortening has occurred, the myosin will bind to an actin monomer further along the filament. If no shortening has occurred, and tropomyosin has not occluded the active site on actin, the myosin may rebind in the same location to continue tension generation (while other myosin S1s are cycling). In regard to its ability to hydrolyze an ATP and unbind from actin, two HMC isoforms exist (α and β) which can combine to form fast (V_1, $\alpha\alpha$), medium (V_2, $\alpha\beta$), or slow (V_3, $\beta\beta$) forms of myosin.[142,143] The latter predominates in cardiac tissue. V_1 and V_2 isoforms are expressed in neonatal animals and in hyperthyroidism,[144] but their importance in human myocardium has not been demonstrated.

actin-myosin interaction and tension generation

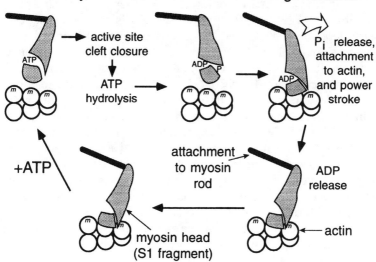

FIGURE 1-9. Schematic of the cycle of the myosin head (S1) in force generation. Dissociation of myosin from actin requires the binding of ATP to the active cleft site on the myosin head near its actin-binding site. Closure of the site and hydrolysis of ATP is accompanied by myosin assuming a "cocked" position, from which it releases P_i and can generate tension upon binding to actin. Following its "power stroke," the cleft opens, permitting ADP to dissociate, but leaving myosin tightly bound to actin. (*Adapted from Rayment I et al. Science 261:58–65, 1993*)

Length (Force)-Dependent Contractile Activation

The force development in a skeletal muscle fiber is largely proportional to the amount of overlap of the sliding filaments of actin and myosin. Skeletal muscle can be stretched to the point where actin-myosin filament overlap begins to decrease and active (and total) tension decreases. Unless shortening is extreme in skeletal muscle, the tension decreases only gradually with shorter sarcomere lengths <1.8 μm. In myocardium, the relationship of active force vs length has a steeper slope: when the sarcomeres are contracted and short (≤1.8 μm) there is very modest active force development for a given [Ca^{2+}], but even small amounts of stretch result in far greater active force development.[145–147]

Substantial evidence suggests that the affinity of troponin C for Ca^{2+} decreases with sarcomere length, i.e., the shorter the muscle length, the more rapidly myofibrils will release Ca^{2+}. As demonstrated by studies using aequorin[148–150] and confirmed by fura-2 [Ca^{2+}] measurements,[151] the rate of decline of Ca^{2+} transients is altered by varying the length and tension development of the myocardium. At a shorter vs longer length (or with quick release of tension), the Ca^{2+} is slightly higher following the peak, but it ultimately declines more rapidly due to decreased troponin affinity for Ca^{2+}. Further work documents that this behavior arises from the myofibrils and is not an artifact due to length-dependent effects on the SR or peculiar to skinned muscle fibers.[152] Conversely, when the same [Ca^{2+}] is present in the myoplasm, more myofibrils appear activated, and more force is generated when cardiac myocytes are stretched.[153] This effect is due to the relation between activation and Ca^{2+} binding to cardiac troponin C, an isoform distinct from skeletal muscle troponin C. Cardiac troponin C demonstrates increased Ca^{2+} sensitivity when sarcomere length[153] and/or force[150,152,154] are greater, so that the same [Ca^{2+}] activates more myosin-actin interaction and cycling. This effect is reduced or not seen when skeletal muscle troponin C (which requires two Ca^{2+} to bind) is substituted for cardiac troponin C.[155,156] Such behavior, in which less Ca^{2+} is required to bind to troponin C when myosin head groups are attached to actin and generating force, can be explained by Ca^{2+} diffusing off of troponin C once a crossbridge, is formed.[157] While the myosin is still bound to actin, Ca^{2+} can thus become available to bind to other troponin C and activate other regions of the actin filament.

Either exclusive force development (isometric shortening or isovolumic contraction) or shortening (unloaded isotonic shortening) can be arranged experimentally. However, the normal physiological situation is some combination of force and shortening. Over the same time period, a longer muscle will shorten more against a given resisting force or afterload because a greater number of myosin units are active at a longer sarcomere length due to the greater troponin C-Ca^{2+} affinity. When the steep length dependence of cardiac contractility is expressed as muscle shortening instead of force development, the result is the classic observation of far greater shortening at greater velocity as clearly delineated by Sonnenblick in isolated muscle (Fig. 1–10C).[158] Furthermore, for any given initial length or resting force, the muscle shortens less rapidly and not as far as the afterload is increased. Cross-bridges cycle to generate greater force but do not cause the myofibrils to shorten as much. This effect has important implications with regard to ventricular function, energy consumption, and perfusion. Relaxation is retarded when there is great resistance to ejection and high intraventricular pressures.[159] It follows that systole and ATP consumption by cycling of myosin with actin will be prolonged, while diastole will be shortened. When there is considerable shortening and less force developed, Ca^{2+} diffuses more readily off of troponin C, and provided that the SR can actively accumulate the Ca^{2+}, then systole is abbreviated.

The length (or force) dependence of myofibril activation also has an important corollary with regard to relaxation, since the change in troponin C Ca^{2+} affinity occurs within a single cardiac cycle. Because tro-

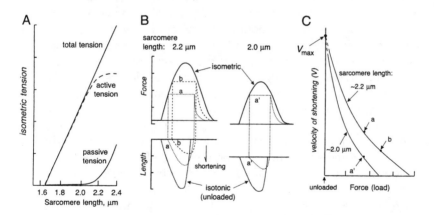

FIGURE 1-10. The interaction of initial length and preload on force development and velocity of shortening. (A) Dependence of active and passive force on muscle length. The difference between the total and passive tension is the active developed tension (*dotted line*). (B) Simultaneous tracings of tension and length from a typical papillary muscle experiment. The *left panel* shows the response at 2.2μm sarcomere length while the right panel shows the response at the shorter 2.0-μ sarcomere length. Once any given force is attained, shortening is a linear function of the initial length. At the shorter length, the muscle can attain less maximum tension (as plotted in A), and also shortens less rapidly. The maximum velocity of shortening is the initial slope of the length tracing and is plotted in C, according to the analysis first described by Sonnenblick.[158]

ponin C Ca^{2+} affinity is decreased when a muscle shortens more, a muscle allowed to shorten relaxes sooner.[160–162] This phenomenon is called length- (or load)-dependent relaxation or shortening deactivation. The decreased Ca^{2+} affinity of troponin C that occurs due to shortening results in a detectably higher cytoplasmic $[Ca^{2+}]$ as it diffuses off of troponin C more rapidly into the myoplasm[148] from which it is reaccumulated into the SR. Consequently, when shortening occurs, the rate of relaxation is dependent upon the rate at which the SR can take up Ca^{2+}. When force or pressure development occurs with little shortening, the decline in $[Ca^{2+}]$ reflects the higher troponin C Ca^{2+} affinity. Such length-dependence of relaxation is a clear demonstration of myocardial economy, since once shortening and ejection of blood has occurred, ATP would be consumed needlessly if myosin continued to cycle.

End-systolic length and tension will strongly influence the rate of relaxation. This effect may explain the apparent dependence of oxygen consumption on cardiac diastolic wall stress. The myocardium is relaxed (Ca^{2+} is accumulated and myofibrils are not interacting) during diastole. It is difficult to reconcile how this state could influence myocardial energy utilization. It seems likely that lower diastolic wall stress (and smaller diameter) will result in a decreased myofibrillar Ca^{2+} sensitivity. If there is the same degree of shortening during the subsequent systole in the presence of a smaller end-systolic diameter, Ca^{2+} will diffuse off of troponin C more rapidly, with a shorter duration of tension development and less energy consumption. This phenomenon may also explain in part the interesting and seemingly contradictory result that dogs whose hearts are depressed by volatile anesthetics have improved diastolic relaxation when extracellular Ca^{2+} is increased, which also increases systolic shortening.[163]

The other component which sharply defines the myocardial length-force relation is the passive behavior mediated by the passive intracellular stress-strain relation and the extracellular connective tissue. Below sarcomere lengths of 2.2 μm, the intrinsic myofibrillar stress-strain relation generated by the polypeptide titin is responsible for the increase in tension with stretch.[9] At longer sarcomere lengths, extracellular collagen fibrils become stretched in intact cardiac muscle which prevents the muscle from being passively stretched beyond that point where total tension declines.[9,146,147] This passive length-force component increases steeply at the muscle length at which active tension development levels off. The contribution of the passive component is evident, for example, when the collagen strands that surround myocytes are enzymatically digested, shifting the passive tension curve to the right.[13] The combination of the steep active length-force relation at short sarcomere lengths due to cardiac troponin C with the steep passive length-force relation at long sarcomere lengths results in a total length-force relation that is virtually linear over the functional range (Fig. 1–10). This linear combination of active and passive components extends to three dimensions in the intact ventricle, providing a simple quantitative description of the heart, particularly when applied to ventricular function and pressure-volume relations.

The myofilament sensitivity to Ca^{2+} and the resulting degree of activation are also modulated by receptor-mediated systems which control troponin I subunit phosphorylation as noted below. While the myofibrils are the primary cellular system responsive to cell dimension or tension, the SR also shows length-dependent behavior. SR Ca^{2+} stores increase following an increase in length.[164] The length-dependent SR effect develops over a number of contractions and appears to account for a more modest component (25 to 25%) of the positive inotropic effect as opposed to the instantaneous effect caused by length dependence of troponin C and Ca^{2+}. The phenomenon is not limited to isolated muscle but is readily demonstrable in intact animals.[165]

EXTRINSIC MODULATION OF CONTRACTILITY

The major mechanism by which the automatic nervous system as well as other hormones and transmitters influence cardiac function is an alteration of the function of the various ion transport pathways in cardiac membranes. Any resulting change in heart rate may in and of itself alter contractile function (see above), but activation of the various pathways exerts a strong, direct modulating effect on the amount of activator Ca^{2+} and also acts upon myofibrillar Ca^{2+} sensitivity and function. The changes in $[Ca^{2+}]$ can in turn influence membrane potential via Na-Ca exchange and certain ion currents. Activation of various processes is appropriately coordinated, so that if the duration of tension development is shortened by enhanced relaxation, the action potential duration will also be decreased. The primary processes and pathways that modulate cardiac function are listed in Table 1–2.

G Protein-Linked Receptor-Mediated Effects

The vast majority of receptors in the heart and peripheral cardiovascular system that modulate function belong to a family of membrane proteins whose actions are mediated by activation of the guanine nucleotide-binding proteins or G proteins. These molecules act as highly specialized intracellular messengers. After they are activated by specific receptors, they in turn activate (or inhibit) a variety of cell effector pathways such as ion channels or second messenger-generating en-

TABLE 1-2. PATHWAYS AND MECHANISMS OF EXTRINSIC MODULATION OF CARDIAC CONTRACTILITY

Ligand	Membrane Receptor	Pathway	Cellular Effect	Action
PGI₂ (prostacyclin)	IP	→G_s protein → adenylyl cyclase→ ↑cAMP→ ↑protein kinase A activity → phosphorylation→	↑Delayed I_K/I_{to} and Cl conductance→	↓AP duration→ sl ↓ duration of Ca²⁺ entry
Serotonin	5-HT₂		↑Myosin "turnover" rate→	↑Contractility
Glucagon Histamine	Glucagon H₂ histamine		↑I_{Ca}(?direct G_s effect) ↑CaRC^a activity→ ↓Phospholamban (Plm) inhibition of SR Ca ATPase→	↑↑Ca²⁺ entry ↑SR Ca²⁺ release ↑SR Ca²⁺ uptake →↑↑Ca²⁺ cycling through the SR
Epinephrine Norepinephrine	β₁-adrenergic			
Isoproterenol Dopamine	β₂-adrenergic		↓TnC Ca²⁺ affinity (via TnI phosphorylation)→	Faster relaxation
Norepinephrine Epinephrine	α₁-adrenergic	→G_q protein → ↑Phospholipase C activity → ↑IP3 and ↑diacylglycerol→ ↑protein kinase C→	↓Transient inward and other K currents → ↑Na⁺,K⁺ ATPase activity → ↑Na⁺/H⁺ exchange→ ??↑CaRC activity and ??↓Plm inhibition →	↑AP duration →↑Ca²⁺ decrease in Ca²⁺ accumulation ↑pH → ↑Ca²⁺ sensitivity of myofilaments ??↑SR Ca²⁺ uptake and release
Angiotensin II Endothelin	Angiotensin II Endothelin			
Adenosine, ?ATP	A1 purinergic	G_i protein→ ↓Adenylyl cyclase → ↓cAMP production	↑$I_{K(Ado,ACh)}$→ Effects opposite to those seen with adenylyl cyclase activation	↓AP duration → ↓Ca²⁺
Acetylcholine	M2 muscarinic		↓I_{Ca} (?) → Certain effects opposite to those seen with ↑cAMP	
NO (from endothelium)	↑Guanylyl cyclase (myoplasmic "soluble") activation	→ ↑cGMP →PDE activation →↓ cAMP		↓Ca²⁺ entry
Atrial naturetic factors	Receptor / → guanylyl cyclase ("particulate")	↑cGMP → PDE activation →↓ cAMP	Activation of Na/K/Cl ion cotransporter	?Altered cell volume

^{a}CaRC, Ca²⁺ release channel; IP3, inositol 1,4,5-trisphosphate; NO, nitric oxide; PDE, phosphodiesterase; Plm, phospholamban; SR, sarcoplasmic reticulum.

zymes.[166–168] The G protein-linked receptors are distinctive in having seven transmembrane alphahelical segments, which create a central cleft (not a channel) on the extracellular surface. Ligands (norepinephrine, histamine, etc.) bind in the cleft of these receptors and cause a conformational change on the intracellular surface of the receptor which promotes dissociation of the heterotrimeric G protein complex. GDP (guanosine diphosphate) and the tightly coupled $\beta\gamma$ subunit dissociate away from the α subunit, which is then free to bind guanosine triphosphate (GTP). The GTP-bound α subunit forms an activating complex which then regulates the membrane effector systems[169] until the GTP is hydrolyzed. The $\beta\gamma$ subunit also appears to play an important signaling role, either by direct interaction with membrane constituents or by binding to and inactivating the α subunits.[170,171]

Cyclic AMP-Dependent Protein Kinase Actions

The most widely studied G protein signal pathway, which is highly relevant to the cardiovascular system, is the regulation of adenylyl cyclase. This produces the second messenger, cyclic adenosine-3',5'-monophosphate (cAMP). Catecholamines (via the β-adrenergic receptor,[172] histamine (via H_2 receptor),[173] prostacyclin (via IP receptor),[174] serotonin (via 5-HT_4 receptor),[175] and glucagon mediate their primary actions by activating G_s, the stimulatory G protein, which in turn activates adenylyl cyclase. The increased intracellular [cAMP] then activates the cAMP-dependent protein kinase (PKA), thus phosphorylating a variety of proteins which leads to an increase in contractility and heart rate.

Ca²⁺ Cycling

The major mechanism by which PKA increases tension is by increasing the amount of Ca^{2+} cycled. This results from PKA-mediated phosphorylation of: 1) the L-type Ca channel; 2) phospholamban; and 3) the Ca release channel. Phosphorylation of the L-type Ca channel alters its gating behavior, changing to a new "mode" in which the open intervals are more sustained so that a greater number of Ca^{2+} ions may enter the cell.[57] Because of the increase in intracellular Ca^{2+} which can contribute to Ca^{2+} mediated inactivation of the channel, the net effect is a marked increase in the peak current and total Ca^{2+} influx. Entering Ca^{2+} is not the primary regulator of activation. Phosphorylation of SR proteins is also critical. Following phosphorylation, phospholamban no longer provides a brake on the SR Ca pump, and Ca^{2+} can be accumulated at a far higher rate.[93] The combination of increased Ca^{2+} entry and SR accumulation results in a greater amount of accumulated Ca^{2+}. The greater amount of SR Ca^{2+} also appears to be released at an enhanced rate following phosphorylation of the cardiac CaRC, the function of which is also enhanced.[176,177] Although the greater amount of entering Ca^{2+} results in greater SR loading, over a sustained period the greater Ca^{2+} influx must be balanced by greater Ca^{2+} efflux. The greater efflux is mediated via the Na-Ca exchanger, which obligates greater Na^+ entry. This demand is matched by phosphorylation and increased activity of the Na-K ATPase which provides for increased Na+ elimination.

Troponin

Phosphorylation of troponin I decreases the affinity of troponin C for Ca^{2+},[178] an effect which would decrease actin-myosin interaction and contractility unless $[Ca^{2+}]_i$ has been increased.

The other actions of PKA noted above serve to markedly enhance the depolarization-induced increase in myoplasmic Ca^{2+} which more than offsets the decreased Ca^{2+} affinity of troponin C for Ca^{2+}, so that contractility is ultimately enhanced.[179] Most importantly, the decreased Ca^{2+} affinity will cause Ca^{2+} to be bound for a shorter time permitting relaxation to occur more quickly. This decreased contractile duration is critical to permitting an adequate distolic period for coronary flow and ventricular filling at higher heart rates (see below). In addition to these actions, β adrenoceptor activation appears to have an independent effect to increase the rate of myosin cross-bridge turnover, an action which will also serve to increase tension development.[180] Myosin fibrils have additional protein present called the C-protein. This protein also appears to phosphorylate in the presence of β adrenoceptor stimulation,[181] possibly contributing to this positive inotropic action[182] by increasing the rate of myosin cross-bridge turnover.

Other Ion Channels

PKA appears to activate a number of channels. A profound action occurs in pacemaking tissue in which the pacemaker current I_f is increased, which enhances the rate of diastolic depolarization and leads to the increased heart rate typical of β-adrenergic activation. The delayed K current[183] as well as the transient outward (I_{to})[184] current are also enhanced by phosphorylation, which will serve to abbreviate the action potential. This is an important electrophysiological effect which ensures that the contractile state is not prolonged. In addition, a Cl^- conductance is activated for which E_{Cl} is about -40 mV. This current will also have a repolarizing action on the plateau and a depolarizing effect during diastole that may contribute to automaticity. The decrease in action potential duration will slightly abbreviate the duration of the Ca^{2+} current but the net effect of β-adrenoceptor stimulation will be an increased Ca^{2+} influx because of the great increase in open Ca channels.

Both $β_1$- and $β_2$-adrenergic receptor subtypes are present in myocardium. $β_2$ receptors appear to be present on both pacemaker tissues and myocytes and are not activated by norepinephrine but by isoproterenol and specific agonists such as Zinterol.[185] The effects noted above apply to the actions of β_1-adrenoceptor stimulation, but not to β_2-stimulation. β_2-adrenoceptor activation does not appear to decrease myofibril Ca^{2+} sensitivity or markedly increase SR Ca^{2+}, and while it does enhance I_{Ca}, the effect is distinct from that of β_1-receptor stimulation.[185] These different actions may depend upon different pools of adenylyl cyclase or compartmentalized cAMP and may have potentially important therapeutic implications. β_2-adrenoceptor activation is not as arrhythmogenic as β_1-receptor stimulation, nor does it shorten the contraction.

Cyclic AMP Regulation by Phosphodiesterase

In addition to regulation of [cAMP] (and PKA protein phosphorylation) by regulation of adenylyl cyclase-mediated cAMP synthesis, there is also hydrolytic breakdown of cAMP governed by alterations in phosphodiesterase activity. A variety of cAMP-phosphodiesterase enzymes exists whose activity can be modulated by intracellular constituents (see below). Inhibition of cAMP hydrolysis by drugs of varying specificity (caffeine, amrinone, milrinone) can be employed to increase cAMP, with its consequent increase in contractile function. Certain phosphodiesterases and phosphatases are also regulated by intracellular messengers (e.g., cyclic GMP), which provide an additional modulatory system of cAMP and PKA phosphorylation.[186,187]

Inhibition of Adenylyl Cyclase

Stimulation of myocardium by acetylcholine (M_2 muscarinic cholinoceptors[188]) and adenosine (A_1-adenosine receptors[189]) causes activation of the adenylyl cyclase-inhibitory G protein, G_i^*. G_i activation can strongly inhibit adenylyl cyclase and thereby reverse the effect of β-receptor stimulation, so that cAMP levels and physiological functions return to nonstimulated levels.[190] Adenosine appears to be more efficiently coupled than acetylcholine in this inhibitory regulatory pathway in human myocardium.[190] The inhibitory actions appear to be mediated at least in part by release of $\beta\gamma$ subunits from $G\alpha_i$, which then bind $G\alpha_s$, resulting in the loss of adenylyl cyclase activation.[171] This action is most obvious in the pacemaker tissues. These tissues appear to possess a very high resting adenylyl cyclase activity, resulting in a high activity of I_f and $I_{Ca,L}$, even in the absence of B-adrenoceptor stimulation. Consequently, muscarinic and A_1 purinergic stimulation by adenosine will depress I_f and $I_{Ca,L}$,[191,192] slowing the diastolic depolarization and action potential contraction velocity. However, even in the absence of β-receptor stimulation, a marked depressant effect on ventricular function may also be present when acetylcholine is directly applied to the myocardium.[193] This is mediated via M_2 receptors present on ventricular myocytes. The effect is due in part to a modest reduction in peak Ca^{2+} current, and more profoundly, to a decrease in action potential duration, which decreases the time for Ca^{2+} influx. Vagal stimulation has a far more modest effect on ventricular contractility, because parasympathetic nerves release acetycholine primarily on sympathetic nerve endings, presynaptically decreasing norepinephrine release.[194] Consequently, vagal stimulation in the presence of enhanced sympathetic activity causes a greater decrease in contractility.

Direct Ion Channel Effects

The G proteins themselves may directly influence ion channel function.[195] G_s activation appears to directly increase Ca channel current[196,197]; however, the importance and relevance of this action to physiological function is unclear.[198] Direct activation by β_2 adrenoceptors might explain observed behavior which differs from that seen with β_1 activation. Likewise, stimulation of P_2-purinergic receptors appears to enhance opening of L-type channels via a pathway involving a G_s pathway exclusive of cAMP production.[199]

An important directly modulated cardiac ion current is that carried by K^+ through a channel which is activated by acetylcholine and adenosine ($I_{K(ACh)}$, $I_{K(Ado)}$, or $I_{K(ACh,Ado)}$). Ligand binding to M_2 muscarinic or A1 adenosine receptors activates G_i which then opens this channel, subsequently causing decreased excitability and even cell hyperpolarization due to the increase in resting K conductance. Activation of this channel is more important in pacemaker tissue and atrial myocytes than in ventricular tissue. While $I_{K(ACh,Ado)}$ is present in human ventricular myocytes, it is largely inactive under normal circumstances and makes only a modest contribution to total K^+ conductance.[200] In the absence of β-adrenoceptor stimulation, the effect of adenosine or acetylcholine on I_{Ca} in ventricular muscle is modest.[193,201] Nevertheless, due to the abbreviated action potential duration when $K_{ACh,Ado}$ channels are activated, the Ca^{2+} current is reduced, elimination by Na-Ca exchange is increased (see above), and contractility decreases significantly.[193]

Effect of Phospholipase C Activation

Another major G protein pathway involves the activation of the phospholipases, enzymes which metabolize phospholipid components of the cell membranes.[202,203] When activated by a G protein (as shown in Fig. 1–11), specifically by G_q (and possibly G_i), phospholipase C cleaves the phosphoester linkage of diphosphoinositide to produce the phosphated sugar, inositol 1,4,5-trisphosphate (IP_3), and leaves a glycerol with two fatty acids (diacylglycerol) in the plasmalemma. Each of these agents can then act as a second messenger. The activity of phosoholi-

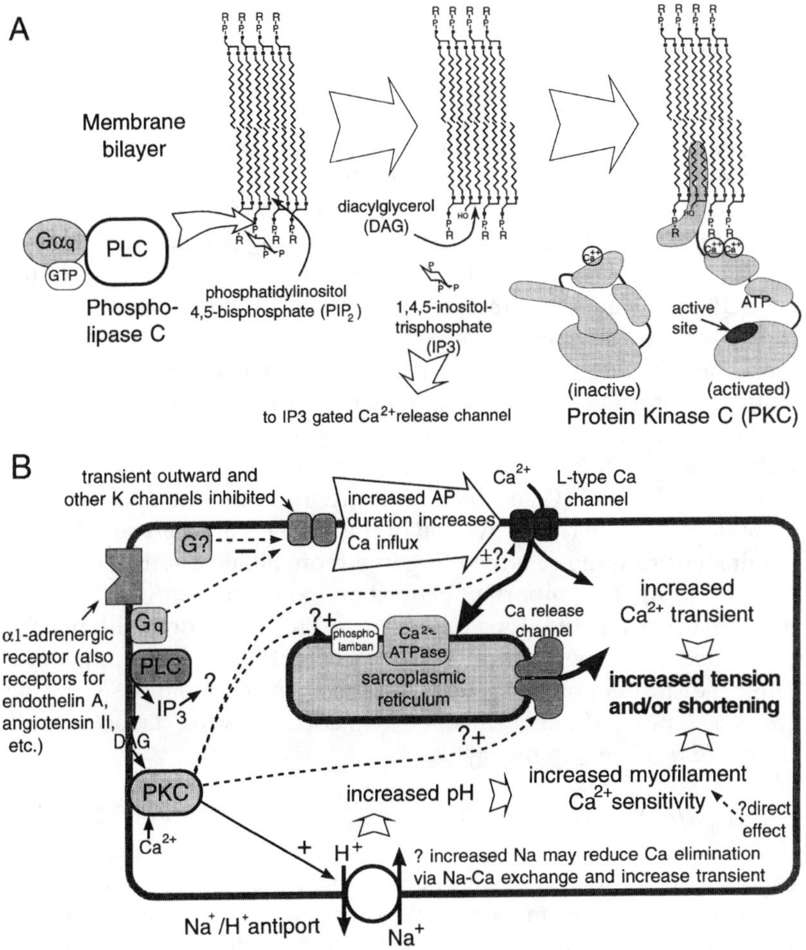

FIGURE 1-11. Phospholipase C (*PLC*) and protein kinase C (*PKC*) cellular activation pathways. (*A*) Proposed membrane molecular pathway for PLC production of diacylglycerol (*DAG*) and inositol 1,4,5-trisphosphate (*IP3*). Activation of PKC appears to involve movement of an autoinhibitory pseudosubstrate region of the molecule to reveal the active site, which occurs when there is intimate association of PKC with the membrane, as well as a requirement for Ca^{2+} (for many PKC subtypes). (*B*) Proposed mechanisms of the positive inotropic effects of α_1-adrenergic stimulation (and other G_q-linked receptors) and PKC activation on cardiac myocytes. PKC causes activation of the Na^+/H^+-antiport, which in turn increases myofilament Ca^{2+} sensitivity, while SR uptake and release may possibly be enhanced. In addition, via a pathway separate from PKC, K channel inhibition causes shorter action potentials with a less positive plateau, resulting in less Ca^{2+} current and less Ca^{2+} elimination via the Na-Ca exchanger (now shown).

pase can also be enhanced by Ca^{2+}, with activity increasing when $[Ca^{2+}]$ increases above resting cellular levels (0.1 μM).[204]

Protein Kinase C and [H]$_i$ Effects

The protein kinase C (PKC) class of over 11 enzymes is dependent on the presence of certain phospholipids such as diacylglycerol, although a number of lipophilic tumor promoters (the phorbol esters) are widely used experimentally to activate these enzymes. A major subgroup of this kinase class is activated by the presence of Ca^{2+}. In its cytoplasmic state, PKC has an autoinhibitory portion which binds to and inhibits the active site, but in the presence of Ca^{2+} and diacylglycerol in the membrane bilayer, the enzyme binds to the plasmalemma with a resulting conformational change which reveals the active site (Fig. 1–11).[205] In cellular homogenates the enzyme can phosphorylate a variety of the molecules activated by PKA, including phospholamban and troponin C.[206–208] PKC also has other important actions. PKC may mediate the α_1-adrenergic activation of the Na^+/H^+ antiport so that H^+ is eliminated from the cell, resulting in a more alkaline intracellular milieu.[209,210] PKC has important actions on ion channels. After an initial increase in activity of L-type Ca channels, PKC activation with phorbol esters decreases their opening.[211] Increased PKC activity appears to blunt the stimulation of I_{Ca} by β-adrenoceptor stimulation[212] and decrease L-type Ca channel currents.[213] In addition, PKC can activate the delayed K+ current in myocytes.

IP$_3$ Effects

IP$_3$ binds to and activates Ca^{2+} flux through a specific intracellular receptor. The IP$_3$ receptor is a homotetrameric protein, smaller in size (2749 amino acids per monomer) yet similar in structure to the CaRC.[214] When IP$_3$ in the myoplasm is increased and binds to this receptor, the protein behaves as a Ca^{2+} channel which releases Ca^{2+} from intracellular sarcoplasmic/endoplasmic reticulum stores. This receptor-activated channel is prominent in smooth muscle and in neuronal, endocrine, and hepatic cells.[215] Several recent investigations suggest that IP$_3$ promotes Ca^{2+} release from cardiac SR[216–218] and that this IP$_3$-induced Ca^{2+} release is enhanced in hypertrophic myocardium.[219] However, the IP$_3$ receptor has a very restricted distribution in myocardium being located near the intercalated discs,[220] and its physiological role in the release of Ca^{2+} in this location or in cardiac tissue in general is unclear.

α_1-Adrenergic Effects

The potential importance of possible PKC-mediated actions are exemplified by the positive inotropic action of α_1-adrenergic receptor stimulation. Phenylephrine, as well as norepinephrine in the presence of β adrenergic blockade, causes an increase in both atrial and ventricular contractility which is associated with an increase in action potential duration,[221,1990,222] effects demonstrable in human ventricular myocardium.[223,224] Following a transient decrease in shortening (variable with species), isolated myocytes showed increased shortening, which correlated with increased intracellular alkalinity and presumed increased myofibrillar Ca^{2+} sensitivity.[222,225] While contractile and pH effects of $α_1$ adrenoceptor stimulation were prevented by blockade of the Na/H antiport with amiloride derivatives, in skinned fibers the inotropic effect of phenylephrine was not prevented by such agents, suggesting some direct phosphorylation of myofilaments.[209,225]

In addition to effects on myofibrillar sensitivity, $α_1$-receptor stimulation also increases the amplitude of the Ca^{2+} transient.[179,226] The mechanism for the increased Ca^{2+} transient is somewhat obscure. As previously noted, $α_1$ adrenoceptor and PKC activation do not cause a marked increase in $I_{Ca,L}$. Likewise, while activated exogenous PKC can mediate phosphorylation of phospholamban[206,207] and CaRC[60] which could enhance SR uptake and Ca^{2+} release,[227] proteins located in the SR membrane do not appear to be influenced by activation of native PKC in the surface membrane. Certain studies suggest that the positive inotropic actions of $α_1$-adrenergic receptor stimulation does not involve PKC.[228] A more likely explanation involves a probable G protein-mediated inhibition of a variety of K^+ currents. Enhancement of delayed K^+ currents by PKC has been demonstrated,[229,230] but the predominant action of $α_1$-adrenoceptor stimulation is a prominent inhibition of the transient outward[221,231] and inwardly rectifying K^+ current, which results in an action potential with a prolonged and more positive plateau.[222,224] This provides a longer period for $I_{Ca,L}$. In addition, because the Na-Ca exchange is very sensitive to membrane potential and $[Na^+]_i$, the greater and longer depolarization will result in slower rate of Ca^{2+} elimination, and a greater compensatory uptake into the SR. These combined effects may account for the significant increase in the Ca^{2+} transient observed during $α_1$-adrenoceptor stimulation. These effects are the opposite of those observed with acetylcholine and adenosine which shorten action potential duration and decrease contractility, even though peak I_{Ca} shows little change.[193]

In spite of increased Ca^{2+}-ATPase activity, the $α_1$-adrenergic receptor-enhanced contractions do not show the enhanced relaxation and shorter duration as seen with $β_1$-receptor stimulation,[179] probably because of the greater Ca^{2+} sensitivity. The tension may in fact be prolonged and in the intact organ, this effect may result in a decreased diastolic interval, potentially reducing time for coronary perfusion. The myocardial inotropic effect of an $α_1$-agonist alone is surprising, but the decrease in cardiac output due to increased vascular resistance may mask its inotropic action. Positive α_1-adrenergic receptor inotropic effects have been documented using methoxamine in human volunteers.[232]

The α_1-receptors have been cloned and divided into four subtypes, α_{1a} to α_{1d}. The α_{1a}-adrenergic receptor is blocked by WB4011 and seems to mediate its actions via phospholipase C activation, with subsequent activation of PKC. The α_{1b}-subtype, defined by its sensitivity to chloroethylclonidine (CEC), appears to act at least in part by increasing the activity of the Na^+,K^+-ATPase,[233] and this pathway also appears to involve phospholipase C activation.[234] The Na^+,K^+-ATPase activation may account for the decrease in ventricular contractility observed initially with α_1-adrenergic stimulation by phenylephrine.[222] Enhancement of Na^+ elimination should ultimately maintain a larger Na^+ gradient, which will increase elimination of Ca^{2+} from the cell.

Distinct from the action of the pure β-agonist isoproterenol, which shortens the duration of the contraction, are the effects of combined β- and α_1-adrenergic receptor activation seen with epinephrine and norepinephrine, the major endogenous sympathetic agonists of the heart. The marked decrease in myofibril Ca^{2+} sensitivity observed with pure β_1-receptor stimulation is far less than with mixed β- and α_1-receptor activation, and the duration of the contraction shows less reduction.[179] Certain aspects of combined β- and α_1-adrenoceptor stimulation may be viewed as complementary; for example, the enhanced Na^+,K^+-ATPase and Na^+ gradient provides a mechanism for removal of the increased Ca^{2+} entry via L-type channels. Recent evidence suggests that α_1-receptor stimulation and increased PKC activity can modulate β-receptor stimulated PKA phosphorylation, which regulates actin-myosin activity.[187]

Calmodulin and Ca^{2+}-Dependent Phosphorylation

In addition to effects of PKA and PKC, channel and enzyme regulation via phosphorylation can also be mediated by a multifunctional Ca-calmodulin-dependent kinase (CaMK II), which is activated when Ca^{2+} combines with calmodulin to form an activating complex. Control of the various Ca^{2+} pathways by this enzyme remains to be fully elucidated, yet it may explain a variety of processes. A major action of CaMK II may be the role by which Ca^{2+} entry facilitates subsequent increases in $I_{Ca,L}$. The Ca^{2+} entry-dependent increase in $I_{Ca,L}$ is markedly reduced when CaMK II is inhibited.[50] Increases in stimulation rate or extracellular Ca^{2+} (and hence peak and mean $[Ca^{2+}]$) not only appear to increase $I_{Ca,L}$ but also increase SR Ca^{2+} uptake, which results in a persistent enhancement of Ca^{2+}-ATPase and the CaRC.[81] Such effects might well be regulated by an enzyme which can respond to the intracellular Ca^{2+} load. Although its physiological significance remains to be delineated, the cardiac CaRC has a site for phosphorylation not present in the skeletal muscle CaRC, which when phosphorylated by CaMK II activates the channel.[80] Such an enzyme system might well be sensitive to an increase in heart rate and the resulting increase in average myoplasmic Ca^{2+} and may account in part for the positive frequency staircase observed in many species. Such a Ca^{2+} dependent phosphorylation system might represent an intrinsic pathway to enhance the contractility of the heart during increases in heart rate.

Endocardial Endothelium, Nitric Oxide and Cyclic GMP

In addition to forming the lining of blood vessels, endothelial cells also line the chambers of the heart, lying directly on the basal membrane and connective tissue which surrounds the endocardial myocytes. Although not as dramatic as the vascular endothelial actions on smooth muscle, this endocardial endothelium does modulate myocardial function (see Chapter 2).[235] Both a negative inotropic effect (myocardial relaxant factor) as well as a stimulatory contractile effect (myocardial contractile factor) are demonstrable. The depressant action is relatively modest, is evidenced primarily by an earlier onset of relaxation, and appears to be mediated by nitric oxide (NO).[235-237] The action can be blocked by inhibition of NO synthase and can be duplicated by sodium nitroprusside.[236,237] Since there is typically improvement in cardiac output due to decreased vascular resistance following administration of nitroprusside in whole animal experiments or clinical settings, the modest myocardial depressant effect of nitroprusside is probably masked. In fact, in isolating ejecting hearts, peak LV pressure and LV-dP/dt were unchanged by nitroprusside, although accelerated ventricular relaxation was observed.[237] The typically modest effect of NO appears to be mediated by activation of a cytoplasmic guanylyl cyclase.[186] Both NO and cyclic GMP (cGMP) have been shown to depress $I_{Ca,L}$. Increased production of cGMP stimulated by NO activates phosphodiesterase (PDE), which degrades cAMP and curtails the stimulatory actions of PKA in the myocyte.

Endothelin

The myocardial contractile factor derived from endocardial endothelium is likely to be an endothelin, a stimulatory vasoconstricting peptide secreted by the endothelium that has been shown to have positive inotropic effects on ventricular myocytes[238] and papillary muscles.[239]

Endothelin receptors appear to activate the G_q-phospholipase C-PKC cascade resulting in intracellular alkalinization.[238] This in turn increases myofilament Ca^{2+} sensitivity,[240] which is sufficient to reverse the effects of an imposed acidosis.[241] There does not appear to be a significant enhancement of $I_{Ca,L}$, whereas effects on the SR may play an important role.[239]

Other Hormonal Effects

Angiotensin

The sequential action of renin (released by juxtaglomerular cells of the kidney) and angiotensin-converting enzyme (present on the endothelial cell membrane) on angiotensinogen produces angiotensin II, which in addition to its effects on the vasculature, also influences the myocardium. Binding to the G protein-linked angiotensin receptor activates the phospholipase C pathway outlined above, causing a positive inotropic effect similar to that of the α_1 adrenergic agonists, without acceleration of relaxation.[242] In the hypertrophied left ventricle of the rat, the IP_3-enhanced release of Ca^{2+}, possibly combined with an enhanced myofibrillar Ca^{2+} affinity, may contribute to impaired relaxation.[242] In addition, increased intracellular Ca^{2+} loading may occur secondary to enhanced Na channel function and Na^+ entry.[243] While these effects lead to an augmented contractile state, they may also delay relaxation and result in impairment of filling seen in pressure overload hypertrophy. This may be especially true in the presence of concomitant myocardial ischemia.[244] Additional major actions of angiotensin II include modulation of cardiac protein synthesis, contributing to myocardial hypertrophy.[245] These actions can be inhibited by pretreatment with an angiotensin-converting enzyme inhibitor. Thus, angiotensin-converting enzyme inhibitors provide an important avenue of treatment for patients with diastolic heart failure beyond the traditional use of these drugs as peripheral vasodilators.

Atrial Naturetic Peptides

The heart secretes and contains receptors for atrial naturetic peptide. Atrial naturetic peptide receptors respond with enzymatic activity when binding ligand and generate cGMP when activated. Unlike the soluble guanylyl cyclases that respond to NO, these receptors are termed "particulate" guanylyl cyclase. The actions of cGMP have been noted, but it is unclear whether the cGMP produced by stimulation of atrial naturetic peptide receptors or stimulated by NO have actions in the same cellular compartments. An effect of atrial naturetic peptide-activated cGMP involves the activation of $Na^+/K^+/2Cl^-$ cotransporter, which is in part responsible for control of myocyte volume.[246]

Thyroid Hormone

The thyroid hormone has profound metabolic consequences in a variety of tissues. The primary alterations in the myocardium are usually attributed to the effects of triiodothyronine (T_3)-involved alterations in nuclear synthetic machinery. These changes involve alteration in myosin isozyme from V_3 toward the faster V_1[144] and greater expression of β-adrenergic receptors.[247,248] These processes contribute dramatically to enhancing tension development. However, in addition to these chronic actions that require time for protein synthesis, T_3 has also been found to have direct effects on a variety of cellular processes which can cause an immediate increase in inotropy. T_3 has direct effects on mitochondrial respiratory rate that do not require protein synthesis,[249,250] which may involve enhanced function of adenine nucleotide translocase.[251] Mitochondria from hypothyroid rats rapidly respond to T_3 with an increase in ATP production and oxygen consumption.[250] T_3 also enhances function of the sarcolemmal Ca-ATPase. Of relevance may also be the direct action of T_3 in increasing I_{Na},[252] since enhanced Na^+ entry would be anticipated to increase intracellular Ca^{2+} stores by reducing its elimination via Na-Ca exchange. Both of these direct effects may be important in the myocardial dysfunction following cardiopulmonary bypass, since a significant decline in T_3 is associated with bypass.[253] Myocardial depression in this setting can be relieved by administration of T_3.[254]

Effects of Ischemia and Hypoxia

ATP stores are rapidly depleted with the loss of delivery of oxygen and/or nutrients to the myocardial cells, and the tissue subsequently undergoes a specific sequence of mechanical and electrophysiological events.[255–258] Within minutes of onset, tension development is reduced by >60%, with an accompanying rise in resting tension (ischemic contracture) as [Ca^{2+}] rises. Contracture is reduced but not eliminated by rest or reduced temperature during hypoxia.[257] In this setting, peak tension and the rate of relaxation is slowed due to impaired SR Ca^{2+} reuptake,[259] and since less Ca^{2+} is accumulated, less is available for release to generate subsequent twitches. Also contributing to the decreased SR release may be a relatively less sensitive response of the CaRC. In studies employing photo-released Ca^{2+}, the cardiac CaRC accommodates higher Ca^{2+} by decreasing Ca^{2+} efflux; the CaRC remains closed until a substantial step increase in Ca^{2+} again activates opening.[260]

Hypoxia in isolated cells is associated with a rise of $[Ca^{2+}]$ to ~200 μM and recovery with reoxygenation, while cells that do not recover show a much greater increase to ~400 μM in both the cytosol and mitochondria.[261] The SR appears to play an important role in postanoxic Ca^{2+} regulation upon reoxygenation.[261,262] However, global ischemia is associated with depressed SR function which persists following reoxygenation.[263,264] This may be secondary to Ca^{2+}-ATPase dysfunction[264] as well as to inappropriate opening of the SR CaRC in certain cases.[263] Decreased Ca^{2+} responsiveness of the myofibrils also appears to contribute to the decreased contractility.[265]

Simultaneous with deterioration of mechanical function, action potential duration is markedly reduced, and the cell typically depolarizes by 10 to 20 mV.[255,258] This effect is associated with a decreased rate of depolarization, an increase in the resting conductance, and a decreased slow inward current.[266] The increase in conductance is due to the activation of a specific K channel which is inactivated by ATP, the K_{ATP} channel.[267] This channel is blocked by the sulfonylurea drugs.[268,269] The K_{ATP} channel appears structurally related to the inward rectifier (G_{K1}), with each subunit having only two transmembrane segments.[23] The K_{ATP} channel also inwardly rectifies due to Mg^{2+} blockade, albeit to a lesser extent than the G_{K1}.[270,271] When ATP is depleted with ongoing ischemia/hypoxia, the channel becomes active, resulting in increased K conductance with less depolarization and decreased action potential duration (Fig. 1–8), an effect which appears to be more prominent in epicardial cells.[272] This K_{ATP} channel activation accounts for the ST segment elevation observed during myocardial ischemia[273] and the increased K^+ efflux and extracellular accumulation seen during hypoxia or ischemia.[274] When $I_{K(ATP)}$ is activated by aprikalim[275] or pinacidil[258] prior to an ischemic insult. Postischemic mechanical dysfunction is reduced. This effect may be mediated in part via coronary vascular effects (see below), but the decreased action potential duration due to $I_{K(ATP)}$ combined with the intracellular acidosis[276] will decrease the duration and intensity of I_{Ca}, thus decreasing the rate of Ca^{2+} entry. The sulfonylurea drug glibenclamide is a specific blocker of the K_{ATP} channel which attenuates the decrease in action potential duration observed during ischemia and worsens the postischemic dysfunction. Sustained (≥ 1 hr) ischemia is also associated with a decrease in G_s protein and its activation of adenylyl cyclase by β-adrenergic receptors, an effect which will also decrease the response to β-adrenoceptor stimulation.[277] During reperfusion, the affinity of β-adrenoceptors shows a compensatory increase in the previously ischemic region.[278]

A byproduct of ischemia is the ultimate breakdown of ATP to adenosine, which has a critical regulatory role not only in coronary flow (see below), but also on myocyte function. Activation of adenosine of A_1 receptors will enhance $I_{K(Ado,ACh)}$ and thereby shorten the action potential. Furthermore, the K_{ATP} channel is also modulated by the G protein $G\alpha_i$, and its activation by ATP deficiency appears to be enhanced in the presence of A_1 activation.[279] Decreased action potential (AP) duration may be beneficial in reducing metabolic demand by decreasing the duration of Ca^{2+} entry and the resulting Ca^{2+} overload, although decreased AP duration may lead to a potential proarrhythmic effect.[280] In addition, adenosine will have dramatic effects on the pacemaker rate via activation of $I_{K(Ado,ACh)}$ channels, which will hyperpolarize nodal tissue and depress diastolic depolarization.

Acidosis

The acidosis that accompanies ischemia contributes to mechanical dysfunction by decreasing myofilament responsiveness to Ca^{2+},[265] as well as by a decrease in I_{Ca}.[276,281–283] The decreased Ca^{2+} entry and myofilament activation serve to decrease ATP consumption. During ischemia and the resulting acidosis, the increased intracellular[H^+] is removed from the cell by the Na/H^+ antiport, causing increased Na^+ entry with an associated rise in [Na^+].[284,285] Na^+ entry is also necessary to eliminate the excessive intracellular Ca^{2+}.[284,286,287] Na-Ca exchange is steeply dependent on [Na^+]$_i$,[288] so that maintenance of the normal [Na^+] of 7 to 10 mM is critical for proper control of intracellular Ca^{2+}. The decreased Na^+ gradient that results from H^+ elimination results in greater Ca^{2+} accumulation and increased cellular dysfunction. Ironically, blockade of the antiport (causing a greater degree of acidosis) as well as blockade of Na^+ entry by other routes proves beneficial.[286,289] While there does not appear to be an increased I_{Na},[290] reduction of Na^+ entry can improve myocardial recovery[289] and prevent ventricular fibrillation.[285] The Na^+ overload can also worsen Ca^{2+} overload upon reperfusion.[284,287] The presence of the added buffering capacity of blood does ameliorate the internal acidification and delay ischemic contracture.[291] Application of extracellular acidosis in the absence of ischemia or hypoxia, however, appears more benign. While there is clearly a myocardial depressant effect associated with decreased I_{Ca}, it is relatively modest above pH 7.1,[281] and the intracellular acidification that results from an elevation of CO_2 shows partial recovery mediated by the Na/H^+ antiport.[292] Decrease in myocardial sensitivity to catecholamine stimulation is frequently suggested, but the magnitude of this effect above pH 7.0 is poorly described. In isolated tissue at pH 6.8 there is a decrease in catecholamine sensitivity; however, the maximal increase in contractility is not depressed.[293]

Stunning

If an episode of ischemia is not sufficient to result in cell death, the myocardium undergoes a period of recovery during which it is "stunned," exhibiting markedly depressed contractility.[294] The scenario of events that leads to this depressed function has been summarized as: a gradual uncontrolled rise in cytoplasmic Ca^{2+} during ischemia; a transient worsening of Ca^{2+} overload upon reperfusion; and a persistent but ultimately reversible decrease in myofibrillar Ca^{2+} sensitivity.[295] The contractile deficit appears to be primarily caused by an alteration in the myofibrillar Ca^{2+} sensitivity since Ca^{2+} regulation is largely restored. This has been demonstrated recently in permeabilized segments of stunned and normal porcine myocardium, in which a significant decrease in Ca^{2+} sensitivity was observed in myocardial biopsies (pCa shifted from 5.88 to 5.69, with no change in maximal tension).[296] Similar changes have not been observed, however, in stunned rat heart.[297]

Preconditioning

If myocardium is subjected to a brief (~5 min) episode of ischemia, the myocytes are "preconditioned," that is, they tolerate subsequent episodes of ischemia for a more sustained period before cell death occurs.[298,299] The protective effect includes improved recovery of contractile function following an ischemic insult and reperfusion, as well as protecting the heart against ischemic arrhythmias.[300] Preconditioning lasts for a relatively brief period (<1 hr), although a more long-term effect may be present.[300] The process seems to require the activity of adenosine, which appears to activate not only $K_{ACh,Ado}$ but also to modulate the function of K_{ATP} channels. Blockade of adenosine receptors appears to largely block the protection elicited by preconditioning,[299,300] while enhancement of adenosine tissue levels with acadesine extends the duration of the preconditioning effect.[301] Support for the notion that the rise in cytoplasmic Ca^{2+} is the initiating cause for stunning[295] (or at least strongly associated with it) comes from the observation that preconditioning partially inhibits the ischemic rise in cytoplasmic Ca^{2+} and attenuates the contractile dysfunction of stunning.[302] The rise in cytoplasmic Na^+ is decreased, suggesting that it may contribute to the development of the Ca^{2+} overload as noted previously.

ANESTHETIC ACTIONS ON SUBCELLULAR PATHWAYS

Inhalational Anesthetics

The volatile anesthetics have long been known to depress myocardial contractility in a dose-dependent fashion (see Chapter 7)[303] although at equianesthetic concentrations the amount of depression varies (halothane>isoflurane).[304,305] Isoflurane, halothane, and enflurane alter a number of specific mechanisms of cardiac EC coupling in an agent-specific fashion.[306] As determined by various investigators,[307–311] the volatile anesthetics directly depress tension development of cardiac myofibrils stimulated by controlled [Ca^{2+}]. However, at relevant clinical levels these actions are usually modest and do not account for the greater contractile depression observed in myocardial tissue with intact membrane systems. When equivalent depression is produced by anesthetics and by decreased external [Ca^{2+}], the effects on the kinetic parameters of isometric and isotonic contractions are reduced to the same extent.[312] The rate of isometric relaxation in particular is increased, suggesting a possible decrease in affinity of troponin C for Ca^{2+}.[312] A greater contribution to myocardial depression appears with reduction of the Ca^{2+} transient which activates myofibrils. Intracellular Ca^{2+} transients and the resulting tension demonstrate similar depression,[313,314] suggesting effects are primarily related to altered activator Ca^{2+} (although at higher isoflurane concentrations this may be less true).[314] A prominent action of the volatile anesthetics is depression of I_{Ca}, via both L- and T-type channels, although it is uncertain whether the degree of depression by halothane and isoflurane is similar at equianesthetic doses.[315] These agents also decrease SR retention of Ca^{2+} as suggested by experiments in whole tissue[304,316–320] and clearly evident in isolated SR vesicles.[321,322] Most prominent is the specific activation of CaRCs by halothane[323,324] and possibly enflurane,[324] depleting the SR Ca^{2+} store as suggested by earlier skinned fiber studies.[309] In addition, a nonspecific "leak" may also contribute. The anesthetics also modify the Ca-ATPase activity. The major action is an enhancement of activity by enflurane,[325] while additional effects are also demonstrable on the Na-Ca exchange current.[326] The effects of a variety of anesthetics on various cellular processes are summarized in Table 1–3.

The volatile anesthetic agents also appear to influence extrinsic modulators of contractility. The "sensitization" by halothane to catecholamines, which may generate dysrhythmias, may also enhance contractility under certain circumstances.[327] This action may be mediated by enhanced β-adrenoceptor coupling, or possibly, by interference with M-cholinoceptors which depress contractile function.[193,328]

TABLE 1-3. MECHANISMS OF ANESTHETIC ACTIONS ON MYOCARDIAL CONTRACTION

	Ca Channel Effects	SR Ca Stores	Relaxation (Ca reuptake)	Contractile Proteins
Volatile anesthetics				
Halothane	Moderate depression	Depleted due to CaRC activation	Ca-ATPase activation	Slightly decreased Ca^{2+} sensitivity
Enflurane	Moderate depression	? CaRC activation, cooling-induced and late release-depressed	Ca-ATPase activation	
Isofluane	Modest-moderate depression	No CaRC activation, cooling-induced and late release-depressed	± Effect	Decreased sensitivity at higher concentrations
Nitrous oxide	? Modest depression	?	?	?
Intravenous agents				
Thiopental	Moderate inhibition; AP prolongation	? Decreased release	? Slightly impaired uptake or release	?
Etomidate	No apparent effect	No apparent effect	No apparent effect	? Increased cross-bridge kinetics
Ketamine	Modest depression	No apparent effect	Slight impaired at very high dose	No apparent effect
Propofol	Modest depression	No apparent effect	? Slightly impaired uptake	No apparent effect
Opiates	? Modest depression	? No apparent effect	? No apparent effect	? No apparent effect

Adapted from various sources including Rusy BF and Komai,[305,306,316,318-320,336,340-342] Riou B et al,[332-334] Housmans PE and Murat I,[312,343,344] Su JY,[308,309,345] Bonsnjak S et al,[313,315] Lynch C III,[304,323,329,346] and others.

Intravenous Anesthetics

Of the intravenous anesthetics, hypnotics and analgesics, thiopental appears to have the most complex actions. Thiopental causes a dose-dependent depression of contractility,[329] and a major mechanism probably involves the depression of $I_{Ca,L}$,[330] which is observed in cardiac myocytes.[331] This effect on Ca channels may be counterbalanced in part by its ability to prolong the cardiac action potential by inhibiting the resting K conductance.[329,331] Thiopental may also have additional effects on the SR Ca^{2+} handling.[320,329]

Depressant actions of other intravenous anesthetics on the myocardium are far less prominent, particularly at clinical concentrations. Most implications regarding subcellular sites of action have been inferred from detailed mechanical studies by Riou and coworkers on the effects of ketamine, etomidate, and propofol in rat heart.[332–334] While these agents generally have minimal effects, ketamine had a slightly positive inotropic action, with possible impairment of SR accumulation at supraclinical levels (≥ 80 μM)[332] as well as depression of I_{Ca}.[335,336] Etomidate had minimal effect, although its propylene glycol vehicle did appear to depress SR function. Propofol at high concentrations depresses the myocardium,[329,334,337] an effect which is compatible with a modest depression of $I_{Ca,L}$,[338] and causes some alteration in SR function at high concentrations.[329,334]

Specific depression of L-type channel I_{Ca} has been observed with stimulation of opiate receptors by leu-enkephalin,[339] although the mechanism is unclear. Whether the synthetic narcotics (fentanyl and congeners) depress I_{Ca} significantly at clinical concentrations, and whether by an opiate receptor or another mechanism, remains to be determined.

Acknowledgments

The author thanks Michael S. Forbes, Ph.D., for providing the micrographs and Anna H. Evans for editorial assistance. Research support for the author was provided by NIH grant R01 GM34411.

References

1. Starling EH: The Linacre Lecture of the Law of the Heart. London, Longmans Green, 1918
2. Forbes MS, Sperelakis N: Ultrastructure of mammalian cardiac muscle. In Sperelakis N (ed): Physiology and Pathophysiology of the Heart, pp. 3–42. Boston, Martinus Nijhoff, 1984
3. Sommer JR, Jennings RB: Ultrastructure of cardiac muscle. In Fozzard HA, Haber E, Jennings RB, Katz AM, Morgan HE (eds): The Heart and Cardio-

vascular System—Scientific Foundations, pp. 3–50. New York, Raven Press, 1992

4. Forbes MS, Sperelakis N: Intercalated discs of mammalian heart: A review of structure and function. Tissue Cell 17:605–648, 1985

5. Bennett MVL, Verselis VK. Biophysics of gap junctions. Semin Cell Biol 3:29–47,1992

6. Lal R, Arnsdorf MF: Voltage-dependent gating and single-channel conductance of adult mammalian atrial gap junctions. Circ Res 71:737–743, 1992

7. Burt JM, Spray DC: Volatile anesthetics block intercellular communication between neonatal rat myocardial cells. Circ Res 65:829–837, 1989

8. Lazrak A, Peres A, Giovannardi S, Peracchia C: Ca-mediated and independent effects of arachidonic acid on gap junctions and Ca-independent effects of oleic acid and halothane. Biophys J 67:1052–1059, 1994

9. Linke WA, Popov VI, Pollack GH: Passive and active tension in single cardiac myofibrils. Biophys J 67:782–792, 1994

10. Fish D, Orenstein J, Bloom S: Passive stiffness of isolated cardiac and skeletal myocytes in the hamster. Circ Res 54:267–276, 1984

11. Engel J, Fechner M, Sowerby AJ, Finch SAE, Stier A: Anisotropc propagation of Ca^{2+} waves in isolated cardiomyocytes. Biophys J 66:1756–1762, 1994

12. Campbell KB, Kirkpatrick RD, Tobias AH, Taheri H, Shroff SG: Series coupled non-contractile elements are functionally unimportant in the isolated heart. Cardiovasc Res 28:242–251, 1994

13. MacKenna D, Omens J, A M, Covell J: Contribution of collagen matrix to passive left ventricular mechanics in isolated rat hearts. Am J Physiol 266:H1007–H1018, 1994

14. Catterall WA: Molecular properties of voltage-sensitive sodium channels. Annu Rev Biochem 55:953–985, 1986

15. Catterall WA, Seagar MJ, Takahashi M: Molecular properties of dihydropyridine-sensitive calcium channels in skeletal muscle. J Biol Chem 263:3535–3538, 1988

16. Mikami A, Imoto K, Tanabe T, et al.: Primary structure and functional expression of the cardiac dihydropyridine-sensitive calcium channel. Nature 340:230–233, 1989

17. Folander K, Smith JS, Antanavage J, Bennett C, Stein RB: Cloning and expression of the delayed-rectifier I_{sK} channel from neonatal rat heart and diethylstilbestrol-primed rat uterus. Proc Natl Acad Sci USA 87:2975–2979, 1990

18. Tamkun MM, Knoth KM, Walbridge JA, Kroemer H, Roden DM, Glover DM: Molecular cloning and characterization of two voltage-gated K^+ channel cDNAs from human ventricle. FASEB J 5:331–337, 1991

19. Tsien RW, Ellinor PT, Horne WA: Molecular diversity of voltage-dependent Ca^{2+} channels. Trends Pharmacol Sci 12:349–354, 1991

20. Miller C: 1990: Annus mirabilis of potassium channels. Science 252:1092–1096, 1991

21. Brehm P, Okamura Y, Mandel G: Ion channel evolution. Semin Neurosci 3:355–367, 1991

22. Kubo Y, Baldwin TJ, Jan YN, Jan LY: Primary structure and functional expression of a mouse inward rectifier potassium channel. Nature 362:127–133, 1993

23. Ho K, Nichols CG, Lederer WJ, et al.: Cloning and expression of an in-

wardly rectifying ATP-regulated potassium channel. Nature 362:31–38, 1993

24. Kubo Y, Reuveny E, Slesinger PA, Jan YN, Jan LY: Primary structure and functional expression of a rat G-protein-coupled muscarinic potassium channel. Nature 364:802–806, 1993

25. Tomaselli GF, Backx PH, Marban E: Molecular basis of permeation in voltage-gated ion channels. Circ Res 72:491–496, 1993

26. Katz AM: Cardiac ion channels. N Engl J Med 328:1244–1251,1993

27. Noda M, Shimizu S, Tanabe T et al: Primary structure of *Electrophorus electricus* sodium channel deduced from cDNA sequence. Nature 312:121–126, 1984

28. Noda M, Ikeda T, Kayano T et al: Existence of distinct sodium channel messenger RNAs in rat brain. Nature 320:188–192, 1986

29. Catterall WA: Molecular properties of voltage-gated ion channels in the heart. In Fozzard HA, Haber E, Jennings RB, Katz AM, Morgan HE (eds): The Heart and Cardiovascular System—Scientific Foundations, pp. 945–962. New York, Raven Press, 1992

30. Bayer R, Kalusche D, Kaufmann R, Mannhold R: Inotropic and electrophysiological actions of verapamil and D600 in mammalian myocardium. III. Effects of optical isomers on transmembrane action potentials. Naunyn Schmiedebergs Arch Pharmacol 290:87–97, 1975

31. Yatani A, Brown AM: The calcium channel blocker nitrendipine blocks sodium channels in neonatal rat cardiac myocytes. Circ Res 56:868–875, 1985

32. Gilliam FR III, Rivas PA, Wendt DJ, Starmer CF, Grant AO: Extracellular pH modulates block of both sodium and calcium channels by nicardipine. Am J Physiol 259:H1178–H1184, 1990

33. Scheuer T, Kass RS: Phenytoin reduces calcium current in the cardiac Purkinje fiber. Circ Res 53:16–23, 1983

34. Scamps F, Undrovinas A, Vassort G: Inhibition of I_{Ca} in single frog cardiac cells by quinidine, flecainide, ethmozin, and ethacizin. Am J Physiol 25:C549–C559, 1989

35. Lynch III C: Depression of myocardial contractility in vitro by bupivacaine, etidocaine, and lidocaine. Anesth Analg 65:551–559, 1986

36. Heinemann SH, Terlau H, Stuhmer W, Imoto K, Numa S: Calcium channel characteristics conferred on the sodium channel by single mutations. Nature 356:441–443, 1992

37. Nilius B, Hess P, Lansman JB, Tsien RW: A novel type of cardiac calcium channel in ventricular cells. Nature 316:443–446, 1985

38. Bean BP: Two kinds of calcium channels in canine atrial cells: Differences in kinetics, selectivity, and pharmacology. J Gen Physiol 86:1–31, 1985

39. Mitra R, Morad M: Two types of Ca^{2+} in guinea pig ventricular myocytes. Proc Natl Acad Sci USA 83:5340–5344, 1986

40. Yang J, Ellinor PT, Sather WA, Zhang J-F, Tsien RW: Molecular determinants of Ca^{2+} selectivity and ion permeation in L-type Ca^{2+} channels. Nature 366:158–161, 1993

41. Lacerda AE, Kim HS, Ruth O, et al: Normalization of current kinetics by interaction between the α_1 and β subunits of the skeletal muscle dihydropyridine-sensitive Ca^{2+} channel. Nature 352:527–530, 1991

42. Kohlhardt M, Bauer B, Krause H, Fleckenstein A: Selective inhibition of the transmembrane Ca conductivity of mammalian myocardial fibres. Pflügers Arch 338:115–123, 1973

43. Lee KS, Tsien RW: Reversal of current through calcium channels in dialysed single heart cells. Nature 297:498–503, 1982
44. Pietrobon D, Hess P: Novel mechanism of voltage-dependent gating in L-type calcium channels. Nature 346:651–655, 1990
45. Yue DT, Herzig S, Marban E: β-Adrenergic stimulation of calcium channels occurs by potentiation of high-activity gating modes. Proc Natl Acad Sci USA 87:753–757, 1990
46. Tseng G-N: Calcium current restitution in mammalian ventricular myocytes is modulated by intracellular calcium. Circ Res 63:468–482, 1989
47. Hryshko LV, Bers DM: Ca current facilitation during postrest recovery depends on Ca entry. Am J Physiol 259:H951–H961, 1990
48. Bates SE, Gurney AM: Ca^{2+}-dependent block and potentiation of L-type calcium current in guinea-pig ventricular myocytes. J Physiol (Lond) 466:345–365, 1993
49. O'Rourke B, Backx PH, Marban E: Phosphorylation-independent modulation of L-type calcium channels by magnesium-nucleotide complexes. Science 257:245–248, 1992
50. Yuan W, Bers DM: Ca-dependent facilitation of cardiac Ca current is due to Ca-calmodulin-dependent protein kinase. Am J Physiol 267:H982–H993, 1994
51. DeFelice LJ: Molecular and biophysical view of the Ca channel: A hypothesis regarding oligomeric structure, channel clustering, and macroscopic current. J Memb Bil 133:191–202, 1993
52. Hadley RW, Lederer WJ: Ca^{2+} and voltage inactivate Ca^{2+} channels in guinea-pig ventricular myocytes through independent mechanisms. J Physiol (Lond) 444:257–268, 1991
53. Nakayama H, Taki M, Striessnig J, Glossmann H, Catterall WA, Kanaoka Q: Identification of 1,4-dihydropyridine binding regions within the α1 subunit of skeletal muscle Ca^{2+} channels by photoaffinity labeling with diazepine. Proc Natl Acad Sci USA 88:9203–9207, 1991
54. Hess P, Lansman JB, Tsien RW: Different modes of Ca channel gating behaviour favoured by dihydropyridine Ca agonists and antagonists. Nature 311:538–544, 1984
55. Kass RS, Arena JP, Chin S: Block of L-type calcium channels by charged dihydropyridines. Sensitivity to side of application and calcium. J Gen Physiol 98:63–75, 1991
56. Hescheler J, Pelzer D, Trube G, Trautwein W: Does the organic channel blocker D600 act from inside or outside on the cardiac cell membrane. Pflügers Arch 393:287–291, 1982
57. McDonald TF, Pelzer S, Trautwein W, Pelzer DJ: Regulation and modulation of calcium channels in cardiac, skeletal, and smooth muscle cells. Physiol Rev 74:365–507, 1994
58. Wagenknecht T, Grassucci R, Frank J, Saito A, Inui M, Fleischer S: Three-dimensional architecture of the calcium channel/foot structure of sarcoplasmic reticulum. Nature 38:167–170, 1989
59. McPherson PS, Campbell KP: The ryanodine receptor/Ca^{2+} release channel. J Biol Chem 268:13765–13768, 1993
60. Coronado R, Morrissette M, Sukhareva M, Vaughn DM: Structure and function of ryanodine receptors. Am J Physiol 266:C1485–C1504, 1994
61. Mészáros LG, Volpe P: Caffeine- and ryanodine-sensitive Ca^{2+} stores of canine cerebrum and cerebellum neurons. Am J Physiol 261:C1048–C1054, 1991
62. Zorzato F, Fujii J, Otsu K et al: Molecular cloning of cDNA encoding hu-

man and rabbit forms of the Ca^{2+} release channel (ryanodine receptor) of skeletal muscle sarcoplasmic reticulum. J Biol Chem 265:2244–2256, 1990

63. Marks AR, Tempst P, Hwang KS et al: Molecular cloning and characterization of the ryanodine receptor/junctional channel complex cDNA from skeletal muscle sarcoplasmic reticulum. Proc Natl Acad Sci USA 86:8683–8687, 1989

64. Otsu K, Willard HF, Khanna VK, Zorzato F, Green NM, MacLennan DH: Molecular cloning of cDNA encoding of the Ca^{2+} release channel (ryanodine receptor) of rabbit cardiac muscle sarcoplasmic reticulum. J Biol Chem 265:13472–13483, 1990

65. Hakamata Y, Nakai J, Takeshima H, Imoto K: Primary structure and distribution of a novel ryanodine receptor/calcium release channel from rabbit brain. FEBS Lett 312:229–235, 1992

66. García J, Tanabe T, Beam KG: Relationship of calcium transients to calcium currents and charge movements in myotubes expressing skeletal and cardiac dihydropyridine receptors. J Gen Physiol 103:125–147, 1994

67. García J, Beam KG: Measurement of calcium transients and slow calcium current in myotubes. J Gen Physiol 103:107–123, 1994

68. Chu A, Fill M, Stefani E, Entman ML: Cytoplasmic Ca^{2+} does not inhibit the cardiac muscle sarcoplasmic reticulum ryanodine receptor channel, although Ca^{2+}-induced Ca^{2+} inactivation of Ca^{2+} release is observed native vesicles. J Memb Biol 135:49–59, 1993

69. Fabiato A: Calcium-induced release of calcium from the cardiac sarcoplasmic reticulum. Am J Physiol 245:C1–C14, 1983

70. Niggli E, Lederer WJ: Voltage-independent calcium release in heart muscle. Science 250:565–568, 1990

71. Cleemann L, Morad M: Role of Ca^{2+} channel in cardiac excitation-contraction coupling in the rat: Evidence from Ca^{2+} transients and contraction. J Physiol (Lond) 432:283–312, 1991

72. Stern MD, Lakatta EG: Excitation-contraction coupling in the heart: The state of the question. FASEB J 6:3092–3100, 1992

73. Lederer WJ, Niggli E, Hadley RW: Sodium-calcium exchange in excitable cells: Fuzzy space. Science 248:371–372, 1991

74. Langer GA, Peskoff A, Post JA: How does the Na^{+}-Ca^{2+} exchanger working the intact cardiac cells? J Mol Cell Cardiol 25:637–639, 1993

75. Post JA, Langer GA: Sarcolemmal calcium binding sites in heart. I. Molecular origin in "gas dissected" sarcolemma. J Memb Biol 129:49–57, 1992

76. Peskoff A, Post JA, Langer GA: Sarcolemmal calcium binding sites in heart. II. Mathematical model for diffusion of calcium release from the sarcoplasmic reticulum into the diadic region. J Memb Biol 129:59–69, 1992

77. Callewaert G: Excitation-contraction coupling in mammalian cardiac cells. Cardiovasc Res 26:923–932, 1992

78. Cheng H, Lederer WJ, Cannell MB: Calcium sparks: Elementary events underlying excitation-contraction coupling in heart muscle. Science 262:740–744, 1993

79. Strand MA, Louis CF, Mickelson JR: Phosphorylation of the porcine skeletal and cardiac muscle sarcoplasmic reticulum ryanodine receptor. Biochim Biophys Acta 1175:319–326, 1993

80. Witcher DR, Kovacs RJ, Schulman H, Cefali DC, Jones LR: Unique phosphorylation site on the cardiac ryanodine receptor regulates calcium channel activity. J Biol Chem 266:11114–11152, 1991

81. Abdelmeguid AE, Feher JJ: Effect of perfusate [Ca^{2+}] on cardiac sarcoplasmic Ca^{2+} release channel in isolated hearts. Circ Res 71:1049–1058, 1992

82. Sitsapesan R, Williams AJ: Mechanisms of caffeine activation of single calcium-release channels of sheep cardiac sarcoplasmic reticulum. J Physiol (Lond) 423:425–439, 1990

83. Pessah IN, Durie EM, Schiedt MJ, Zimanyi I: Anthraquinone-sensitized Ca^{2+} release channel from rat cardiac sarcoplasmic reticulum: Possible receptor-mediated mechanism of doxorubicin cardiomyopathy. Molec Pharmacol 37:503–514, 1990

84. Boucek RJ Jr, Buck SH, Scott F et al: Anthracycline-induced tension in permeabilized cardiac fibers: Evidence for the activation of the calcium release channel of sarcoplasmic reticulum. J Mol Cell Cardiol 25:249–259,1993

85. Jayaraman T, Brillantes A, Timerman A et al: FK506 binding protein associated with the calcium release channel (ryanodine receptor). J Biol Chem 267:9474–9477, 1992

86. Grover AK, Khan I: Calcium pump isoforms: Diversity, selectivity and plasticity. Cell Calcium 13:9–17, 1992

87. Brandl CJ, Green NM, Korczak B, MacLennan DH: Two Ca^{2+}-ATPase genes: Homologies and mechanistic implication of deduced amino acid sequences. Cell 44:597–607, 1986

88. Brandl CJ, de Leon S, Martin DR, MacLennan DH: Adult forms of the Ca^{2+}-ATPase of the sarcoplasmic reticulum. J Biol Chem 262:3768–3774, 1987

89. Hasselbach W, Oetlicker H: Energetics and electrogenicity of the sarcoplasmic reticulum calcium pump. Annu Rev Physiol 43:325–339, 1983

90. MacLennan DH: Molecular tools to elucidate problems in excitation-contraction coupling. Biophys J 58:1355–1365, 1990

91. Simmerman HKB, Collins JH, Theibert JL, Wegener AD, Jones LR: Sequence analysis of phospholamban. J Biol Chem 261:13333–13341, 1986

92. Fujii J, Ueno A, Kitano K, Tanaka S, Kadoma M, Tada M: Complete complementary DNA-derived amino acid sequence of canine cardiac phospholamban. J Clin Invest 79:301–304, 1987

93. Kim HW, Steenart NAE, Ferguson DG, Kranias EG: Functional reconstitution of the cardiac sarcoplasmic reticulum Ca^{2+}-ATPase with phospholamban in phospholipid vesicles. J Biol Chem 265:1702–1709, 1990

94. Balke CW, Egan TM, Wier WG: Processes that remove calcium from the cytoplasm during excitation-contraction coupling in intact rat heart cells. J Physiol (Lond) 474:447–462, 1994

95. Kijima Y, Ogunbunmi E, Fleischer S: Drug action of thapsigargin on the Ca^{2+} pump protein of sarcoplasmic reticulum. J Biol Chem 266:22912–22918, 1991

96. Janczewski AM, Lakatta EG: Thapsigargin inhibits Ca^{2+} uptake, and Ca^{2+} depletes sarcoplasmic reticulum in intact cardiac myocytes. Am J Physiol 265:H517–H522, 1993

97. Hove-Madsen L, Bers DM: Sarcoplasmic reticulum Ca^{2+} uptake and thapsigargin sensitivity in permeabilized rabbit and rat ventricular myocytes. Circ Res 73:820–828, 1993

98. Baudet S, Shaoulian R, Bers DM: Effects of thapsigargin and cyclopiazonic acid on twitch force and sarcoplasmic reticulum Ca^{2+} content of rabbit ventricular muscle. Circ Res 73:813–819, 1993

99. Mitchell RD, Simmerman HKB, Jones LR: Ca^{2+} binding effects on protein conformation and protein interactions of canine cardiac calsequestrin. J Biol Chem 263:1376–1381, 1988

100. Scott BT, Simmerman HKB, Collins JH, Nadal-Ginard B, Jones LR: Com-

plete amino acid sequence of canine cardiac calsequestrin deduced by cDNA cloning. J Biol Chem 263:8958–8964, 1988

101. Franzini-Armstrong C, Kenney LJ, Varriano-Marston E: The structure of calsequestrin in triads of vertebrate skeletal muscle: A deep-etch study. J Cell Biol 105:49–56, 1987

102. Ikemoto N, Ronjat M, Mészáros L, Koshita M: Postulated role of calsequestrin in the regulation of calcium release from sarcoplasmic reticulum. Biochemistry 28:6764–6771, 1989

103. Knudson CM, Stang KK, Jorgensen AO, Campbell KP: Biochemical characterization and ultrastructural localization of a major junctional sarcoplasmic reticulum glycoprotein (triadin). J Biol Chem 268:12637–12645, 1993

104. Bridge JHB, Smolley JR, Spitzer KW: The relationship between charge movements associated with I_{Ca} and I_{Na-Ca} in cardiac myocytes. Science 248:376–378, 1990

105. Bers DM, Bassani JWM, Bassani RA: Competition and redistribution among calcium transport systems in rabbit cardiac myocytes. Cardiovasc Res 27:1772–1777, 1993

106. Nicoll DA, Longoni S, Philipson KD: Molecular cloning and functional expression of the cardiac sarcolemmal Na^+-Ca^{2+} exchanger. Science 250:562–565, 1990

107. Mullins LJ: The generation of electric currents in cardiac fibers by Na/Ca exchange. Am J Physiol 236:C103–C110, 1979

108. Bridge JHB, Bassingthwaighte JB: Uphill sodium transport driven by an inward calcium gradient in heart muscle. Science 219:178–180, 1983

109. Crespo LM, Grantham CJ, Cannell MB: Kinetics, stoichiometry and role for the Na-Ca exchange mechanism is isolated cardiac myocytes. Nature 345:618–621, 1990

110. Kimura J, Akinori A, Irisawa H: Na-Ca exchange current in mammalian heart cells. Nature 319:596–597, 1986

111. Blaustein MP: Sodium/calcium exchange and the control of contractility in cardiac muscle and vascular smooth muscle. J Cardiovasc Pharmacol 12(suppl 5):S56–S68, 1988

112. LeBlanc N, Hume JR: Sodium current-induced release of calcium from cardiac sarcoplasmic reticulum. Science 248:372–376, 1990

113. Levesque PC, Leblanc N, Hume JR: Release of calcium from guinea pig cardiac sarcoplasmic reticulum by sodium-calcium exchange. Cardiovasc Res 28:370–378, 1994

114. Nuss HB, Houser SR: Sodium-calcium exchange-mediated contractions in feline ventricular myocytes. Am J Physiol 263:H1161–H1169, 1992

115. Levi AJ, Brooksby P, Hancox JC: One hump or two? The triggering of calcium release from the sarcoplasmic reticulum and the voltage dependence of contraction in mammalian cardiac muscle. Cardiovasc Res 27:1743–1757, 1993

116. Lipp P, Niggli E: Sodium current-induced calcium signals in isolated guinea-pig ventricular myocytes. J Physiol (Lond) 474:439–446, 1994

117. Sham J, Cleemann L, Morad M: Gating of the cardiac Ca^{2+} release channel: The role of Na^+ current and Na^+-Ca^{2+} exchange. Science 255:850–853, 1992

118. Callewaert G, Cleeman L, Morad M: Caffeine-induced Ca^{2+} release activates Ca^{2+} extrusion via Na^+-Ca^{2+} exchanger in cardiac myocytes. Am J Physiol 257:C147–C152, 1989

119. Arlock P, Katzung BG: Effects of sodium substitutes on transient inward

current and tension in guinea-pig and ferret papillary muscle. J Physiol (Lond) 360:105–120, 1985

120. Lynch C III: Cellular electrophysiology of the heart. In Lynch C III (ed): Clinical Cardiac Electrophysiology: Perioperative Considerations, pp. 1–52. Philadelphia, JB Lippincott, 1994

121. Horisberger J-D, Lemas V, Kraehenbuhl J-P, Rossier B: Structure-function relationship of Na,K-ATPase. Annu Rev Physiol 53:565–584, 1991

122. Wang K, Villalobo A, Roufogalis B: The plasma membrane calcium pump: A multiregulated transporter. Trends Cell Biol 2:46–51, 1992

123. Langer GA: Calcium and the heart: Exchange at the tissue, cell, and organelle levels. FASEB J 6:893–902, 1992

124. Baum VC, Klitzner TS: Excitation-contraction coupling in neonatal myocardium: Effects of halothane and isoflurane. Dev Pharmacol Ther 16:99–107, 1991

125. Wendt-Gallitelli MF, Jacob R: Rhythm-dependent role of different calcium stores in cardiac muscle: X-ray microanalysis. J Mol Cell Cardiol 14:487–492, 1982

126. Shattock MJ, Bers DM: Rat vs. rabbit ventricle: Ca flux and intracellular Na assessed by ion-selective microelectrodes. Am J Physiol 256:C813–C822, 1989

127. Bers DM, Bridge JHB: Relaxation of rabbit ventricular muscle by Na-Ca exchange and sarcoplasmic reticulum calcium pump—ryanodine and voltage sensitivity. Circ Res 65:334–342, 1989

128. Negretti N, O'Neill SC, Eisner DA: The relative contributions of different intracellular and sarcolemmal systems to relaxation in rat ventricular myocytes. Cardiovasc Res 27:1826–1830, 1993

129. Kieval R, Bloch R, Lindenmayer G, Ambesi A, Lederer W: Immunofluorescence localization of the Na-Ca exchanger in heart cells. Am J Physiol 163:C545–C550, 1992

130. Frank JS, Mottino G, Reid D, Molday RR, Philipson KD: Distribution of the Na-Ca exchange protein in mammalian cardiac myocytes: An immunofluorescence an dimmunocolloidal gold-labelling study. J Cell Biol 117: 337–345, 1992

131. Miura Y, Kimura J: Sodium-calcium exchange current. Dependence on internal Ca and Na and competitive binding of external Na and Ca. J Gen Physiol 93:1129–1145, 1989

132. Yue DT, Burkhoff D, Franz MR, Hunter WC, Sagawa K: Postextrasystolic potentiation of the isolated canine left ventricle. Circ Res 56:340–350, 1985

133. Egan TM, Noble D, Noble SJ, Powell T, Spindler AJ, Twist VW: Sodium-calcium exchange during the action potential in guinea-pig ventricular cells. J Physiol (Lond) 411:639–661, 1989

134. Barcenas-Ruiz L, Beukelmann DJ, Wier WG: Sodium-calcium exchange in heart: Membrane currents and changes in $[Ca^{2+}]_i$. Science 238:1720–1722, 1987

135. Scarpa A, Graziotti P: Mechanisms for intracellular calcium regulation in heart. I. Stopped-flow measurements of Ca uptake by cardiac mitochondria. J Gen Physiol 62:756–772, 1973

136. Bassani JWM, Bassani RA, Bers DM: Ca^{2+} cycling between sarcoplasmic reticulum and mitochondria in rabbit cardiac myocytes. J Physiol (Lond) 460:603–621, 1993

137. Wertman K, Drubin D: Actin constitution: Guaranteeing the right to assemble. Science 258:750–60, 1992

138. Wang Z, Gergely J, Tao T: Characterization of the Ca^{2+}-triggered confor-

mational transition in troponin C. Proc Natl Acad Sci USA 89:11814–11817, 1992

139. Tao T, Gong BJ, Leavis P: Calcium-induced movement of troponin-I relative to actin in skeletal muscle thin filaments. Science 247:1339–1341, 1990

140. Potter JD, Gergely J: Troponin, tropomyosin, and actin interactions in the Ca²⁺ regulation of muscle contraction. Biochemistry 13:2697–2703, 1974

141. Rayment I, Holden HM, Whittaker M, et al: Structure of the actin-myosin complex and implications for muscle contraction. Science 261:58–65, 1993

142. McNally EM, Kraft R, Bravo-Zehnder M, Taylor DA, Leinwand LA: Full-length rat alpha and beta cardiac myosin heavy chain sequences: Comparisons suggest a molecular basis for functional differences. J Mol Biol 210:665–671, 1989

143. Pagani E, Julian F: Rabbit papillary muscle myosic isozymes and the velocity of muscle shortening. Circ Res 54:586–594, 1984

144. Litten RZ, Martin BJ, Low RB, Alpert NR: Altered myosin isozyme patterns from pressure-overloaded and thyrotoxic hypertrophied rabbit hearts. Circ Res 50:856–864, 1982

145. Julian FJ, Sollins MR: Sarcomere length-tension relations in living rat papillary muscle. Circ Res 37:299–308, 1975

146. Julian FJ, Sollins MR, Moss RL: Absence of a plateau in length-tension relationship of rabbit papillary muscle when internal shortening is prevented. Nature 260:340–342, 1976

147. ter Kurs HEDJ, Rijnsburger WH, van Heuningen R, Nagelsmit MJ: Tension development and sarcomere lengths in rat cardiac trabeculae. Evidence of length dependent activation. Circ Res 46:703–714, 1980

148. Housmans PD, Lee NKM, Blinks JR: Active shortening retards the decline of the intracellular calcium transient in mammalian heart muscle. Science 221:159–161, 1983

149. Lab MJ, Allen DG, Orchard CH: The effects of shortening on myoplasmic calcium concentration and on the action potential in mammalian ventricular muscle. Circ Res 55:825–829, 1984

150. Allen DG, Eisner DA, Pirolo JS, Smith GL: The relationship between intracellular calcium concentration and contraction in calcium-overloaded ferret papillary muscles. J Physiol (Lond) 364:169–182, 1985

151. Backx PH, ter Keurs HEDJ: Fluorescent properties of rat trabeculae microinjected with fura-2 salt. Am J Physiol 264:H1098–H1110, 1993

152. Saeki Y, Kurihara S, Hongo K, Tanaka E: Alterations in intracellular calcium and tension of activated ferret papillary muscle in response to step length changes. J Physiol (Lond) 463:291–306, 1993

153. Kentish JC, ter Keurs HEDJ, Ricciardi L, Bucx JJJ, Noble MIM: Comparison between the sarcomere length-force relations of intact and skinned trabeculae from rat right ventricle: Influence of calcium contractions on these relations. Circ Res 58:755–768, 1986

154. Hofmann P, Fuchs F: Evidence for a force-dependent component of calcium binding to cardiac troponin C. Am J Physiol 22:C541–C546, 1987

155. Babu A, Sonnenblick E, Gulati J: Molecular basis for the influence of muscle length on myocardial performance. Science 240:74–76, 1988

156. Gulati J, Sonnenblick E, Babu A: The role of troponin C in the length dependence of Ca²⁺-sensitive force of mammalian skeletal and cardiac muscle fibers. J Physiol (Lond) 444:305–324, 1990

157. Landesberg A, Sideman S: Mechanical regulation of cardiac muscle by coupling calcium kinetics with cross-bridge cycling: A dynamic model. Am J Physiol 267:H779–H795, 1994

158. Sonnenblick EH: Determinants of active state in heart muscle; force, velocity, instantaneous muscle length, time. Fed Proc 24:1396–1409, 1964
159. Burkoff D, de Tombe PP, Hunter WC: Impact of ejection on magnitude and time course of ventricular pressure-generating capacity. Am J Physiol 265:H899–H909, 1993
160. Brutsaert DL, De Clerck NM, Goethals MA, Housmans PR: Relaxation of ventricular cardiac muscle. J Physiol (Lond) 283:469–480, 1978
161. Brutsaert DL, Housmans PR, Goethals MA: Dual control of relaxation: Its role in the ventricular function in the mammalian heart. Circ Res 47:637–652, 1980
162. Pery-man N, Chemla D, Coirault C, Suard I, Riou B, Lecarpentier Y: A comparison of cyclopiazonic acid and ryanodine effects on cardiac muscle relaxation. Am J Physiol 265:H1364–H1372, 1993
163. Pagel PS, Kampine JP, Schmeling WT, Warltier DC: Reversal of volatile anesthetic-induced depression of myocardial contractility by extracellular calcium also enhances left ventricular diastolic function. Anesthesiology 78:141–154, 1993
164. Allen DG, Kurihara S: The effects of muscle length on intracellular calcium transients in mammalian cardiac muscle. J Physiol (Lond) 327:79–94, 1982
165. Lew WYW: Mechanisms of volume-induced increase in left ventricular contractility. Am J Physiol 265:H1778–H1786, 1993
166. Birnbaumer L: G Proteins in signal transduction. Annu Rev Pharmacol Toxicol 30:675–705, 1990
167. Holmer SR, Homcy CJ: G proteins in the heart: A redundant and diverse transmembrane signaling network. Circulation 84:1891–1902, 1991
168. Lynch C III, Jaeger JM: The G protein cell signalling system. In Lake C (ed): Advances in Anesthesia 11, pp. 65–112. Chicago, Mosby-Year Book, 1994
169. Hepler JR, Gilman AG: G proteins. Trends Biochem Sci 17:383–387, 1992
170. Iñiguez-Lluhi J, Kleuss C, Gilman AG: The importance of G-protein βγ subunits. Trends Cell Biol 3:230–236, 1993
171. Iyengar R: Molecular and functional diversity of mammalian Gs-stimulated adenylyl cyclases. FASEB J 7:768–775, 1993
172. Schwinn DA, Caron MG, Lefkowitz RJ: The beta-adrenergic receptor as a model for molecular structure-function relationships in G-protein-coupled receptors. In Fozzard HA (ed): The Heart and Cardiovascular System. New York, Raven Press, 1992
173. McNeill JH, Muschek LD: Histamine effects on cardiac contractility, phosphorylase and adenyl cyclase. J Mol Cell Cardiol 4:611–624, 1972
174. Alloatti G, Serazzi L, Levi EC: Prostaglandin $I_2(PGI_2)$ enchances calcium current in guinea-pig ventricular heart cells. J Mol Cell Cardiol 23:851–860, 1991
175. Ouadid H, Seguin J, Dumuis A, Bockaert J, Nargeot J: Serotonin increases calcium current in human atrial myocytes via the newly described 5-hydroxytryptamine$_4$ receptors. Molec Pharmacol 41:346–351, 1992
176. Takasago T, Imagawa T, Shigekawa M: Phosphorylation of the cardiac ryanodine receptor by cAMP-dependent kinase. J Biochem (Tokyo) 106:872–877, 1989
177. Yoshida A, Takahashi M, Imagawa T, Shigekawa M, Takisawa H, Nakamura T: Phosphorylation of ryanodine receptors during β-adrenergic stimulation. J Biochem (Tokyo) 111:186–190, 1992
178. Robertson S, Johnson J, Holroyde M, Kranias E, Potter J, Solaro R: The effect of troponin I phosphorylation on the Ca^{2+}-binding properties of the Ca^{2+}-regulatory site of bovine cardiac troponin. J Biol Chem 257:260–263, 1982

179. Endoh M, Blinks JM: Actions of sympathomimetic amines on the Ca^{2+} transients and contractions of rabbit myocardium: Reciprocal changes in myofibrillar responsiveness to Ca^{2+} mediated through α- and β-receptors. Circ Res 62:247–265, 1988

180. Hoh J, Rossmanith G, Kwan L, Hamilton A: Adrenaline increases the rate of cycling of crossbridges in rat cardiac muscle as measured by pseudo-random binary noise-modulated perturbation analysis. Circ Res 62:452–461, 1988

181. Garvey J, Kranias E, Solaro R. Phosphorylation of C-protein, troponin I and phospholamban in isolated rabbit hearts. Biochem J 249:709–714, 1988

182. Hartzell HC, Titus L: Effects of cholinergic and adrenergic agonists on the phosphorylation of a 165,000 dalton myofibrillar protein in intact cardiac muscle. J Biol Chem 257:2111–2120, 1982

183. Walsh KB, Begenisich TB, Kass RS: β-Adrenergic modulation in the heart: Independent regulation of K and Ca channels. Pflügers Arch 411:232–234, 1988

184. Nakayama T, Fozzard H: Adrenergic modulation of the transient outward current in isolated canine purkinje cells. Circ Res 62:162–172, 1988

185. Xiao P-P, Lakatta EG: β_1-Adrenoceptor stimulation and β_2-adrenoceptor stimulation differ in their effects on contraction, cytosolic Ca^{2+}, and Ca^{2+} current in single rat ventricular cells. Circ Res 73:286–300, 1993

186. Chinkers M, Garbers D: Signal transduction by guanylyl cyclases. Annu Rev Biochem 60:553–575, 1991

187. McClellan G, Weisberg A, Winegrad S: cAMP can raise or lower cardiac actomyosin ATPase activity depending on α-adrenergic activity. Am J Physiol 267:H431–H442, 1994

188. Barnard EA: Separating receptor subtypes from their shadows. Nature 335:301–302, 1988

189. Shryock J, Song Y, Wang D, Baker SP, Olsson RA, Belardinelli L: Selective A_2-adenosine receptor agonists do not alter action potential duration, twitch shortening, or cAMP accumulation in guinea pig, rat, or rabbit isolated ventricular myocytes. Circ Res 72:194–205, 1993

190. Böhm M, Gierschik P, Schwinger RHG, Uhlmann R, Erdmann E: Coupling of M-cholinoceptors and A_1 adenosine receptors in human myocardium. Am J Physiol 266:H1951–H1958, 1994

191. DiFrancesco D, Ducouret P, Robinson RB: Muscarinic modulation of cardiac rate at low acetylcholine concentrations. Science 243:669–671, 1989

192. Petit-Jacques J, Bescond J, Bois P, Lenfant J: Particular sensitivity of the mammalian heart sinus node cells. News Physiol Sci 9:77–79, 1994

193. Boyett MR, Kirby MS, Orchard CH, Roberts A: The negative inotropic effect of acetylcholine on ferret ventricular myocardium. J Physiol (Lond) 404:613–635, 1988

194. Löffelholz K, Pappano AJ: The parasympathetic neuroeffector junction of the heart. Pharmacol Rev 37:1–24, 1985

195. Brown AM, Birnbaumer L: Ion channels and their regulation by G protein subunits. Ann Rev Physiol 52:197–213, 1990

196. Yatani A, Codina J, Imoto Y, Reeves JP, Birnbaumer L, Brown AM: A G protein directly regulates mammalian cardiac calcium channels. Science 238:1288–1292, 1987

197. Yatani A, Brown AM: Rapid β-adrenergic modulation of cardiac calcium channel currents by a fast G protein pathway. Science 245:71–74, 1989

198. Hartzell HC, Fischmeister R: Direct regulation of cardiac Ca^{2+} channels by

G proteins: Neither proven nor necessary? Trends Pharmacol Sci 13:380–385, 1992

199. Scamps F, Nilius B, Alvarez J, Vassort G: Modulation of L-type Ca channel activity by P_2 purinergic agonist in cardiac cells. Pflügers Arch 422:465–471, 1993

200. Koumi S-I, Wasserstrom JA: Acetylcholine-sensitive muscarinic K^+ channels in mammalian ventricular myocytes. Am J Physiol 266:H1812–H1821, 1994

201. Isenberg G, Belardinelli L: Ionic basic for the antagonism between adenosine and isoproterenol on isolated mammalian ventricular myocytes. Circ Res 55:309–325, 1984

202. Sternweis PC, Smrcka AV: Regulation of phospholipase C by G proteins. Trends Biochem Sci 17:502–506, 1992

203. Smrcka AV, Hepler JR, Brown KO, Sternweiss PC: Regulation of polyphosphoinositide-specific phospholipase C activity by purified G_q. Science 251:804–807, 1991

204. Rhee SG, Kim H, Shuh P-G, Choi WC: Multiple forms of phosphoinositide-specific phospholipase C and different modes of activation. Biochem Soc Trans 19:337–341, 1991

205. Sando JJ, Maurer MC, Bolen EJ, Grisham CM. Role of cofactors in protein kinase C activation. Cell Signal 4:595–609, 1992

206. Iwasa Y, Hosey MM: Phosphorylation of cardiac sarcolemma proteins by the calcium activated phospholipid-dependent kinase. J Biol Chem 259:534–540, 1984

207. Movsesian MA, Nishikawa M, Adelstein RS: Phosphorylation of phospholamban by calcium-activated, phospholipid-dependent protein kinase. J Biol Chem 259:8029–8032, 1984

208. Noland TA Jr, Kuo JF: Protein kinase C phosphorylation of cardiac troponin I and troponin T inhibits Ca^{2+}-stimulated MgATPase activity in reconstituted actomyosin and isolated myofibrils, and decreases actin-myosin interactions. J Mol Cell Cardiol 25:53–65, 1993

209. Terzic A, Pucéat M, Clément O, Scamps F, Vassort G: α_1-adrenergic effects on intracellular pH and calcium and on myofilaments in single rat cardiac cells. J Physiol (Lond) 447:275–292, 1992

210. Gambassi G, Spurgeon HA, Lakatta EG, Blank PS, Capogrossi MC: Different effects of α-and β-adrenergic stimulation on cytosolic pH and myofilament responsiveness to Ca^{2+} in cardiac myocytes. Circ Res 71:870–882, 1992

211. Lacerda AE, Rampe D, Brown AM: Effects of protein kinase C activators on cardiac Ca^{2+} channels. Nature 335:249–251, 1988

212. Zheng J-S, Christie A, Levy M, Scarpa A: Ca^{2+} mobilization by extracellular ATP in rat cardiac myocytes: Regulation by protein kinase C and A. Am J Physiol 263:C933–C940, 1992

213. Boutjdir M, Restivo M, Wei Y, El-Sherif N: α_1-β-adrenergic interactions on L-type calcium current in cardiac myocytes. Pflügers Arch 421:397–399, 1992

214. Furuichi T, Yoshikawa S, Miyawaki A, Kentaroh W, Maeda N, Mikoshiba K: Primary structure and functional expression of the inositol 1,4,5-triposphate-binding protein P_{400}. Nature 342:32–38, 1989

215. Ferris C, Snyder S: Inositol 1,4,5-trisphosphate-activated calcium channels. Annu Rev Physiol 54:469–488, 1992

216. Baker KM, Aceto JA: Characterization of avian angiotensin II cardiac re-

ceptors: Coupling to mechanical activity and phosphoinositide metabolism. J Mol Cell Cardiol 21:375–382, 1989

217. Dösemeci A, Dhallan RS, Cohen NM, Lederer WJ, Rogers TB: Phorbol ester increases calcium current and simulates the effects of angiotensin II on cultured neonatal rat heart myocytes. Circ Res 62:347–357, 1988

218. Nosek TM, William MF, Zeigler ST, Godt RE: Inositol triphosphate enhances calcium release in skinned cardiac and skeletal muscle. Am J Physiol 250:C807–C811, 1986

219. Kawaguchi H, Shoki M, Sano H et al: Phospholipid metabolism in cardiomyopathic hamster heart cells. Circ Res 69:1015–1021, 1991

220. Kijima Y, Saito A, Jetton TL, Magnuson MA, Fleischer S: Different intracellular localization of inositol 1,4,5-triphosphate and ryanodine receptors in cardiomyocytes. J Biol Chem 268:3499–3506, 1993

221. Fedida D, Shimoni Y, Giles WR: α-Adrenergic modulation of the transient outward current in rabbit atrial myocytes. J Physiol (Lond) 423:257–277, 1990

222. Ertl R, Jahnel U, Nawrath H, Carmeliet E, Vereecke J: Differential electrophysiologic and inotropic effects of phenylephrine in atrial and ventricular heart muscle preparations from rats. Naunyn Schmiedebergs Arch Pharmacol 344:574–581, 1992

223. Schümann HJ, Wagner J, Knorr A, Reidemeister JC, Sadon V, Schramm G: Demonstration in human atrial preparations of α-adrenoceptors mediating positive inotropic effects. Naunyn Schmiedebergs Arch Pharmacol 302:333–338, 1978

224. Brückner R, Meyer W, Mügge A, Schmitz W, Scholz H: α-Adrenoceptor-mediated positive inotropic effect of phenylephrine in isolated human ventricular myocardium. Eur J Pharmacol 99:345–347, 1984

225. Fedida D, Braun AP, Giles WR: α₁-Adrenoceptors in myocardium: Functional aspects and transmembrane signalling mechanisms. Physiol Rev 73:469–487, 1993

226. O'Rourke B, Reibel DK, Thomas AP: α-Adrenergic modification of the Ca^{2+} transient and contraction in single rat cardiomyocytes. J Mol Cell Cardiol 24:809–820, 1992

227. Edes I, Kranias E. Phospholamban and troponin I are substrates for protein kinase C in vitro but not in intact beating guinea pig hearts. Circ Res 67:394–400, 1990

228. Endou M, Hattori Y, Tohse N, Kanno M: Protein kinase C is not involved in alpha₁-adrenoceptor mediated positive inotropic effect. Am J Physiol 260:H27–H36, 1991

229. Walsh KB, Kass RS: Regulation of a heart potassium channel by protein kinase A and C. Science 242:67–69, 1988

230. Tohse N, Kameyama M, Sekiguchi K, Shearman MS, Kanno M: Protein kinase C activation enhances the delayed rectifier potassium current in guinea-pig heart cells. J Mol Cell Cardiol 22:725–734, 1990

231. Fedida D, Bouchard RA: Mechanisms for the positive inotropic effect of α₁-adrenoceptor stimulation in rat cardiac myocytes. Circ Res 71:673–688, 1992

232. Curiel R, Pérez-González J, Brito N et al: Positive inotropic effects mediated by α₁-adrenoceptors in intact human subjects. J Cardiovasc Pharmacol 14:603–615, 1989

233. Williamson AP, Kennedy RH, Seifen E, Lindemann JP, Stimers JR: α₁ᵦ-Adrenoceptor-mediated stimulation of Na-K pump current in adult rat ventricular myocytes. Am J Physiol 264:H1315–H1318, 1993

234. Lazou A, Fuller SJ, Bogoyevitch MA, Orfali KA, Sugden PH: Characterization of stimulation of phosphoinositide hydrolysis by α_1-adrenergic agonists in adult rat hearts. Am J Physiol 267:H970–H978, 1994

235. De Hert SG, Gillebert TC, Andries LJ, Brutseart DL: Role of the endocardial endothelium in the regulation of myocardial function. Physiologic and pathophysiologic implications. Anesthesiology 79:1354–1366, 1993

236. Brady AJB, Warren JB, Poole-Wilson PA, Williams TJ, Harding SE: Nitric oxide attenuates cardiac myocyte contraction. Am J Physiol 265:H176–H182, 1993

237. Grocott-Mason R, Fort S, Lewis M, Shah A: Myocardial relaxant effect of exogenous nitrous oxide in isolated ejecting hearts. Am J Physiol 266:H1699–H1705, 1994

238. Kohmoto O, Ikenouchi H, Hirata Y, Momomura S-I, Serizawa T, Barry WH: Variable effects of endothelin-1 on $[Ca^{2+}]_i$ transients, pH_i, and contraction in ventricular myocytes. Am J Physiol 265:H793–H800, 1993

239. Tohse N, Hattori Y, Nakaya H, Endou M, Kanno M: Inability of endothelin to increase Ca^{2+} current in guinea-pig heart cells. Br J Pharmacol 99:437–438, 1990

240. Wang J, Morgan JP: Endothelin reverses the effects of acidosis on the intracellular Ca^{2+} transient and contractility in ferret myocardium. Circ Res 71:631–639, 1992

241. Wang J, Paik G, Morgan JP: Endothelin 1 enhances byofilament Ca^{2+} responsiveness in aequorin-loaded ferret myocardium. Circ Res 69:582–589, 1991

242. Moravec CS, Schluchter MD, Paranandi L et al: Inotropic effects of angiotensin II on human cardiac muscle in vitro. Circulation 82:1990, 1990

243. Moorman JR, Kirsch GE, Lacerda AE, Brown AM: Angiotensin II modulates cardiac Na^+ channels in neonatal rat. Circ Res 65:1804–1809, 1989

244. Eberli FR, Apstein CS, Ngoy S, Lorell BH: Exacerbation of left ventricular ischemic diastolic dysfunction by pressure-overload hypertrophy: Modification by specific inhibition of cardiac angiotensin converting enzyme. Circ Res 70:931–943, 1992

245. Unger T, Gohlke P: Coverting enzyme inhibitors in cardiovascular therapy: Current status and future potential. Cardiovasc Res 28:146–158, 1994

246. Clemo HF, Feher JJ, Baumgarten CM: Modulation of rabbit ventricular cell volume and $Na^+/K^+/2Cl^-$ cotransport by cGMP and atrial naturetic factor. J Gen Physiol 100:89–114, 1992

247. Williams TL, Lefkowitz RJ: Thyroid hormone regulation of β-adrenergic receptors number. J Biol Chem 252:2787–2789, 1977

248. Disatnik MH, Shainberg A: Regulation of beta-adrenoceptors by thyroid hormone and amiodarone in rat myocardiac cells in culture. Biochem Pharmacol 41:1039–1044, 1991

249. Sterling K, Lazarus JH, Milch PO, Sakurada T, Brenner MA: Mitochondrial thyroid hormone receptor: Localization and physiological significance. Science 201:1126–1129, 1978

250. Sterling K, Brenner MA, Sakurada T: Rapid effect of triiodothyronine on the mitochondrial pathway in rat liver in vivo. Science 210:340–342, 1980

251. Dyke CM, Yeh T Jr, Lehman JD et al: Triiodothyronine-enhanced left ventricular function after ischemic injury. Ann Thorac Surg 52:14–19, 1991

252. Dudley JSC, Baumgarten CM: Bursting of cardiac sodium channels after acute exposure to 3,5,3'-triiodo-L-thyronine. Circ Res 73:301–313, 1993

253. Bremner W, Taylor K, Baird S: Hypothalamo-pituitary-thyroid axis func-

tion during cardiopulmonary bypass. J Thorac Cardiovasc Surg 75:392–399, 1978

254. Novitsky D, Human PA, Cooper DKC: Inotropic effect of triiodothyronine following myocardial ischemia and cardiopulmonary bypass: An experimental study in pigs. Ann Thorac Surg 45:500–505, 1988

255. Brooks WW, Struckow B, Bing OHL: Myocardial hypoxia and reoxygenation: Electrophysiologic and mechanical correlates. Am J Physiol 226:523–527, 1974

256. Carmeliet E: Cardiac transmembrane potentials and metabolism. Circ Res 42:577–587, 1978

257. Lewis MJ, Grey AC, Henderson AH: Determinants of hypoxic contracture in isolated heart muscle preparations. Cardiovasc Res 13:86–94, 1979

258. Cole W, McPherson CD, Sontag D: ATP-regulated K⁺ channels protect the myocardium against ischemia/reperfusion damage. Circ Res 69:571–581, 1991

259. Sys SU, Housmans PR, Van Ocken ER, Brutsaert DL: Mechanisms of hypoxia-induced decrease of load dependence of relaxation in cat papillary muscle. Pflugers Arch 401:368–373, 1984

260. Györke S, Fill M: Ryanodine receptor adaptation: Control mechanism of Ca^{2+}-induced Ca^{2+} release in heart. Science 260:807–809, 1993

261. Miyata H, Lakatta EG, Stern MD, Silverman HS: Relation of mitochondrial and cytosolic free calcium to cardiac myocyte recovery after exposure to anoxia. Circ Res 71:605–613, 1992

262. Siegmund B, Zude R, Piper HM: Recovery of anoxic-reoxygenated cardiomyocytes from severe Ca^{2+} overload. Am J Physiol 263:H1262–H1269, 1992

263. Davis MD, Lebolt W, Feher JJ: Reversibility of the effects of normothermic global ischemia on the ryanodine-sensitive and ryanodine-insensitive calcium uptake of cardiac sarcoplasmic reticulum. Circ Res 70:163–171, 1992

264. Kaplan P, Hendrikx M, Mattheussen M, Mubagwa K, Flameng W: Effect of ischemia and reperfusion on sarcoplasmic reticulum calcium uptake. Circ Res 71:1123–1130, 1992

265. Hajjar R, Gwathmey J: Direct evidence of changes in myofilament responsiveness to Ca^{2+} during hypoxia and reoxygenation in myocardium. Am J Physiol 259:H784–H795, 1990

266. Vleugels A, Vereeke J, Carmeliet E: Ionic currents during hypoxia in voltage-clamped cat ventricular muscle. Circ Res 47:501–508, 1980

267. Noma A: ATP-regulated K⁺ channels in cardiac muscle. Nature (Lond) 305:147–148, 1983

268. de Weille JR: Modulation of ATP sensitive potassium channels. Cardiovasc Res 26:1017–1020, 1992

269. Edwards G, Weston AH: The pharmacology of ATP-sensitive potassium channels. Annu Rev Pharmacol Toxicol 33:597–637, 1993

270. Horie M, Irisawa H, Noma A: Voltage-dependent magnesium blockade of adenosine-triphosphate-sensitive potassium channel in single guinea-pig ventricular cells. J Physiol (Lond) 287:251–272, 1987

271. Matsuda H: Magnesium gating of the inwardly rectifying K⁺ channel. Annu Rev Physiol 53:289–298, 1991

272. Furukawa T, Kimura S, Furukawa N, Bassett AL, Myerburg RJ: Role of cardiac ATP-regulated potassium channels in differential responses of endocardial and epicardial cells to ischemia. Circ Res 68:1693–1702, 1991

273. Kubota I, Yamaki M, Shibata T, Ikeno E, Hosoya Y, Tomoike H: Role of ATP-sensitive K⁺ channel on ECG ST segment elevation during a bout of

myocardial ischemia: A study of epicardial mapping in dogs. Circulation 88:1845–1851, 1993

274. Weiss JN Vankatesh, N, Lamp, ST: ATP-sensitive K+ channels and cellular K+ loss in hypoxic and ischaemic mammalian ventricle. J Physiol (Lond) 447:649–673, 1992

275. Auchampach JA, Maruyama M, Cavero I, Gross GJ: Pharmacological evidence for a role of ATP-dependent potassium channels in myocardial stunning. Circulation 86:311–319, 1992

276. Vogel S, Sperelakis N: Blockade of myocardial slow inward current at low pH. Am J Physiol 233:C99–C103, 1977

277. Susanni EE, Manders WT, Vatner DE, Vatner SF, Homcy CJ: One hour of myocardial ischemia decreases the activity of the stimulatory guanine-nucleotide regulatory protein G_s. Circ Res 65:1145–1150, 1989

278. Vatner D, Kiuchi K, Manders W, Vatner S: Effects of coronary arterial reperfusion on β-adrenergic receptor-adenylyl cyclase coupling. Am J Physiol 264:H196–H204, 1993

279. Kirsch GE, Codina J, Birnbaumer L, Brown AM: Coupling of ATP-sensitive K+ channels to A_1 receptors by G proteins in rat ventricular myocytes. Am J Physiol 28:H820–H826, 1990

280. Wilde AAM, Janse MJ: Electrophysiological effects of ATP sensitive potassium channel modulation: Implications for arrhythmogenesis. Cardiovasc Res 28:16–24, 1994

281. Fry CH, Poole-Wilson PA: Effects of acid-base changes on excitation-contraction coupling in guinea-pig and rabbit cardiac ventricular muscle. J Physiol (Lond) 313:141–160, 1981

282. Klöckner U, Isenberg G: Calcium channel current of vascular smooth muscle cells: Extracellular protons modulate gating and single channel conductance. J Gen Physiol 103:665–678, 1994

283. Klöckner U, Isenberg G: Intracellular pH modulates the availability of vascular L-type Ca^{2+} channels. J Gen Physiol 103:647–663, 1994

284. Tani M, Neely JR: Role of intracellular Na+ in Ca^{2+} overload and depressed recovery of ventricular function of reperfused ischemic rat hearts: Possible involvement of H+-Na+ and Na+-Ca^{2+} exchange. Circ Res 65:1045–1056, 1989

285. Neubauer S, Newell JB, Ingwall JS: Metabolic consequences and predictability of ventricular fibrillation in hypoxia: a ^{31}P- and ^{23}Na-magnetic resonance study of the isolated rat heart. Circulation 86:302–310, 1992

286. Scholz W, Albus U, Linz W, Martorana P, Lang HJ, Schölkens BA: Effects of Na+/H+ exchange inhibitors in cardiac ischemia. J Mol Cell Cardiol 24:731–740, 1992

287. Haigney MCP, Miyata H, Lakatta EG, Stern MD, Silverman HS: Dependence of hypoxic cellular calcium loading on Na+-Ca^{2+} exchange. Circ Res 71:547–557, 1992

288. Wier WG: Cytoplasmic $[Ca^{2+}]$ in mammalian ventricle: Dynamic control by cellular processes. Annu Rev Physiol 52:467–485, 1990

289. Ver Donck L, Borgers M, Verdonck F: Inhibition of sodium and calcium overload pathology in the myocardium: A new cytoprotective principle. Cardiovasc Res 27:349–357, 1993

290. Mejía-Alvarez R, Marban E: Mechanism of the increase in intracellular sodium during metabolic inhibition—direct evidence against mediation by voltage-dependent sodium channels. J Mol Cell Cardiol 24:1307–1320, 1992

291. Yan G-X, Kléber AG: Changes in extracellular and intracellular pH in ischemic rabbit papillary muscle. Circ Res 71:460–470, 1992

292. Cingolani H, Koretsune Y, Marban E: Recovery of contractility and pH_i during respiratory acidosis in ferret hearts: Role of Na^+-H^+ exchange. Am J Physiol 259:H843–H848, 1990

293. Than H, Orchard CH: The effect of acidosis and hypoxia on the response of cardiac muscle isolated from ferret hearts to noradrenaline. J Physiol (Lond) 435:98P, 1991

294. Braunwald E, Kloner RA: The stunned myocardium: Prolonged, postischemic ventricular dysfunction. Circulation 66:1146–1149, 1982

295. Kusuoka H, Marban E: Cellular mechanisms of myocardial stunning. Annu Rev Physiol 54:243–256, 1992

296. Hofmann PA, Miller WP, Moss RL: Altered calcium sensitivity of isometric tension in myocyte-sized preparations of porcine postischemic stunned myocardium. Circ Res 72:50–56, 1993

297. Dietrch DLL, van Leeuwen GR, Stienen GJM, Elzinga G: Stunning does not change the relation between calcium and force in skinned rat trabeculae. J Mol Cell Cardiol 25:541–549, 1993

298. Murray CE, Jennings RB, Reimer KA: Preconditioning with ischemia: A delay of lethal cell injury in ischemic myocardium. Circulation 74:1124–1136, 1986

299. Lawson C, Downey J: Preconditioning: State of the art myocardial protection Cardiovasc Res 27:542–550, 1993

300. Parratt JR: Protection of the heart by preconditioning: Mechanisms and possibilities for pharmacologic exploitation. Trends Pharmacol Sci 15:19–25, 1994

301. Tsuchida A, Yang X-M, Burckhartt B, Mullane KM, Cohen MV, Downey JM: Acadesine extends the window of protection afforded by ischemic preconditioning. Cardiovasc Res 28:379–383, 1994

302. Steenbergen C, Perlman ME, London RE, Murphy E: Mechanism of preconditioning-ionic alterations. Circ Res 72:112–125, 1993

303. Brown BR, Crout JR: A comparative study of the effects of five general anesthetics on myocardial contractility: Isometric conditions. Anesthesiology 34:236–245, 1971

304. Lynch C III: Differential depression of myocardial contractility by halothane and isoflurane *in vitro.* Anesthesiology 64:620–631, 1986

305. De Traglia MC, Komai H, Rusy BF: Differential effects of inhalational anesthetics on myocardial potentiated-state contractions *in vitro.* Anesthesiology 68:534–540, 1988

306. Rusy BF, Komai H: Anesthetic depression of myocardial contractility: A review of possible mechanisms. Anesthesiology 67:745–766, 1987

307. Su JY, Kerrick WGL: Effects of halothane on Ca^{2+}-activated tension development in mechanically disrupted rabbit myocardial fibers. Pflügers Arch 375:111–117, 1978

308. Su JY, Kerrick WGL: Effects of enflurane on functionally skinned myocardial fibers from rabbits. Anesthesiology 52:385–389, 1980

309. Su JY, Bell JG: Intracellular mechanism of action of isoflurane and halothane on striated muscle of the rabbit. Anesth Analg 65:457–462, 1986

300. Murat I, Ventura-Clapier R, Vassort G: Halothane, enflurane, and isoflurane decrease calcium sensitivity and maximal force in detergent-treated rat cardiac fibers. Anesthesiology 69:892–899, 1988

311. Herland JS, Julian FJ, Stephenson DG: Effects of halothane, enflurane, and isoflurane on skinned rat myocardium activated by Ca^{2+}. Am J Physiol 264:H224–H232, 1993

312. Housmans PE: Negative inotropy of halogenated anesthetics in ferret ventricular myocardium. Am J Physiol 259:H827–H834, 1990
313. Bosnjak ZJ, Kampine JP: Effects of halothane on transmembrane potentials, Ca++ transients, and papillary muscle tension. Am J Physiol 251: H374–H381, 1986
314. Bosnjak ZJ, Aggarwal A, Turner LA, Kampine JM, Kampine JP. Differential effects of halothane, enflurane, and isoflurane and papillary muscle tension in guinea pigs. Anesthesiology 76:123–131, 1992
315. Bosnjak ZJ, Supan FD, Rusch NJ: The effects of halothane, enflurane and isoflurane on calcium currents in isolated canine ventricular cells. Anesthesiology 74:340–345, 1991
316. Komai H, Rusy BF: Differences in the myocardial depressant action of thiopental and halothane. Anesth Analg 63:313–318, 1984
317. Komai H, Rusy BF: Calcium and thiopental-induced spontaneous activity in rabbit papillary muscle. J Mol Cell Cardiol 18:73–79, 1986
318. Komai H, Rusy BF: Negative inotropic effects of isoflurane and halothane in rabbit papillary muscles. Anesth Analg 66:29–33, 1987
319. Komai H, Rusy BF: Direct effect of halothane and isoflurane on the function of the sarcoplasmic reticulum in intact rabbit atria. Anesthesiology 72:694–698, 1990
320. Komai H, Redon D, Rusy BF: Effects of thiopental and halothane on spontaneous contractile activity induced in isolated ventricular muscles of the rabbit. Acta Anaesthiol Scand 35:373–379, 1991
321. Casella ES, Suite DA, Fisher YI, Blanck TJJ: The effect of volatile anesthetics on the pH dependence of calcium uptake by cardiac sarcoplasmic reticulum. Anesthesiology 67:386–390, 1987
322. Frazer MJ, Lynch C III: Halothane and isoflurane effects on Ca²⁺ fluxes of isolated myocardial sarcoplasmic reticulum. Anesthesiology 77:316–323, 1992
323. Lynch C III, Frazer MJ: Anesthetic alteration of ryanodine binding by cardiac calcium release channels. Biochim Biophys Acta 1194:109–117, 1994
324. Connelly TJ, Coronado R: Activation of the Ca²⁺ release channel of cardiac sarcoplasmic reticulum by volatile anesthetics. Anesthesiology 81:459–469, 1994
325. Miao N, Frazer MJ, Lynch C III: Anesthetic actions on Ca²⁺ uptake and Ca-ATPase activity of cardiac sarcoplasmic reticulum. In Bosnjak ZJ, Kampine JP (eds): Anesthesia and Cardiovascular Disease. Advances in Pharmacology 31, pp. 145–165. San Diego, Academic Press, 1994
326. Baum VC, Wetzel GT: Sodium-calcium exchange in neonatal myocardium: Reversible inhibition by halothane. Anesth Analg 78:1105–1109, 1994
327. Böhm M, Schmidt U, Schwinger RHG, Böhm S, Erdmann E: Effects of halothane on β-adrenoceptors and M-cholinoceptors in human myocardium: Radioligand binding and functional studies. J Cardiovasc Pharmacol 21:296–304, 1993
328. Durieux ME: Effects of halothane on muscarinic transmission. Anesthesiology, 82:174–182, 1995
329. Park WK, Lynch C III: Propofol and thiopental depression of myocardial contractility—a comparative study of mechanical and electrophysiologic effects in isolated guinea pig ventricular muscle. Anesth Analg 74:395–405, 1992
330. Ikemoto Y: Reduction by thiopental of the slow-channel-mediated action potential of canine papillary muscle. Pflugers Arch 372:285–286, 1977

331. Pancrazio JJ, Frazer MJ, Lynch C III: Barbiturate anesthetics depress the resting K^+ conductance of myocardium. J Pharmacol Exp Therap 265:358–365, 1993

332. Riou B, Lecarpentier Y, Chemla D, Viars P: Inotropic effect of ketamine on rat cardiac papillary muscle. Anesthesiology 71:116–125, 1989

333. Riou B, Lecarpentier Y, Chemla D, Viars P: *In vitro* effects of etomidate on intrinsic myocardial contractility in rat. Anesthesiology 72:330–340, 1990

334. Riou B, Besse S, Lecarpentier Y, Viars P. *In vitro* effects of propofol on rat myocardium. Anesthesiology 76:609–616, 1992

335. Baum VC, Tecson ME: Ketamine inhibits transsarcolemmal calcium entry in guinea pig myocardium: Direct evidence by single cell voltage champ. Anesth Analg 73:804–807, 1991

336. Rusy BF, Amuzu JK, Bosscher HA, Redon D, Komai H: Negative inotropic effect of ketamine in rabbit ventricular muscle. Anesth Analg 71:275–278, 1990

337. Cook DJ, Housmans PR. Mechanism of the negative inotropic effect of propofol in isolated ferret ventricular myocardium. Anesthesiology 80:859–871, 1994

338. Olcese R, Usai C, Maestrone E, Nobile M: The general anesthetic propofol inhibits transmembrane calcium current in chick sensory neurons. Anesth Analg 78:955–960, 1994

339. Xio R-P, Spurgeon HA, Capogrossi MC, Lakatta EG: Stimulation of opioid receptors on cardiac ventricular myocytes reduces L type Ca^{2+} channel current. J Mol Cell Cardiol 25:661–666, 1993

340. Komai H, Rusy BF: Effect of halothane on rested-state and potentiated state contraction in rabbit papillary muscle relationship to negative inotropic effect. Anesth Analg 61:403–409, 1982

341. Komai H, Redon D, Rusy BF: Effects of isoflurane and halothane on rapid cooling contractures in myocardial tissue. Am J Physiol 257:H1804–H1811, 1989

342. Rusy BF, Thomas-King PY, King GP, Komai H: Effects of propofol on the contractile state of isolated rabbit papillary rabbit muscles under various stimulation conditions. Anesthesiology 73:A559, 1990

343. Housmans PE, Murat I: Comparative effects of halothane, enflurane, and isoflurane at equipotent anesthetic concentrations on isolated ventricular myocardium of the ferret. I. Contractility. Anesthesiology 69:451–463, 1988

344. Housmans PE, Murat I: Comparative effects of halothane, enflurane, and isoflurane at equipotent anesthetic concentrations on isolated ventricular myocardium of the ferret. II. Relaxation. Anesthesiology 69:464–471, 1988

345. Su JY, Kerrick WGL: Effects of halothane on caffeine-induced tension transients in functionally skinned myocardial fibers. Pflugers Arch 380:29–34, 1979

346. Lynch C III: Differential depression of myocardial contractility by volatile anesthetics *in vitro:* Comparison with uncouplers of excitation-contraction coupling. J Cardiovasc Pharmacol 15:655–665, 1990

347. Takeshima H, Nishimura S, Matsumoto T et al: Primary structure and expression from complementary DNA of skeletal muscle ryanodine receptor. Nature 339:439–445, 1989

348. Stern MD: Theory of excitation-contraction coupling in cardiac muscle. Biophys J 63:497–517, 1992

Stefan G. De Hert

The Role of Cardiac Endothelium in the Regulation of Ventricular Function

2

In the cardiovascular system, the endothelium has long been regarded as a passive barrier between the blood and underlying muscular and connective tissues. This view was considerably changed in 1980 when Furchgott and Zawadski reported on the role of vascular endothelium in the modulation of contractility of subjacent vascular smooth muscle cells.[1] Their finding introduced a new approach in vascular physiology, with endothelium becoming an important subject of research in cardiovascular physiology, pathophysiology, and pharmacology.

The endothelium covers a total surface of about 700 m² and constitutes a continuous structure in arteries, capillaries, and veins. Nevertheless, these three types of vascular endothelium have several distinct morphological and physiological properties. Endothelium not only covers the inner surface of the vascular tree but also the inner surface of the heart. This endocardial endothelium forms a continuous layer with the vascular endothelium, but, until recently, little was known of its morphological and physiological properties. The finding of Brutsaert et al,[2] that endocardial endothelium also modulated contractility of subjacent myocardium introduced a new direction of research in the physiology and pharmacology of cardiac function.

A review of the current knowledge of the role of the endothelium in the regulation of myocardial function is presented in this chapter. First, several aspects of the role and importance of the endocardial en-

Ventricular Function, edited by David C. Warltier. Williams & Wilkins, Baltimore © 1995.

dothelium during embryological and phylogenetic development will be reviewed. Secondly, some important morphological properties of endocardial endothelium and the differences with other types of vascular endothelium will be discussed. Then, experimental data on the functional role of endocardial and coronary endothelium in the regulation of myocardial function will be presented. Finally, possible implications of cardiac endothelium for human physiology and pathophysiology will be speculated upon.

ROLE OF CARDIAC ENDOTHELIUM DURING EMBRYOLOGICAL AND PHYLOGENETIC DEVELOPMENT

The primary tubular heart, consisting of a single midline tube, is formed during the 19th and 20th day of human embryological development. Initially, the cellular layers of the original endocardial and myocardial tubes remain separated by a space filled with extracellular matrix, termed cardiac jelly. Cardiac jelly is gradually reduced in thickness during further development, and the endocardium comes in close proximity to the myocardium. The myocardium develops in an outer compact zone and an inner spongy zone with extensive intercellular spaces. During subsequent trabeculation of the inner surface of the heart, endocardial endothelial cells invade the inner spongy myocardium, and eventually all intertrabecular spaces are lined by endocardial endothelium. At discrete sites, endocardial endothelial cells invade spaces between individual myocardial cells, including cells of the more compact outer myocardial zone. In this way, endocardial endothelium forms a plexus of sinusoids that are in contiguity with the ventricular lumen and which may penetrate deep into the myocardium. These invaginations of endocardium are believed to function as primitive nutrient vessels before the establishment of a true coronary circulation.[3]

Other cell types, including cells derived from the epicardial layer make their appearance in the myocardium as development proceeds. The epicardium gives rise to adjacent connective tissue and to a network of true coronary blood vessels during its formation. Following the formation of these first capillaries in the subepicardial layer during the fourth week of embryological development, a venous connection is established between capillaries and the coronary sinus. Buds of true coronary arteries become evident in the subepicardium in the fifth week of development. Later, these arteries interconnect with the preexisting capillaries. In humans, the coronary arteries usually open at about day 39 of embryological development. Before the onset of true coronary vascularization in the embryo, the myocardium is thus characterized by extensive intercellular spaces or sinusoids, lined by endocardial endothelium, through which substances diffuse to the adjacent myocardium. The intertrabecular spaces regress during further development of the coronary circulation. These spaces are either reduced to strands of endothelium without lumen or they may give rise to capillaries in the central and inter portions of the myocardium with persistence of ventricular communication through the thebesian and arteriosinusoidal vessels.[4]

A similar evolution in the role and importance of endocardium and coronary circulation for the supply and function of subjacent myocardium is present in the phylogenetic development of species.[5,6] Most primitive vertebrates possess endocardial endothelium that forms one continuous layer at the inner surface of the heart and through which exchange of substances is accomplished between the luminal blood and the myocardium. The coronary system makes its first appearance in Chondrichthyes (cartilaginous fish). Interestingly, the occurrence and the extent of coronary vasculature do not only depend on the phylogenetic stage of the species but are also related to ecophysiological factors such as the weight of the heart and the activity of the species. In sluggish sharks, for instance, only a few branches of coronary vessels are present which are usually restricted to the epicardial side of the heart. The inter myocardial layer of the ventricle is spongy with many trabeculae covered by a continuous layer of endocardial endothelial cells. In contrast, there is a tendency towards intramyocardialization of the ventricular branches of the coronary vessels in fast-swimming sharks. The ventricular wall of other fast swimming fish, such as trout and tuna, also consists of two distinct layers. The internal spongy layer is supplied by diffusion from the intertrabecular spaces, whereas the outer compact layer has a vascular supply. The heart of some smaller and less active species of the same or even higher phylogenetic development has a ventricular wall which is trabeculated. The endocardial endothelium which lines these trabeculations is formed by a continuous layer of cells which appears to be metabolically very active. The myocardium in these fish is exclusively supplied by diffusion from the ventricular chamber.[7]

The ventricular wall of hearts in small amphibia (*Rana temporaria* and *Rana ridibunda*) consists of a spongy myocardium without a coronary circulation. Larger frogs have a thin layer of compact outer myocardium with branches of the epicardial network of coronary vessels. Reptiles also have a ventricular wall with an internal spongy trabecular layer and an outer compact layer of myocardium which is supplied by coronary vessels. In the trabeculae of the spongy layer, some myocardial capilliaries may be found, but the greatest part of this spongy myocardial layer is supplied by the endocardial endothelium.[7]

The higher metabolical turnover of homeothermic animals requires a higher supply of oxygen and a higher efficiency of the heart. In birds and mammals, the outer compact layer of myocardium is much thicker than in poikilothermic or cold-blooded animals, and the coronary vascular system becomes more important for the supply of oxygen and nutrients than the endocardial endothelium. The coronary and the intertrabecular systems are not entirely separated. Not only in lower vertebrates but also in mammals—including man—communicating or Thebesian vessels have been demonstrated. Such connections exist especially between the right ventricular lumen and the coronary veins. In some human pathological specimens, wide intertrabecular spaces persist and open into coronary vessels.[8,9]

These data suggest that endocardial endothelium has—at least during a certain part of embryological and phylogenetic development—a key role in the supply of oxygen and nutrients of subjacent myocardium and hence in the regulation of myocardial function. During further development, a portion of the role of endocardial endothelium is replaced by the coronary circulation and autonomic innervation of the heart. This evolution, however, does not necessarily imply that the function of endocardial endothelium in later stages of development is reduced to a mere passive barrier between the superfusing blood and underlying myocardium. Earlier speculation on the physiological role of the endocardium has focused on a possible mechanical function in preventing cardiac overdistension, supporting elastic recoil during relaxation, acting as an elastic buffer to prevent compression of the subendocardial vasculature, and controlling the patency of the Thebesian vessels.[10] The endocardium has also been suggested to have electrophysiological, anticoagulant, and fibrinolytic properties, as well as a role in water and ion exchange and in ATP and glycogen metabolism.[10,11] However, experimental evidence for these proposed physiological roles is scarce. Growing evidence has been gathered demonstrating that a functional role for the endocardial endothelium is not limited to a certain stage of embryological and phylogenetic development but that endocardial endothelium also has a physiological role in the regulation of myocardial function in adult mammalian species.

FUNCTIONAL MORPHOLOGY

In mammalia, the cavitary side of the heart has a complex structure with sinuses, papillary muscles, numerous fissures, and cylinder-like membranous trabeculae carneae. Complex trabeculations have been described which are generally more pronounced in the right than in the left ventricle of the human heart.[12] The entire ventricular wall, trabeculae, and papillary muscles all consist of myocardium, covered on the cavitary side by endocardium. The endocardium in a normal heart can be macroscopically discerned from the subjacent myocardium as a thin transparent to white layer. The endocardium can be divided into two layers: the endocardium proprium and the subendocardium. The subendocardium lies between the endocardium proprium and the myocardium (Fig. 2–1). The term, "subendocardium," is also used to describe the innermost layer of myocardium by some investigators. Its usage in this chapter is distinct and refers to a region not of myocardium lying adjacent to the innermost layer of heart muscle. The endocardium proprium consists of a thin luminal layer of cells, the endocardial endothelium, and a subendothelial fibroelastic layer. The endocardial endothelium lies on a basement membrane, which consists of a basal lamina and a reticular lamina with fine collagen fibers. These fibers diffuse into the fibroelastic layer. The fibroelastic layer consists of a matrix of collagen and elastic fibers containing fibroblasts or myofibroblasts. The elastic material in the endocardium is formed by elastinic microfibrils which are attached to the amorphous masses of elastin. It contains glycoproteins with a high concentration of disulfide groups. The elastic

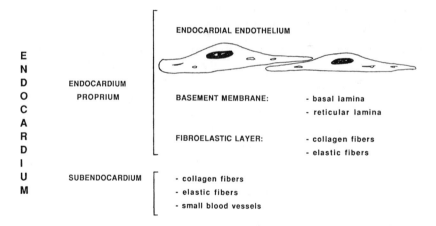

MYOCARDIUM

FIGURE 2-1. Schematic drawing of the subsequent layers in the endocardium. The endocardium can be divided into the endocardium proprium and the subendocardium. The subendocardium lies between the endocardium proprium and the myocardium. The endocardium proprium consists of a thin luminal layer of cells, the endocardial endothelium, and a subendothelial fibroelastic layer. The endothelial cells lie on a basement membrane, which consists of a basal and a reticular lamina.

fibers in the fibroelastic layer increase in size and complexity near the subendocardium. The fibroelastic layer is of a variable thickness, with especially large differences between atria and ventricles. Usually, the endocardium in the left atrium is much thicker than in the right atrium, but the thinnest endocardium is found in both ventricles.[13] In humans, the thickness of the endocardium ranges from 600 to 900 μm in the left atrium, 50 to 800 μm in the right atrium and 50 to 300 μm in the ventricles.[13] Species differences exist in the thickness of the endocardium which may influence interpretation of results of experimental studies. In cat papillary muscles, for instance, the endocardium is much thinner (20 μm) than in the human heart. The endocardium is also thicker in the outflow tract and near the atrioventricular orifices. There is no clear-cut border between endocardium and subendocardium. The subendocardium is mainly characterized by the presence of thick collagen fibers and small blood vessels. This connective tissue layer also contains some elastic fibers, fibroblast-like cells, and unmyelinated nerve fibers. In mammals, the conducting Purkinje fibers lie immediately under the subendocardium. The subendocardium is continuous with the perimysium of the myocardium.[14]

Endocardial Endothelium

The endocardial endothelium is composed of a continuous layer of closely apposed cells in the mammalian heart (Fig. 2–2). These cells are characterized by a thick region around the nucleus, where most organelles can be found, and a thin part towards the periphery. Endocardial endothelial cells are generally reported to contain a small number of mitochondria with few cristae, a small Golgi complex, and a poorly developed endoplasmic reticulum which consists of both granular and agranular tubular profiles. Like many vascular endothelial cells, endocardial endothelial cells contain numerous vesicles lying free in the cytoplasm or attached to the luminal or basal plasmalemma. Smooth vesicles in endocardial endothelium which are probably involved in the transport of macromolecules appear to be less numerous than in myocardial capillary endothelium.[6,15,16]

Cell shape and surface area of endocardial endothelial cells appear to be highly variable in different areas of the heart. Shear stress might explain this phenomenon. Cells are polygonal in the endocardium of the apex, probably an area of low shear stress, and endocardial endothelial cells are elongated in the outflow tract of the left and right ventricles, which are presumably areas of high shear stress.[6,15] Shear stress is probably not the only explanation for the differences in cell shape and cell surface. Experiments have demonstrated that vascular endothelial cells respond to cyclical stretch by acquiring a more elon-

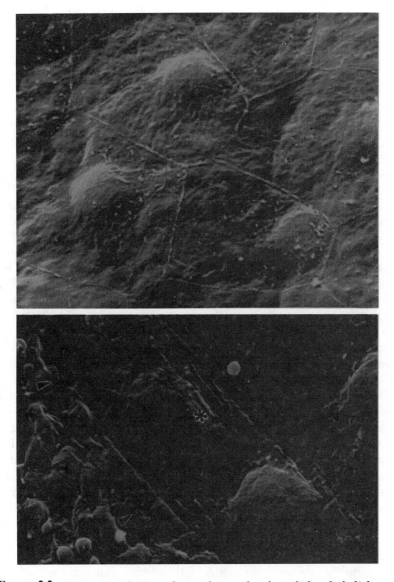

FIGURE 2-2. (*Upper panel*) View of an undamaged endocardial endothelial surface. This surface sample was obtained near the tendon end of a dog right ventricular papillary muscle. The smooth polygonal endocardial endothelial cells and the thin intercellular borders are clearly visible. The cells show bulging nuclei and have a smooth surface with only a few short microvilli. (*Lower panel*) View of a damaged endocardial endothelial surface obtained from dog right ventricular papillary muscle. This figure shows the transition between normal and damaged endocardial endothelial surface. The wound edge is indicated by the *arrowheads*. The intact endocardial endothelium (*asterisk*) shows a smooth surface with bulging nuclei. Along the wound edge, the endocardial endothelium is damaged, and a peripheral part of an endocardial endothelial cell has folded over. Platelets partially cover the denuded basal lamina.

gated cell shape and by a reorientation of the endothelial cells perpendicular to the stretch direction. Cardiac valves, especially the atrioventricular valves, are highly elastic structures, which are also subjected to shape variations during the cardiac cycle. In different species, cardiac valves were demonstrated to possess small valvular endocardial endothelial cells. It was therefore suggested that the presence of endocardial endothelial cells with a small surface area on highly elastic structures was an adaptation of endothelial cells to withstand large variations in shape during cyclic stretching. However, it should be noted that variations of endocardial endothelial cell shape and cell surface area were not only noticed between different species but also in similar structures within the same heart and in similar areas between different hearts. Part of the variability might result from the highly variable macro- and microstructure of the ventricular wall.[6,15]

The surface of vascular and endocardial endothelial cells is usually characterized either by a smooth surface or by the presence of microvilli. Microvilli occur as scattered or grouped protrusions with a globular or hair-like appearance. The function of these endothelial surface structures is not well understood. Microvilli may increase surface area and enhance interaction with the circulating blood by reducing blood flow over the cell surface. The number of microvilli on the cells not only depends on the region of the heart but also shows considerable differences between species.[6,15]

A characteristic feature of endocardial endothelium is the complex intercellular contact zone with overlapping membranous folds and extensive interdigitations.[17] Apparently endocardial endothelial cells possess a similar organization of tight junctions as myocardial capillaries. Variable numbers and sizes of gap junctions have been reported in endocardial endothelium, depending upon the area of the heart, the species studied, and the methodology of fixation and microscopic analysis. The presence of gap junctions in endocardial endothelium suggests that intercellular communication is an important function of endocardial endothelial cells. The gap junctions might allow biochemical and electrophysiological communication between cells, which further amplifies the sensory function of the endocardial endothelium.[5,6,15] Remarkably, gap junctions appear to be absent in capillary endothelium, and junctional communication in cell cultures is lower between microvascular endothelial cells than between macrovascular cells.[18] This heterogeneity in the occurrence of gap junctions in different vessel segments might indicate that macrovascular endothelium and endocardial endothelium have a more global sensory role than endothelium of capillaries, where the regulation of local physiological conditions might not require the existence of extensive intercellular communication by gap junctions.[15] Intercellular clefts are deeper in endocardial endothelium than in capillary endothelium. In addition, endocardial endothelial cells usually have a larger surface area, resulting in a lower total length of intercellular clefts per μm^2 than myocardial capillary endothelial cells. The organization of the tight junctions is similar to myocardial capillary endothelium. All of these structural features of the endocardial endothelium suggest that it might be less permeable than adjacent myocardial capillaries. Contrary to this assumption, however, it appeared experimentally that intravenously injected dextran (mw 10,000) coupled to lucifer yellow first penetrated the endocardial endothelium and only thereafter the myocardial capillary endothelium. This difference was not related to a less developed junctional structure in endocardial endothelium vs capillary endothelium, but, instead, seemed to result from differences in hydrostatic pressure. Indeed the fluorescent tracer was found to penetrate earlier through capillary endothelium in subepicardial myocardium than in subendocardial myocardium, and this was in accordance with the differences in blood flow and fluid pressure between subepicardial and subendocardial coronary vessels. Fluid pressure was thus an important physiological determinant of permeability of endocardial endothelium. The large surface area of most endocardial endothelial cells, the deep intercellular clefts, and perhaps even the low number of smooth vesicles might be adaptations of the endocardial endothelium to withstand transendothelial transport driven by the high hydrostatic ventricular pressures.[6,15]

Molecular charge may be another important physiological determinant of transendocardial endothelial permeability. Dextrans with a molecular weight of 40,000 did not penetrate through either endocardial endothelium or coronary vascular endothelium, whereas horseradish peroxidase, which has a similar molecular weight, did penetrate myocardial capillary endothelium in beating hearts. These dissimilarities in permeability are probably caused by the presence of positively charged isoenzymes in horseradish perioxidase which may penetrate more rapidly through endothelium than tracers having only a negative charge such as dextrans coupled to lucifer yellow. Ionic charge may be important especially in endocardial endothelium with its deep intercellular clefts, since glycoproteins in the intercellular clefts probably form a negatively charged matrix with properties of a molecular sieve. From recent data it appeared that solutes can diffuse from the ventricular lumen to the subendocardial myocardium. Substances released by the endocardial endothelium can thus interact directly with subendocardial myocytes and do not require prior transport through the coronary system.[6,15]

The cytoskeleton in endocardial endothelial cells contain F-actin, intermediate filaments, and microtubules. In endocardial endothelium of both ventricles, F-actin staining was usually restricted to the periphery of endocardial endothelial cells, forming in a manner similar to vascular endothelium, the peripheral actin band. This peripheral band has been demonstrated to be involved in the regulation of paracellular permeability. In vascular endocardial cells, especially in arterial endothelium, F-actin also forms centrally located microfilament bundles or stress fibers. These structures are thought to enhance cell-substrate adhesion, and their presence was correlated with exposure to shear stress. Hence, the lack of stress fibers in most endocardial endothelial cells can be explained by the absence of shear stress in large endocardial endothelial regions of both ventricles. Both other components of the cytoskeleton, microtubules and intermediate filaments, are also involved in the maintenance of cell structure and endothelial integrity.[6,15]

Subendothelial Layer

Limited information is known about the cells in the endocardial interstitial tissue. Only a few fibroblasts or myofibroblasts are present in the connective tissue between the endocardial endothelium and the elastic layer. More cells are found between the elastic layer and the myocardium. The connective tissue cells have long and arborized cytoplasmic processes. Cytoplasmic organelles of these fibroblast-like cells, in particular the Golgi complex and the endoplasmic reticulum, are well developed. Smooth muscle cells can be present in the fibroelastic layer and can form a discontinuous layer in the atria.[14] Interstitial cells constitute a large part, up to 30% of the total interstitial volume in heart valves. The cells have numerous thin and long processes which form a complex cellular network. Similar to smooth muscle cells, the valvular interstitial cells contain numerous bundles of actin filaments and cGMP protein kinase. Valvular cells are extensively coupled by gap junctions. Epinephrine and angiotensin II stimulate contraction of these cells. In valves, another cell type with less smooth muscle actin, a prominent Golgi apparatus and distinct endoplasmatic reticulum is also present. Interstitial cells from porcine cardiac valves can be stimulated to release as much prostacyclin as aortic endothelial cells. Valvular interstitial cells thus appear to be very active cells.[19] Their specific structure might be correlated with the cyclic forces acting on valves during systole and diastole. Valvular interstitial cells are closely associated with motor nerve terminals. In contrast, nearly all nerve fibers in ventricular and atrial endocardium are probably sensory axons.

Morphologic Changes of Endocardium in Cardiac Pathology

Changes in the structure of the endocardium have been noticed in different experimentally produced pathological states. For example, in chronically volume-loaded canine hearts, the endocardium was significantly thicker than in controls.[20] The subendothelial tissue showed a thickening of the basement membrane and elastofibrosis. Changes in endocardial endothelium were also noticed. The number of microvilli increased, and microfilament bundles appeared in the cytoplasm, while the number of pinocytotic vesicles decreased. These changes in endocardial endothelial structure have been attributed to an increase in wall tension or in wall shear stress.[19] Isoproterenol has been shown to induce cardiac necrosis and reparative fibrosis.[21] It also damaged endocardial endothelium by formation of intercellular gaps and rapid loss of endocardial endothelial cells in certain areas, with subsequent deposition of platelets and adherence of granulocytes.[21] After isoproterenol treatment, regenerating endocardial endothelial cells were distinguished from normal endothelial cells by the appearance of desmosomes, long and thin microvilli, hypertrophy of the Golgi complex, and an increase of the rough endoplasmatic reticulum.[22] Following in vitro exposure to high concentrations of phenylephrine[23] or 5-hydroxytryptamine[24], formation of intercellular gaps and selective destruction of endocardial endothelium have also been demonstrated. Whether high concentrations of these substances (for instance, 5-hydroxytryptamine concentration in blood of patients with carcinoid syndrome) also damage endocardial endothelium in vivo remains to be established. Cardiac tissue from patients with tropical hypereosinophilic endomyocardial fibrosis (Loeffler's endocarditis) was shown to have areas with a thick thrombus or fibrin strands where endocardial endothelium was absent. The remaining endocardial endothelial cells had a swollen appearance with many cytoplasmic organelles.[25] Eosinophils from patients with Loeffler's syndrome have indeed been shown to selectively damage endocardial endothelium in isolated papillary muscles.[26] Recently, the presence of eosinophilic peroxidase was demonstrated on the endocardial endothelium of patients with hypereosinophilic endocarditis.[27] This protein can generate cytotoxic oxidants, indicating that endocardial endothelium might be involved in the pathogenesis of this disease. Changes in the endocardium have also been described in the aging heart. A marked thickening of the endocardium has been noticed with changes in the stratification of the elastic layer, basement irregularities, reduplication of endocardial collagen, acellularity of the fibroelastic layer, appearance of adipose tissue, focal hypertrophy of smooth muscle cells in the left atrium, and loss of cohesion with the subendocardium so that the endocardium can easily be detached from the subendocardial tissue.[13]

FUNCTIONAL ROLE OF ENDOCARDIAL ENDOTHELIUM

Brutsaert et al. first demonstrated that the endocardial endothelium constitutes a structure that actively regulates myocardial performance.[2]

This evidence was first gathered from in vitro studies on isolated papillary muscles of the cat heart and was later confirmed by other groups in a similar experimental model. Recently, it has been demonstrated in an open chest dog model that endocardial endothelium might also be implicated in the regulation of myocardial performance in vivo.[29] Continuing research is presently directed toward further elucidation of this phenomenon and to its possible underlying mechanisms.

In Vitro Studies

Selective removal of the endocardial endothelium from isolated papillary muscles resulted in an immediate and irreversible abbreviation of isometric twitch duration and was accompanied by a decline in peak isometric twitch tension, with no significant changes in the early phase of the twitch.[2] In other words, the presence of an intact endocardial endothelium modulated performance of myocardium with a prolongation of isometric twitch duration and concomitant increase in peak twitch performance but without significantly affecting V_{max} (V_{max} is the maximal velocity of unloaded muscle shortening and is widely used as a measurement of contraction velocity) [Fig. 2–3]. These observations were done in isolated cardiac muscles from different animal species and used many different techniques to selectively impair the endocardial endothelium. Among these techniques, gentle abrasion of the muscle surface with a plastic blade or short immersion of the muscle in a detergent (Triton X-100) is the most frequently used. Damage by all techniques was limited to the endocardial endothelium, without injury of the underlying myocardium. The observed changes in myocardial contraction after damage of the endocardial endothelium were not accompanied by changes in V_{max} at any calcium concentration or by changes of peak myocardial performance at 7.5 mM calcium. As true myocardial depression is manifested by a diminished peak twitch tension at 7.5 mM calcium and by a fall in V_{max} at all calcium concentrations, these findings suggest preservation of intact myocardial function. Morphological examination of the papillary muscles by light microscopy and transmission electron microscopy showed a selective damage of endocardial endothelium without morphological change of the underlying myocardium.[2]

The endocardial endothelium has been shown to participate in the inotropic response to a variety of agents. Atrial natriuretic peptide has a direct effect on isolated cardiac muscle. Similar to the removal of a functional endocardium, atrial natriuretic peptide induced early tension decline and diminished peak twitch tension with no changes in V_{max}. This effect was selectively mediated through endocardial en-

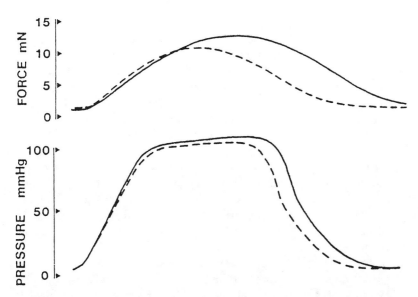

FIGURE 2-3. (*Upper panel*) Isometric twitch contraction of cat papillary muscle before (*solid lines*) and after (*dashed lines*) selective removal of endocardial endothelium in vitro. Removal of the endocardial endothelium results in a decrease in peak isometric twitch tension and in twitch duration with no significant changes in the early phase of the twitch. In other words, the presence of an intact endocardial endothelium modulates myocardial function with a prolongation of isometric twitch duration and an increase in peak twitch performance. (*Lower panel*) Left ventricular pressure tracing before (*solid lines*) and after (*dashed lines*) selective damage of the endocardial endothelium in vivo. Damaging the endocardial endothelium shortens ventricular ejection duration and decreases systolic ventricular performance with no significant changes in early contractile hemodynamics. In other words, the presence of an intact endocardial endothelium modulates ventricular function by prolonging ejection duration and slightly increasing systolic peak performance.

dothelium as it was abolished after impairment of the endocardial surface.[30] This suggested that atrial natriuretic peptide acts on myocardium indirectly through receptors localized on the endocardial endothelium. The involvement of atrial natriuretic peptide in the modulation of myocardial performance is not surprising. Immunohistochemical and in situ hybridization studies have demonstrated the presence of specific receptors for atrial natriuretic peptide on endocardial endothelial cells in left and right ventricles, whereas only few receptors were detected in ventricular myocardium.[31,32] These receptors could mediate the observed response, possibly through release by the endocardial endothelium of a factor that alters the pattern of myocardial contraction. In vascular smooth muscle the action of atrial natriuretic peptide is accompanied by an increase in intracellular cyclic guanosine monophosphate (cGMP). The similarities between the effects on myocardial performance caused by the removal of functional endothelium and those produced by dibutyryl cGMP (a cGMP analogue known to cross cell membranes) by sodium nitroprusside (a drug that increases intracellular cGMP) or by atrial natriuretic peptide suggest that alterations in intracellular cGMP might somehow be implicated in the endothelial-mediated control of cardiac performance.[5,6,30]

There is also experimental evidence that at least a portion of the effects of catecholamines on myocardial muscle are mediated through the endocardial endothelium. Low concentrations of the α_1-agonist, phenylephrine, in the presence of β-adrenergic blockade have been demonstrated to produce a marked positive inotropic response with typical prolongation of the twitches but with no change in V_{max}. This response was opposite to the effects of atrial natriuretic peptide and similar to what would be expected from positive activation of the endocardium-mediated control of cardiac performance. The α_1-agonist positive inotropic effect was abolished after treatment with prazosin (an α_1-adrenergic receptor antagonist) or after damaging the endocardial surface endothelium. This suggested that cardiac α_1-agonist activity seemed to be mediated—at least in part—through endocardial endothelium.[24]

In muscles with an intact endocardial endothelium, vasopressin (ADH) has been shown to decrease peak twitch tension and to abbreviate twitch duration with concomitant premature tension decline during relaxation. In contrast, following damage of the endocardial endothelium, vasopressin produced a positive inotropic effect characterized by increases in peak twitch tension and V_{max} but without prolongation of twitch duration. These findings indicated that the inotropic effects of vasopressin depended upon the presence of an intact endocardial endothelium.[33] Serotonin (5-hydroxytryptamine) and adenosine triphosphate caused a more pronounced positive inotropic effect in muscles with damaged endocardial endothelium than in preparations with an intact endocardial endothelium.[25] Apparently, the presence of an intact endocardial endothelium prevents or attenuates the expression of the positive inotropic effects of vasopressin, serotonin, and adenosine triphosphate.

The interaction of angiotensin I and II with endocardial endothelium appears to be more complex.[34] A positive inotropic action was observed with angiotensin I and II in the presence and in the absence of an intact endocardial endothelium. In muscle with intact endocardial endothelium, addition of the angiotensin-coverting enzyme inhibitor, captopril, significantly diminished the response to angiotensin II. In muscle with a damaged endocardial endothelium, a captopril-induced potentiation of the response was observed. Hence, the presence of an intact endocardial endothelium prevented the potentiation of the inotropic effect of angiotensin II by captopril. This phenomenon of captopril-induced sensitization and desensitization of the inotropic effects of angiotensin II was abolished by indomethacin. This may indicate that stimulation of prostaglandin synthesis was the mediator of this phenomenon, but this is only an hypothesis and requires further investigation.

Aggregation of platelets was demonstrated to increase contractile performance in the absence of an intact endocardial endothelium.[35] How an intact endocardial endothelium suppresses and modifies the direct effect of aggregating platelets on subjacent myocardium is unknown. The modulatory role of endocardial endothelium could not be explained by the synthesis of arachidonic acid metabolites such as prostacyclin because cyclooxygenase inhibition with indomethacin failed to alter the inhibitory effects of an intact endocardium. Platelet aggregation results in the release of several substances including serotonin, adenosine triphosphate, calcium, and thromboxane A_2. Inotropic responses to serotonin and to adenosine triphosphate were found to be significantly greater in the absence of an intact endocardium.[25] The possible mechanisms involved in the modulatory role of the endocardial endothelium in the observed platelet-myocardial cell interaction, however, remain speculative.

In conclusion, these different studies in isolated papillary muscle have revealed that endocardial endothelium modulates performance of subjacent myocardium, and the endocardial endothelium senses and mediates some of the inotropic effects of different circulating substances and formed elements in the blood.

In Vivo Studies

Although all of these in vitro studies have revealed an interesting aspect of the role of endocardial endothelium, their implications for mammalian or human cardiac physiology and pathophysiology remained limited. Based on the data obtained in vitro, it was hypothetized that the presence of an intact endocardial endothelium might play a role in the regulation of cardiac performance in vivo. It could be expected from in vitro effects that the presence of an intact endocardial endothelium would modulate ventricular performance by prolonging systole with a slight increase in peak performance but with no significant change in early contractile dynamics.

The major problem in extending the in vitro observations to an in vivo situation was the lack of a suitable method to selectively damage endocardial endothelium in vivo. However, the development of a novel technique using high-power, high-frequency continuous wave ultrasound for selective damage of the endocardial endothelium made it possible to extend in vitro observations to the in vivo condition. Irradiation of the endocardial surface of the heart with a source of high-power (5 W/cm^2, high-frequency (0.9 MHz), continuous wave ultrasound has been shown in vitro to induce selective damage of the endocardial endothelium, with subsequent effects on myocardial performance.[36] This method of damaging the endocardial endothelium has been applied in vivo. It appeared that selective inactivation of normal endocardial endothelial function by intracavitary irradiation of the ventricular wall by high-power, high-frequency, continuous wave ultrasound affected in vivo ventricular performance, shortening ejection duration and decreasing systolic function. This was accompanied by a pronounced early reextension of various parts of the ventricular wall. Early contractile hemodynamics were not significantly affected. In other words, presence of an intact endocardial endothelium prolonged ejection duration and delayed relaxation. This regulation of myocardial performance by the endocardial endothelium was similar to the effects observed in vitro (Fig. 2–3).[29] Hence, endocardial endothelial cells both in vitro and in vivo directly modulate or control the performance of subjacent myocardium.

These observations indicated the existence of an endocardial endothelial-mediated autoregulation of cardiac performance. The next question was whether such regulation of myocardial performance by endocardial endothelium acted as an independent regulator of myocardial function or whether it functioned in continuous interplay with other modulators of ventricular function, such as regulation by volume loading (heterometric autoregulation) and regulation through neurohumoral activation (homeometric autoregulation). From our experiments it appeared that regulation of ventricular function by endocardial endothelium interacted with heterometric autoregulation. The effects of inactivation of normal endocardial endothelial function were more pronounced at low ventricular volumes. At a left ventricular end-diastolic pressure (LVEDP) of 4.0 mm Hg, inactivation of endocardial endothelium with ultrasound decreased left ventricular ejection duration (time from end-diastole to peak $-dP/dt$) by 7.8%. The decrease in ejection duration by ultrasound was 4.4 and 1.9% when LVEDP was raised to 10.6 and 17.9 mm Hg, respectively. This interaction between regulation of ventricular performance by volume loading and by endocardial endothelium indicated that ventricular function could be particularly dependent on endocardial integrity when circulating volume was decreased (Fig. 2–4).[37] The reasons why the magnitude of the modulation of myocardial function by endocardial endothelium depends on the prevailing ventricular volume are, as yet, speculative. A

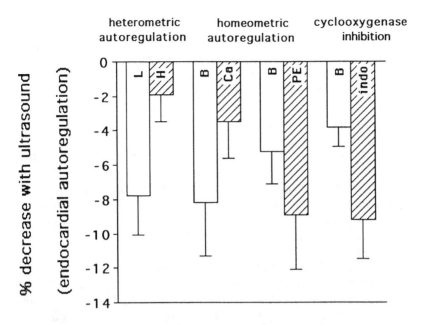

FIGURE 2-4. Magnitude of effects of selective transient inactivation of normal endocardial endothelial function (by intracavitary irradiation with a source of high-power, high-frequency, continuous wave ultrasound) in different experimental conditions. The effects of endocardial autoregulation of ventricular performance are evaluated as changes in time interval from end-diastole to peak − dP/dt. The magnitude of endocardial autoregulation is compared in different conditions of heterometric and homeometric autoregulation. Data are expressed as mean ± 1 SD. *Heterometric autoregulation:* The effects of selective inactivation of normal endocardial endothelial function in different conditions of LV volume (low (L): LVEDP = 4.1 ± 0.3 mm Hg, and high (H): LVEDP = 17.9 ± 1.8 mm Hg). The effects on time interval from end-diastole to peak − dP/dt were significantly more pronounced at low LVEDP (L: decrease in time interval with 7.8 ± 2.3% and H: decrease in time interval with 1.9 ± 1.6%; P < 0.001). *Homeometric autoregulation:* The effects of selective inactivation of normal endocardial endothelial function in different conditions of ventricular inotropism in two different protocols. In a first protocol, the effects of calcium were evaluated. In baseline conditions (B), selective inactivation of normal endocardial endothelial function decreased the time interval from end-diastole to peak − dP/dt by 8.4 ± 3.1%, whereas after administration of calcium (Ca), this effect was only 3.5 ± 2.1% (P<0.001). In a second protocol, the effects of selective α_1-agonism with phenylephrine (PE) were evaluated: in baseline conditions (B), selective inactivation of normal endocardial endothelial function decreased the time interval from end-diastole to peak − dP/dt by 5.3 ± 1.9%, whereas after administration of PE, this effect was 8.9 ± 3.2% (P <0.001). *Cyclooxygenase inhibition:* The effects of selective inactivation of normal endocardial endothelial function before and after administration of the cyclooxygenase inhibitor indomethacin (indo). In baseline conditions (B), selective inactivation of normal endocardial endothelial function decreased the time interval from end-diastole to peak − dP/dt with 3.8 ± 1.1%, whereas after indomethacin this effect was 9.2 ± 2.3% (P < 0.001).

common underlying mechanism has been suggested.[2] It is possible that, similar to mechanisms of length modulation of myocardial function,[38,39] endocardial modulation of cardiac performance may be mediated through changes in the sensitivity of the contractile proteins for calcium. This hypothesis has been supported by experiments demonstrating that endocardial endothelium altered the calcium responsiveness of myocardial filaments.[40] If length and endocardial regulation act via the same mechanism, it is conceivable that when length modulation of myocardial performance is maximized, the effects of endocardial modulation would become less pronounced.[37,41]

Regulation of ventricular performance by endocardial endothelium also interacts with homeometric autoregulation. The functional effects of inactivation of the endocardial endothelium were more pronounced at lower calcium concentrations. Ultrasound decreased ejection duration by 8.4% during control conditions, whereas this effect was only 3.5% after administration of calcium (Fig. 2–4).[37] The mechanism of this action of calcium remains to be established. Calcium has been shown to have a role in the preservation of functional and structural integrity of cellular membranes and intercellular connections. Cellular sealing processes also appear to depend largely on calcium.[42,43] Therefore, it is possible that the protective action of calcium may be based on its membrane-stabilizing properties. Whether this is the only effect of calcium, or whether some interaction is involved between the endocardial endothelium and calcium kinetics downstream from endothelial cells, is still under investigation.[37,41]

The effects of inactivation of normal endocardial endothelial function also appeared to be more pronounced in the presence of α_1-adrenoceptor activation (Fig. 2–4).[37] Ultrasound decreased ejection duration by 5.2% during control conditions. In the presence of phenylephrine and concomitant β-blockade, ejection duration decreased by 8.9%. It was therefore suggested that at least a part of the inotropic activity of phenylephrine might be mediated through the endocardial endothelium.[24,37] How the positive inotropic effects of phenylephrine could be part of a cascade of events dependent upon the endocardial endothelium still remains to be elucidated.

The functional effects of inactivation of the endocardial endothelium were also more pronounced in the presence of inhibitors of cyclooxygenase.[44,45] Ultrasound decreased ejection duration by 9.2% after indomethacin, compared to a decrease of 3.8% during baseline conditions. Similar effects were produced by acetylsalicylic acid. These findings indicated that the functional effects of the endocardial endothelium were greater in the presence of cyclooxygenase inhibitors and that prostaglandins might be involved in the modulation of myocardial performance by endocardial endothelium. Whether prostaglandins play a direct role as a myocardial contracting or relaxing factor released from endothelium or merely function as a trigger for the release of another contracting or relaxing factor is unknown.

These in vivo data confirm findings of in vitro experiments. Endocardial endothelium modulates ventricular performance. The endocardial endothelium interacts with heterometric and homeometric autoregulation of ventricular function. In addition, endocardial endothelium mediates—at least in part—the inotropic effects of phenylephrine.

Mechanisms of Endocardial Function

The previously discussed data have demonstrated that the endocardial-endothelium modulates myocardial performance both in vitro and in vivo. The next intriguing question is by which possible mechanisms this modulation may act. It is conceivable that the endocardial endothelium may act as a finely tuned modulator of permeability between superfusing blood and myocardium.[5,6] An adjustable physiochemical barrier might selectively regulate the exchange of particles, hormones, and other active macromolecules between the superfusing blood and the interstitial microenvironment of the cardiac muscle cells. Endocardial endothelium is in anatomical contiguity with vascular endothelium. It is now well recognized that vascular endothelium plays many functional roles, including that of regulating vascular smooth muscle tone through the release of vasoactive agents. The endocardial endothelium might be expected to have some properties in common with those of endothelium lining the vascular tree. Thus, it is possible that endocardial endothelium also releases substances with inotropic properties which might influence performance of myocardium.[2,5] At least two possible mechanisms involved in the endocardial endothelial modulation of myocardial function can be hypothesized. Endocardial endothelium may act as an electrochemical barrier between the superfusing blood and the underlying myocardium; it may release chemical substances or messengers; or it may exert its influence on underlying myocardium by a combination of both these mechanisms (Fig. 2–5).[5,6,41]

Physicochemical Control

It appears that the endocardial endothelium may offer specific permeability features. Differences in tracer permeability between endocardial and subendocardial vascular endothelium have been attributed to differences in hydrostatic pressure. Transport of tracers through the en-

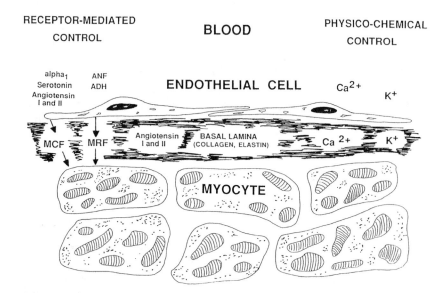

| RECEPTOR-MEDIATED CONTROL | BLOOD | PHYSICO-CHEMICAL CONTROL |

FIGURE 2-5. Schematic representation of the hypothesized mechanisms of regulation of myocardial function by endocardial endothelium. Endocardial endothelium may exert its effect through physicochemical control, by establishing an electrochemical gradient for various ions; or through receptor-mediated control, by releasing myocardial contracting (*MCF*) and myocardial relaxing factors (*MRF*) in response to various circulating substances in the blood. (*Reproduced with permission of the J.B. Lippincott Company from De Hert SG et al. Anesthesiology 79:1354,1993*)

docardial endothelium also depended on molecular charge of the tracers. Data on the differences in permeability between endocardial endothelium and coronary endothelium of the subendocardium indicated that the endocardium might have characteristic electrochemical properties.[6,15,16] As an electrochemical barrier with variable permeability, the endocardium could control homeostasis of the microenvironment of the interstitial fluid surrounding myocytes. Ion channels and transmembrane potential have been described in vascular endothelial cells.[46] Some preliminary results also suggest existence of a transmembrane potential and of ion channels in endocardial endothelial cells.[41] The presence of gap junctions between the endocardial endothelial cells indicated the possibility of electrochemical coupling between these cells.[6] Although all of these features suggest a possible role for the endocardium to act as an electrochemical barrier between the blood and underlying myocardium, definitive experimental evidence is lacking.

Release of Endocardial Substances with Inotropic Properties

Vascular endothelium releases vasoactive agents which modulate vascular smooth muscle tone. It was therefore hyposthesized that the endocardial endothelium might have similar properties.[2] The presence of an intact functional endocardial endothelium delays the onset of isometric tension decline and shifts the $[Ca]_0$-tension curves and the length-tension curves upward and to the left. This effect is irreversibly abolished after removal of the endothelium. It was postulated that this observation might indicate that endocardial endothelium releases a positive inotropic factor that would increase the sensitivity of contractile proteins for calcium. Similarly, the endocardial endothelium might produce and release another factor that decreases sensitivity of the contractile proteins for calcium and induces relaxation.[2] These factors were provisionally called myocardial contracting factor (MCF) and myocardial relaxing factor (MRF), respectively. The relative amount of these factors would represent the contribution of the endocardial endothelium to the shape and duration of the muscular twitch or the ventricular contraction. This hypothesis has been supported by experimental evidence that the endocardial endothelium releases substances with inotropic properties. Bioassay experiments have demonstrated that effluent from superfused cultured endocardial endothelial cells contains both an agent which prolongs myocardial contraction (an MCF which has been termed endocardin) and an MRF which is an endothelium-derived relaxing factor (EDRF)-like agent that shortens the duration of contraction.[47] Nitric oxide (NO) accounts for the biological activity of EDRF.[48] There is now evidence that endocardial endothelial cells do produce and release NO. Endocardial endothelial cells of cardiac valves have been shown to continuously release an EDRF-like substance.[49] Furthermore, constitutive NO synthase can be isolated from cultured porcine ventricular endocardial cells.[50]

Removal of endocardial endothelium shortens the duration of contraction and decreases twitch tension, indicating that in isolated papillary muscle under basal conditions the tonic actions of MCF or endocardin predominate. Similarly, in the intact heart, damage of the endocardial endothelium shortens ejection duration also indicating that MCF exerts a tonic effect on left ventricular contraction. Tonic EDRF activity in endocardial endothelial cells appears to be low since blockade of EDRF synthesis with L-N^G- monomethyl arginine (L-NMMA) does not prolong contraction in papillary muscle preparations.[51] EDRF activity in endocardial endothelium appears to be low in these preparations, but it has been suggested that it might be greater in vivo where it could be increased by the shear stress of blood flow along the endocardial endothelium,[51] as was shown for pulsatile flow and vascular endothelium.[52,53] EDRF and other sources of NO stimulate soluble guanylyl cyclase to increase intracellular cGMP levels.[47] Briefly, the NO signalling pathway in the endothelium starts with the production of NO from L-arginine by enzymes called NO-synthase(s). These enzymes are activated by the binding of calcium and calmodulin, often in response to agonist-receptor interaction leading to an increased intracellular calcium concentration. After its production, NO binds to the heme moiety of guanylyl cyclase, which catalyzes the production of cGMP (Fig. 2–6). Increasing myocardial cGMP levels by stimulation of particulate guanylate cyclase with atrial natriuretic peptide or stimulation of soluble guanylyl cyclase with other NO donors such as nitrovasodilator drugs has been shown to shorten muscle twitch contrac-

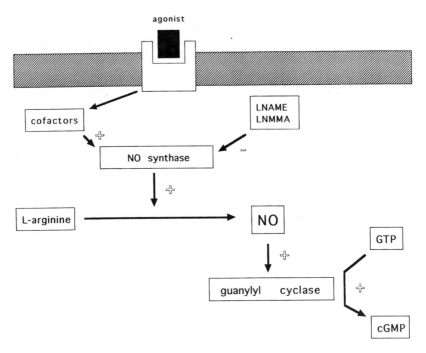

FIGURE 2-6. Schematic representation of the nitric oxide (NO) pathway. NO is formed from *L*-arginine by enzymes called NO synthase(s). NO synthase is activated by the binding of cofactors, mainly calcium and calmodulin. This activation occurs often in response to an agonist-receptor interaction leading to an increased cytosolic calcium. NO synthase is competitively inhibited by specific analogs of *L*-arginine such as nitro-*L*-argine methyl ester (*LNAME*) and I-N[G]-monomethyl arginine (*LNMMA*). After its production, NO binds to guanylyl cyclase, and this enzyme catalyzes the formation of cyclic 3′,5′-guanosine monophosphate (*cGMP*) from guanosine triphosphate (*GTP*).

tions.[47] How cGMP mediates its effect on myocardial contraction has not been entirely established. The characteristic response to elevation of myocardial cGMP, a shortened duration of contraction, is similar to the response following a reduction in resting muscle length, which has been attributed to a length-dependent decrease in contractile protein affinity for calcium.[38,39] It was therefore hypothesized that a similar mechanism might underlie the effect of increasing cGMP.[51] Increasing cGMP might activate a cGMP-dependent protein kinase which mediates phosphorylation of cardiac troponin I with a consequent reduction in the affinity of troponin C for calcium (see chapter 1).[54,55] However, it should be noted that under certain circumstances, cGMP has also been reported to increase affinity of the contractile proteins for calcium.[56]

Recently, it has been suggested that the presence of an intact endocardial endothelium may play a crucial role in the manifestation of the myocardial effects of NO donors. In isolated papillary muscles with an intact endocardial endothelium, NO donors caused a reduction of peak isometric tension associated with a shortening of the twitch and no changes in velocity of contraction (an effect that mimics the functional effects of removal of endocardial endothelium). When the endocardial endothelium was selectively damaged, NO donors caused an inotropic response characterizedd by an increase in peak twitch tension and in velocity of contraction but with no change in twitch duration.[57] These results indicated that the endocardial endothelium can influence cGMP regulation in subjacent myocardium. The mechanisms of this dual response to cGMP in myocardium are not completely clear. In isolated ventricular myocytes, relatively low concentrations (0.1 to 10 μmol/liter) of cGMP have been reported to have a stimulatory effect on the cAMP-elevated L-type calcium channel current (I_{Ca}), leading to an increase in calcium availability. Higher concentrations of cGMP have either no effect or reduce I_{Ca}. It was suggested that stimulation of this cAMP-elevated I_{Ca} by low concentrations of cGMP was due to a participation of cGMP-inhibitable cAMP-phosphodiesterase, whose presence in the heart has been well documented.[58,59] The higher concentrations of cGMP have been reported to inhibit cAMP-elevated I_{Ca} via cGMP-mediated protein kinase (cGMP-PK) in myocytes.[60] In addition to its direct effects on the calcium channel, cGMP-PK may also decrease the calcium sensitivity of the myofilaments through phosphorylation of the inhibitory subunits of troponin.[61] The precise level of cGMP at which the direction of the inotropic response changes from positive to negative may depend on the basal cGMP levels. Basal cGMP levels in turn may be determined by the state of the overlying endocardial endothelium.[57] It would thus seem that cGMP has more than one mode of action in cardiac muscle. With respect to the role of endocardial endothelium in the modulation of the inotropic response to NO, it should be mentioned that there are also myocardial effects of NO which act independently of the endocardial endothelium. For example, cytokines have a negative inotropic effect on myocardium, effects attributed to enhanced activity of a constitutive NO synthase. Removal of endocardial endothelium did not alter this response, indicating that this phenomenon occurred independently of the endocardial endothelium.[62]

The MCF or endocardin has not yet been identified. Removal of endocardial endothelium and the tonic influence of MCF does not alter action potential duration.[63] One of the possible candidates for MCF could be endothelin. Endothelin receptors have been found on cardiomyocytes,[64,65] and endocardial endothelial cells have been shown to synthetize and release endothelin-1.[66] However, endothelin produces prolongation of the action potential and induces a symmetrical increase in isometric twitch contraction. Both effects are unlike those of endocardin, which causes primarily prolongation of contraction without changing action potential duration.[67] These data indicate that factors other than endothelin are involved in MCF activity. The most likely mode of action of MCF presently appears to be on the sensitivity of the contractile proteins to calcium.[51] This hypothesis has recently been endorsed by experiments in isolated, aqueorin-loaded ferret papillary muscle preparations.[40]

Prostanoids are a major product by which vascular endothelium affects smooth muscle. It might therefore be suspected that prostanoids are also involved in the regulation of myocardial function by endocardial endothelium. Tissue cyclooxygenase was found to be twice as high in the endocardium than in the myocardium and was specifically localized in endothelial cells.[68] In addition, endocardial endothelium from isolated cardiac valves[49] as well as valvular endocardial endothelial cells in culture produce prostacyclin.[69] Recently, it was demonstrated that ventricular endocardial endothelial cells also exhibited a sustained production of prostacyclin and PGE_2.[70] These results indicate the possibility that endocardial prostanoid release could modulate myocardial function. The hypothesis that prostaglandins might be involved in the regulation of myocardial function by endocardial endothelium is concordant with our experimental observation that the functional effects of endocardial endothelium were sensitized in the presence of cyclooxygenase inhibitors.[44]

The exact physiological roles of MCF (endocardin, endothelin, and possibly other substances) and MRF (EDRF-like substance, prostacyclin, and possibly other substances) remain to be clearly established, and further research is needed to reveal their exact nature and mechanisms of action. Whether in addition to the release of these factors, the endocardial endothelium also modulates the function of subjacent myocardium through electrotonic control by means of a variable electrochemical gradient has yet to be established.

MODULATION OF MYOCARDIAL FUNCTION BY CORONARY VASCULAR ENDOTHELIUM

Because of an extensive vascularity, the heart also contains large quantities of coronary vascular endothelium which lies in close proximity to the myocardium. It might therefore be hypothesized that myocardial function is also regulated by substances released from coronary vascular endothelium.[71] This hypothesis has recently been confirmed by experimental evidence demonstrating that coronary vascular endothelial cells directly affect contractile performance of adjacent myocardium, in a manner similar to the control of subjacent cardiomyocytes by endocardial endothelium.[72-74] In Langendorff perfusion experiments, coronary vascular endothelial modulation of myocardial performance was shown to involve changes in contraction duration with no effects on early contraction dynamics. These changes were shown to be additive to those effects mediated by endocardial endothelium.[72] The relative production of inotropic factors by coronary vascular endothelium depended in part on oxygen tension and coronary blood flow. However, it is not yet clear to which extent oxygen tension acts directly on the endothelial cells and/or on other cells in the myocardium. The endothelial cells may release substances with inotropic properties in response to coronary flow and local oxygen tension, and the cardiac myocytes may influence endothelial function in accordance with the metabolic state of the myocytes. Under conditions of high ventricular work relative to energy supply, such a negative feed back loop would serve to downregulate contractility and decrease energy requirements. When energy supply is relatively high, upregulation of contractility could occur. This system of interaction would constitute a form of autoregulation of cardiac function.[73,74] From these findings it would seem that all endothelial cells, regardless of whether they are endocardial or coronary vascular in origin, may directly control or modulate the contractile state of the subjacent cardiomyocytes. This would imply that, in addition to the regulation of myocardial function by endocardial endothelium, there is also a mechanism of regulation of myocardial function by coronary vascular endothelium as well. Both types of regulation function through alterations in the duration of contraction by altering the onset of ventricular relaxation and rapid filling and probably act in close interplay with each other.[71]

The relative contribution of both types of regulation (modulation by endocardial and coronary vascular endothelium) may, at least in part, depend upon the relative amount of endocardial and coronary vascular endothelial cells per tissue weight of cardiomyocytes in any given region of the cardiac wall.[71] Equally important may be the relative amount of blood constituents that can be exposed at any time to these two endothelial structures. All circulating blood passes through the cardiac cavities, at least once every 2 minutes at rest, and is continuously exposed to the endocardial endothelium. The prominent trabecular structure of the cavitary side of the heart is covered with endothelial cells resulting in a large endocardial surface area. When one adds to this the specific surface characteristics of endocardial endothelial cells, such as the numerous microvilli and membrane invaginations, this will offer a relatively high ratio of endocardial endothelial surface to ventricular volume. In contrast, only about 4 to 5% of the cardiac output flows through the coronary circulation, where this relatively small amount of blood is distributed over a widely branched coronary microcirculation. It is, therefore, difficult to predict how much of the blood is directly exposed to the total mass of endocardial endothelial cells and how much to the vascular coronary endothelial cells. On theoretical grounds, it may be speculated that in regions of the heart where the ventricular wall is thinnest and/or highly trabeculated (for example, in the right ventricle or at the apex or posterior wall of the left ventricle), autoregulation mediated by endocardial endothelium could be relatively more important.[71]

IMPLICATIONS FOR CARDIAC PHYSIOLOGY

Performance of the heart relies largely on autoregulatory mechanisms. It has long been assumed that autoregulation of the heart is accomplished through intrinsic feedback mediated by length changes of each myocyte (heterometric autoregulation) and through extrinsic feedback or neurohumoral control mediated by the coronary circulation and the autonomic nervous system (homeometric autoregulation). Experimental evidence now indicates that there might be a third autoregulatory mechanism of cardiac performance, i.e., regulation of myocardial function by endothelium (both endocardial and coronary vascular endothelium).

With these data in mind, it might be appropriate to complement somewhat the traditional picture of cardiac performance.[71] From phylogenesis and embryology of the heart, we have learned that development of endocardial endothelium precedes differentiation and contraction of myocytes. Autoregulation mediated by endocardial endothelium and heterometric autoregulation probably constitute the earliest and most primitive controlling mechanisms of heart function. The coronary circulation and cardiac innervation, including the Purkinje network, are relatively late phylogenetic and embryological developments. The contribution of the latter regulatory mechanisms, at first probably merely complementary, will in later evolution have a more substantial role, eventually becoming equally important or even more important than regulation of myocardial function by endocardial endothelium.

Cardiac performance is thus modulated by three main autoregulatory mechanisms: heterometric autoregulation, homeometric autoregulation, and endothelium-mediated autoregulation, the latter depending on the functional effects of coronary vascular endothelium and endocardial endothelium (Fig. 2–7). Heterometric autoregulation or regulation by cardiac muscle length or ventricular volume involves increased peak performance with prolongation of contraction duration and an increase in contraction velocity. Homeometric autoregulation or regulation by neurohumoral control primarily involves an increase in contraction velocity with a decrease in contraction duration. This decrease is substantial during administration of β-adrenergic agonists but is less pronounced during administration of calcium.[75] Regulation by endothelium involves a decrease in contraction duration with little ef-

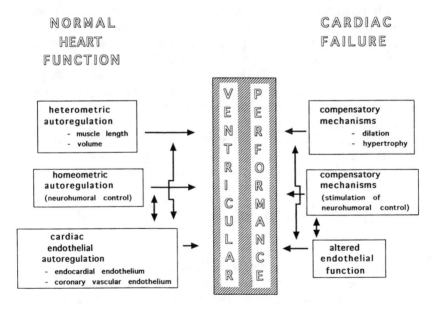

FIGURE 2-7. Schematic representation of the autoregulatory mechanisms of ventricular performance. Three autoregulatory mechanisms of myocardial function can be discerned: heterometric autoregulation, homeometric autoregulation, and cardiac endothelial autoregulation, which depends on normal function of both endocardial endothelium and coronary vascular endothelium. Regulation by endocardial endothelium interacts with heterometric and homeometric autoregulation. In the course of cardiac failure, several compensatory mechanisms are elicited. The possible role of cardiac endothelium in this process remains to be elucidated.

fect on peak performance and no effect on contraction velocity. Effects of coronary and endocardial endothelium on myocardial function appear additive.[72] Regulation of myocardial performance by endocardial endothelium interacts with regulation by Starling's law in such a way that when one regulation mechanism becomes maximized, the functional effects of the other mechanism become less important.[37,41] There is also experimental evidence, both in vitro and in vivo, that the endocardial endothelium mediates, either fully or partially, the inotropic actions of several substances involved in the neurohumoral regulation of contractile function. Hence, regulation of contractility by endothelium interacts with the two other mechanisms of autoregulation of myocardial function.[41,71]

How significant is regulation by endocardial endothelium in day-to-day adaptations of ventricular function of the heart compared with the two other control mechanisms of cardiac performance? In isolated cardiac muscles, the magnitude of modulation by endocardial endothelium (measured as changes in twitch duration from stimulus to one-half isometric relaxation (RT1/2)) reaches mean values ranging from 10.6 to 13%. In the canine left ventricle, the magnitude of modulation by endocardial endothelium (measured as change in time from end-diastole to peak $-dP/dt$ or, in other words, time from stimulus to peak rate of pressure decline) ranges from 3.5 to 9.2%, depending on the experimental conditions. Under those experimental conditions in which in vivo modulation by endocardial endothelium was maximized (at low ventricular volumes, reduced inotropism, or after addition of phenylephrine or indomethacin), shortening of systole by impairment of endocardial endothelium was found to be higher, ranging between 7.8 and 9.2% (Fig. 2-4). When the effects of damage to the endocardial endothelium were evaluated by alterations in ventricular output and stroke volume, decreases up to 19% were found.[45]

What is the importance and magnitude of regulation of ventricular function by endocardial endothelium compared to regulation by changes in ventricular volume? In an experimental model, when LVEDP was increased with volume loading (10.6 ± 1.5 to 17.9 ± 1.8 mm Hg), the time interval from end-diastole to peak $-dP/dt$ increased by 4.3%. The increase in time interval to peak $-dP/dt$ with an increase in LVEDP from low (4.1 ± 0.9 mm Hg) to baseline (10.6 ± 1.5 mm Hg) values was 12.2%.[37,71] Comparison of the variations in systolic duration by heterometric autoregulation and autoregulation via endocardial endothelium suggests that both types of autoregulation may, with respect to effects on systolic duration, be nearly as powerful in day-to-day adaptations of cardiac performance. The magnitude of the effects of endocardial endothelium on modulation of systolic duration resembles the magnitude of the effects of heterometric autoregulation.[71]

There are also other important actions of the endocardial endothelium. Endocardial endothelium forms a continuous layer and may, as such, play a role in the prevention of mural thrombus formation.[51] EDRF, for example, increases platelet cGMP and acts synergistically with agents which increase cyclic adenosine monophosphate (e.g., prostacyclin, adenosine) to inhibit platelet activation, aggregation, and adhesion.[76,77] It has now been reported that stimulation of EDRF from cultured porcine endocardial endothelial cells, (similar to vascular endothelial cells) inhibits platelet adhesion to these cells.[51] There is growing interest too in a possible role of cGMP as a growth inhibitor under appropriate conditions.[51]

The actions of substances released by endocardial endothelium is not necessarily limited to the cardiomyocytes. Substances released by the endocardial endothelium may also have a potentially significant effect in the downstream modulation of ventricular afterload. The half-life of NO is probably too short to account for such an action, but this is not the case for prostanoids. The vascular effects of prostacyclin and PGE_2 in the pulmonary and systemic circulations are well recognized. It has been suggested that endocardial prostanoid release could also modulate vascular tone downstream from the ventricles, attributing a role of the endocardium in ventricular-arterial coupling by an endocrine mechanism.[70]

From the evidence which is presently available, it appears that endocardial endothelium plays a substantial role in cardiac physiology. It acts as a modulator of cardiac performance in close interaction with heterometric and homeometric autoregulation of cardiac function. There is now growing evidence that the endocardial endothelium has antithrombotic action and may also participate in the regulation of tone of the pulmonary and systemic vasculature.

IMPLICATIONS FOR CARDIAC PATHOPHYSIOLOGY

Several compensatory mechanisms are elicited during the course of evolving myocardial dysfunction. These include compensatory mechanisms based on activation of various neurohumoral systems and compensatory mechanisms based on adaptations in structure of the cardiac muscle, such as hypertrophy and ventricular dilation (Fig. 2–7).[78] The response of ventricular performance to myocardial hypertrophy appears grossly similar to the response observed during venticular volume loading and overloading.[79-81] Whether the resemblance between the adaptations of ventricular performance through Starling's law, volume overloading, and myocardial hypertrophy also implies a possible interaction with regulation of myocardial function by the endocardial endothelium in pathological conditions is an intriguing question which remains unanswered. Plasma levels of several hormones are elevated during cardiac dysfunction.[82–86] These include not only vasoconstrictive hormones, such as catecholamines, vasopressin, and renin, and angiotensin but also vasorelaxing substances, such as atrial natriuretic peptide. In addition to their vasoactive effects, these substances also have effects on contraction and relaxation. The myocardial effects of several of these agents have been shown to be mediated, at least in part, by an intact endocardial endothelium. To what extent the role of the endocardial endothelium in the responsiveness to myocardium to these different substances is altered in different pathological conditions is unknown. However, it might be expected that damage to the endocardium with failure of the endothelium to fulfill its normal functions may have serious consequences especially when other forms of autoregulation are impaired.[41]

Endocardial endothelium itself may show evidence of morphological damage. Endocardial lesions have been described in various forms of parietal endocarditis such as hypereosinophylic endomyocardial fibrosis and endocardial fibroelastosis.[25–27] Endocardial endothelium is also altered with increasing age,[13] in the presence of mural thrombi after myocardial infarction, in ventricular aneurysms, and in dilated cardiomyopathy.[87,88] Endocardial endothelial function may also be impaired in a variety of experimental conditions. Acute exposure of isolated papillary muscle preparations to high concentrations of α-adrenoceptor agonists, 5-hydroxytryptamine, vasopressin, angiotensin II, or activated eosinophils structurally damaged endocardial endothelium with subsequent impairment of function.[22–25] Morphological changes were also observed in the endocardium in chronically volume-loaded canine hearts.[20] How these abnormalities of endothelial function might contribute to cardiac pump dysfunction in disease states such as heart failure, carcinoid syndrome, or hypereosinophilia remains to be determined. Because, no functional role had been attributed to the endocardial endothelium until a few years ago, any possible role of endocardial endothelium in cardiac pathophysiology had not been considered. Further evidence of morphological and/or functional damage to the endocardial endothelium in various disease states is necessary to elucidate the role of endocardial endothelium in different pathological conditions and to determine whether regional or generalized dysfunction of endocardial endothelium exists in vivo and whether this dysfunction is secondary to the evolution of underlying diseased myocardium or, instead, constitutes a primary cause of cardiac disease.

EDRF activity in the coronary vasculature is known to be impaired in many pathological conditions such as hypercholesterolemia, hypertension, diabetes, and heart failure.[51] Whether a similar impairment contributes to endocardial endothelium-related cardiac pump dysfunction has to be studied. Some recent evidence has indeed suggested impairment of endocardial endothelial function in the course of heart failure. In dogs with pacing-induced heart failure, evidence of endocardial damage was reported. This damage was associated with a reduction in myocardial α-adrenergic responsiveness.[89] In another observation, pathological overproduction of NO/EDRF was demonstrated to occur as a result of immune activation of an inducible NO synthase in a number of different cell types including cardiac myocytes and endothelial cells. The potential for deleterious myocardial effects, as in endotoxic shock, was supported by the finding in isolated papillary muscles that acute exposure to cytokines caused marked NO-dependent abbreviation of contractile twitch tension.[51]

Nitrovasodilator drugs are the pharmacological counterpart of endogenous EDRF. These drugs also possess inotropic effects which may be mediated through the endocardial endothelium. The influence of nitrovasodilator drugs on intrinsic myocardial performance certainly merits close attention because of potential clinical implications. In a recent preliminary study, we found that patients undergoing coronary artery bypass graft surgery showed a variable inotropic response to a short-lasting low-dose infusion of sodium nitroprusside. Four types of responses could be discerned (Fig. 2–8). In 21 of 60 patients (35%, group 1), nitroprusside caused a positive inotropic response before extracorporeal circulation (ECC) with an incrase in peak left ventricular pressure, an increase in peak +dP/dt, and a slight increase in systolic ejection duration (time from end-diastole to peak −dP/dt). Interestingly, after the end of ECC, the same infusion of nitroprusside had the opposite effect. A negative inotropic response was found with a decrease in peak left ventricular pressure, a decrease in peak +dP/dt, and no significant change in systolic ejection duration. In 14 of 60 patients (23%, group 2), nitroprusside had a positive inotropic response before ECC, but after ECC left ventricular hemodynamics were not significantly altered. In 7 of 60 patients (12%), nitroprusside had no significant effect on left ventricular hemodynamics before ECC, but after ECC infusion of nitroprusside produced a negative inotropic effect. Finally, in 18 of 60 patients (30%, group 4), infusion of nitroprusside did not alter left ventricular hemodynamics before nor after ECC. The underlying mechanisms of this phenomenon are still under investigation. Whether these different inotropic responses to sodium nitroprusside are caused by a different functional state of underlying myocardium or whether they might be a reflection of altered endocardial endothelial function represents an important area of research.

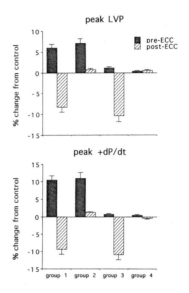

FIGURE 2-8. Effects of a short-lasting (5 min), low-dose (0.5 μg/kg/min) infusion of sodium nitroprusside before and after extracorporeal circulation (ECC) in 60 patients undergoing coronary artery bypass grafting. All patients were paced in atrioventricular sequential mode during the protocol. Left ventricular end-diastolic pressures were kept constant during infusion of nitroprusside. The effects of sodium nitroprusside on peak left ventricular pressure (*LVP*) and peak +dP/dt are displayed as the percentage of change after nitroprusside compared to the baseline value before the start of the infusion of nitroprusside. Based on the different effects of nitroprusside before (*pre-ECC*) and after (*post-ECC*) extracorporeal circulation, four different types of response could be discerned. Data are expressed as mean ± SD. *Group 1:* In 21 of 60 patients (35%), nitroprusside induced a positive inotropic response before ECC. Peak LVP increased by 6.0 ± 0.9%, peak +dP/dt increased by 10.6 ± 1.2%, and time interval from end-diastole to peak −dP/dt (systolic ejection duration) increased with 3.6 ± 0.4%. After ECC, nitroprusside induced a negative inotropic response in these patients. Peak LVP decreased with 8.2 ± 1.2%, peak +dP/dt decreased with 9.3 ± 1.4%, whereas systolic ejection duration was not significantly altered (increase of 0.4 ± 0.2%). *Group 2:* In 14 of 60 patients (23%), nitroprusside induced a positive inotropic response before ECC but did not alter left ventricular hemodyanmics after ECC. Before ECC, peak LVP increased with 7.1 ± 1.1%, peak +dP/dt increased with 11.1 ± 1.7%, and systolic ejection duration increased with 3.7 ± 0.6%. After ECC, peak LVP increased with 0.8 ± 0.3%, peak +dP/dt increased with 1.3 ± 0.2%, and ejection duration increased with 0.9 ± 0.4%. *Group 3:* In 7 of 60 patients (12%), nitroprusside did not alter left ventricular hemodynamics before ECC, but after ECC it induced a negative inotropic response. Before ECC, peak LVP increased with 1.2 ± 0.3%, peak +dP/dt increased with 0.7 ± 0.3%, and systolic ejection duration increased with 0.6 ± 0.2%. After ECC, peak LVP decreased with 10.3 ± 1.4%, peak +dP/dt decreased with 10.8 ± 1.5%, and systolic ejection duration increased with 0.3 ± 0.2%. *Group 4:* In 18 of 60 patients (30%), nitroprusside did not alter left ventricular hemodynamics before nor after ECC. Before ECC peak LVP increased with 0.4 ± 0.2%, peak +dP/dt increased with 0.5 ± 0.2%, and systolic ejection duration increased with 0.5 ± 0.2%. After ECC, peak LVP increased with 0.6 ± 0.2%, peak LVP decreased with 0.4 ± 0.2%, and systolic ejection duration increased with 0.7 ± 0.3%.

Cardioprotection (during cardiac surgery or in preservation for cardiac transplantation) and alteration of myocardial function in the period after cardiac surgery are subjects of current intensive research. The role of the endocardial endothelium in myocardial function highlights the need to direct attention also toward the preservation of endocardial endothelial function as an important part of improving cardiac function after cardiac surgery.

Regulation of myocardial function by endocardial endothelium has been shown to interact with the actions of calcium and it has been suggested that calcium homeostasis might play a role in the modulation of function by endocardial endothelium. Endocardial endothelium also has a role in mediating the myocardial effects of a number of agents with inotropic properties. In view of this information, it is of interest to know whether the effects of drugs used in the treatment of cardiac disorders are different in the presence of dysfunctional endocardial endothelium. This question has implications far beyond basic cardiac physiology or clinical cardiology. Because of the large number of patients with cardiac disease presenting for surgery and anesthesia, it would be of special interest to know whether any of the drugs used during anesthetic practice has a deleterious effect in the presence of a damaged or dysfunctional endocardial endothelium.[41]

IMPLICATIONS FOR ANESTHESIA

The finding that endothelium modulates vascular tone and that EDRF/NO acts as signal transduction mechanism for the activation of soluble guanylyl cyclase has led to a new approach in the study of the effects of anesthetic agents. Several investigations have examined the role of the endothelium in mediating the vascular responses of anesthetics or the effects of anesthetics on endothelium-dependent responses. The potent inhalational anesthetics (halothane, enflurane, and isoflurane) appear to inhibit endothelium-dependent vasodilation in response to a number of receptor-mediated agonists.[90–94] Recently it has been demonstrated that these volatile anesthetics can also inhibit nonreceptor-mediated EDRF/NO release.[94] There are multiple sites at which anesthetics may, potentially, inhibit EDRF/NO production or release. These possible mechanisms have recently been reviewed by Johns.[95] It has been suggested that one of the potential actions of inhalational anesthetics might be based on interference with the receptor activation.[91,96] Volatile anesthetics have been shown to have specific effects on calcium homeostasis (see chapter 1) and may decrease calcium availability for NO synthase activation. There is also some experimental evidence that inhalational anesthetics may interact with the availability of one of several cofactors (calmodulin) for NO synthase.[95] NO synthase is 80–90% membrane-associated in endothelial cells.[97,98] This provides an additional potential mechanism for anesthetic interaction. Volatile anesthetics could impair endothelial NO synthase activity through interaction with the enzyme or by altering the fluidity or structure of the enzyme-associated membrane. It is also possible that inhalational anesthetics may inactivate EDRF after its production, either via a direct interaction, or indirectly, by enhancing free radical activity within the endothelial cell, leading to an inactivation of EDRF by superoxide.[99] Finally, anesthetics might also act by altering activation of guanylyl cyclase. It was recently demonstrated that halogenated anesthetics are attracted to the same ferrous heme-binding site used by NO to activate guanylyl cyclase.[100]

Propofol has been shown to stimulate the production and release of NO, suggesting that its vasodilatory properties might be secondary to NO.[101] Others, however, failed to confirm this finding and concluded that vasodilation with propofol was not endothelium-dependent but probably resulted from blockade of voltage-gated influx of extracellular calcium.[102] In another study, however, the intravenous anesthetics thiopental, ketamine, and propofol were shown to have no direct effect on the tone of large and small canine coronary arteries at concentrations used in routine clinical practice.[103] Recently, experimental data were published suggesting that the inhibitory action of the barbiturates, thiopental and pentobarbital, on endothelium-dependent relaxation in arteries is mediated by inhibiting the action of NO or by inactivating NO in vascular smooth muscle and not by inhibition of endothelial NO synthesis.[104] The local anesthetics bupivacaine, lidocaine, etiodocaine, and 2-chloroprocaine selectively inhibit endothelium-dependent vasodilation at a site distal to receptor activation at the endothelial cell but proximal to guanylyl cyclase in smooth muscle.[105]

It is clear that anesthetic agents may interfere with regulation of vascular smooth muscle tone through actions on the endothelium, but the underlying mechanisms for this phenomenon remain to be definitively elucidated. Based on these findings, it has been hypothesized that a number of myocardial effects of anesthetic agents could also be mediated through endocardial endothelium.[41] This hypothesis has recently been tested (Fig. 2–9). In isolated cat papillary muscles, we found the negative inotropic effect of thiopental in low concentrations (1.5 to 6 μg/ml) to be dependent on the presence of an intact endocardial endothelium. Thiopental caused a dose-dependent decrease in total isometric twitch tension and in time from stimulus to half isometric twitch relaxation in the presence of an intact endocardial endothelium. After damage of the endocardial endothelium, thiopental (1.5 to 6 μg/ml) did not alter total tension and time to half relaxation. At concentrations ≥ 9 μg/ml, the negative inotropic effect of thiopental was similar in the

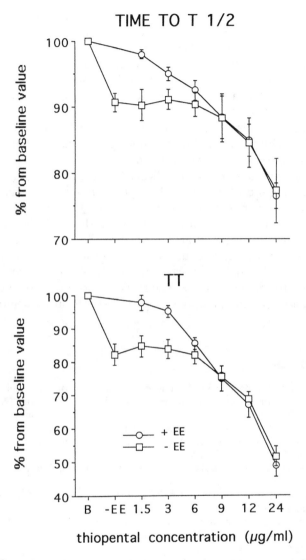

FIGURE 2-9. Effect of increasing doses of thiopental on the time interval from stimulus to half isometric twitch relaxation (upper panel, time to T1/2) and on total isometric twitch tension (lower panel, TT) in cat papillary muscle in the presence of endocardial endothelium (EE) (n = 7) and after selective removal of EE (n = 7). The effects are evaluated as percentage of change from the baseline value. In the presence of EE, thiopental induces a dose-dependent decrease in time to T1/2 and in TT. Selective removal of EE decreases contraction duration and developed tension. Interestingly, increasing concentrations of thiopental in the range of 1.5 to 6 mg/ml did not alter time to T1/2 and TT any more. Only at concentrations of 9 mg/ml and more was a negative inotropic effect similar to that seen in the presence of EE noticed. These data suggest that the negative inotropic effect of thiopental in the concentration range of 1.5 to 6 mg/ml might depend on the presence of an intact EE. Data are expressed as mean ± 1 SD bar.

presence or absence of an intact endocardial endothelium. This dual dose-dependent inotropic response of thiopental in the absence of endocardial endothelium suggests that in the concentration range from 1.5 to 6 $\mu g/ml$, the negative inotropic response of thiopental depends upon the presence of an intact endocardial endothelium. The negative inotropic response at higher concentrations (9 $\mu g/ml$ and more) are probably caused by a direct myocardial effect. The possible underlying mechanisms for this phenomenon and the possible role of the endocardial endothelium in mediating the inotropic effects of other anesthetic agents are presently under investigation.

These experimental data indicate that the endocardial endothelium plays an important role in the regulation of myocardial function. The concept of endocardial endothelial autoregulation has important implications. Impairment of normal endocardial endothelial function may profoundly alter myocardial function. The possible involvement of the endocardial endothelium in different cardiac diseases might introduce an additional approach to the study of cardiac pathophysiology. Our current knowledge of the role of endocardial function in cardiac physiology and pathophysiology represents only a beginning.

References

1. Furchgott RF, Zawadski JV: The obligatory role of endothelial cells in the relaxation of arterial smooth muscle by acetylcholine. Nature 288: 373, 1980
2. Brutsaert DL, Meulemans AL, Sipido KR, Sys SU: Effects of damaging the endocardial surface on the mechanical performance of isolated cardiac muscle. Circ Res 62:357, 1988
3. Manasek FJ: Histogenesis of the embryonic myocardium. Am J Cardiol 25:149, 1970
4. Manasek FJ: The ultrastructure of embryonic myocardial blood vessels. Dev Biol 26:42, 1971
5. Brutsaert DL: The endocardium. Annu Rev Physiol 51:263, 1989
6. Brutsaert DL, Andries LJ: The endocardial endothelium. Am J Physiol 263:H985, 1992
7. Ostadal B: Phylogenetic and ontogenetic development of the terminal vascular bed in the heart muscle and its effect on the development of experimental cardiac necrosis. In Proceedings of the 2nd Annual Meeting of the International Study Group for Research in Cardiac Development, pp. 111–132, 1969
8. Howse HD, Ferrans VJ, Hibbs RG: A comparative histochemical and electron microscopic study of the surface coatings of cardiac muscle cells. J Mol Cell Cardiol 1:157, 1970
9. Grant RT, Regnier M: The comparative anatomy of the cardiac coronary vessels. Heart 13:285, 1926
10. Becker BJ: Studies of the human mural endocardium. J Pathol Bacteriol 88:541, 1964

11. Anversa P, Giacomelli F, Wiener J: Intercellular junctions of the endocardium in adult rats. Anat Rec 183:477, 1975
12. Boyd MT, Sewards JB, Tajik AJ, Edwards WD: Frequency and location of prominent left ventricular trabeculations at autopsy in 474 normal human hearts: Implications for evaluation of mural thrombi by two-dimensional echocardiography. J Am Coll Cardiol 9:323, 1987
13. McMillan JB, Lev M: The aging heart. I. Endocardium. J Gerontol 14:268, 1959
14. Klein W, Böck P: Elastica-positive material in atrial endocardium. Light an electron microscopic identification. Acta Anat 116:106, 1983
15. Andries LJ: Endocardial Endothelium: RG Landes Publishing Cie, Functional Morphology. Austin, TX, 1994
16. Andries LJ, Brutsaert DL: Differences in functional structure between endocardial endothelium and vascular endothelium. J Cardiovasc Pharmacol 17(S3):S243, 1991
17. Melax H, Leeson TS: Fine structure of the endocardium in adult hearts. Cardiovasc Res 1:349, 1967
18. Kumar S, West DC, Ager A. Heterogeneity in endothelial cells from large vessels and microvessels. Differentiation 36:57, 1987
19. Johnson CM, Hanson MN, Helgeson SC: Porcine cardiac valvular subendothelial cells in culture: Cell isolation and growth characteristics. J Mol Cell Cardiol 19:1185, 1987
20. Masuda M, Kawamura K, Tohda K, Shozawa T, Sageshima M, Honma M: Endocardium of the left ventricle in volume-loaded canine heart. Acta Pathol Jpn 39:111, 1989
21. Jalil JE, Janicki JS, Pick R, Abrahams C, Weber KT. Fibrosis-induced reduction of endomyocardium in the rat after isoproterenol treatment. Circ Res 65:258, 1989
22. Norhona-Dutra AA, Steen EM, Woolf N: The early changes induced by isoproterenol in the endocardium and adjacent myocardium. Am J Pathol 114:231, 1984
23. Turcotte H, Bazin M, Boutet M: Junctional complexes in regenerating endocardium. J Ultrastruct Res 79:133, 1982
24. Meulemans AL, Andries LJ, Brutsaert DL: Endocardial endothelium mediates positive inotropic response to alpha$_1$-adrenoreceptor agonist in mammalian heart. J Mol Cell Cardiol 22:267, 1990
25. Shah AM, Andries LJ, Meulemans AL, Brutsaert DL: Endocardium modulates inotropic response to 5-hydroxytryptamine. Am J Physiol 257:H1790, 1989
26. Krishnaswami H, Data A, Bhaktaviziam A, Krishnaswami S, Cherian G: Electron microscopic changes in tropical endomyocardial fibrosis. Trans R Soc Trop Med Hyg 78:205, 1984
27. Shah AM, Brutsaert DL, Meulemans AL, Andries LJ, Capron M: Eosinophils from hypereosinophylic patients damage endocardium of isolated feline heart preparations. Circulation 81:1081, 1990
28. Slungaard A, Mahoney JR: Bromide-dependent toxicity of eosinophil peroxidase for endothelium and isolated working rat hearts: A model for eosinophilic endocarditis. J Exp Med 173:117, 1991
29. Gillebert TC, De Hert SG, Andries LJ, Jagenau AH, Brutsaert DL: Intracavitary ultrasond impairs left ventricular performance: Presumed role of endocardial endothelium. Am J Physiol 263:H857, 1992
30. Meulemans AL, Andries LJ, Brutsaert DL: Atriopeptin III induces early relaxation of isolated mammalian papillary muscle. Circ Res 62:1171, 1988

31. Bianchi C, Gutkowska K, Thibault G, Garcia R, Genest J, Cantin M: Radioautographic localization of ^{125}I-atrial natriuretic factor (ANF) in rat tissues. Histochemistry 82:441, 1985
32. Wilcox JN, Augustine A, Goeddel DV, Lowe DG: Differential regional expression of three natriuretic peptide receptor genes within primate tissues. Mol Cell Biol 11:3454, 1991
33. Shoemaker IE, Meulemans AL, Andries LJ, Brutsaert DL: Role of the endocardial endothelium in the positive inotropic action of vasopressin. Am J Physiol 259:H1148, 1990
34. Meulemans AL, Andries LJ, Brutsaert DL: Does endocardial endothelium mediate positive inotropic response to angiotensin I and angiotensin II? Circ Res 66:1594, 1990
35. Shah AM, Meulemans AL, Brutsaert DL: Myocardial inotropic responses to aggregating platelets and modulation by the endocardium. Circulation 79:1315, 1989
36. Andries LJ, Meulemans AL, Brutsaert DL: Ultrasound as a novel method for selective damage of the endocardial endothelium. Am J Physiol 261: H1636, 1991
37. De Hert SG, Gillebert TC, Brutsaert DL: Alteration of left ventricular endocardial function by intracavitary high power ultrasound interacts with volume, inotropic state and alpha$_1$-adrenergic stimulation. Circulation 87: 1275, 1993
38. Allen DG, Kentish JC: The cellular basis of the length-tension relation in cardiac muscle. J Mol Cell Cardiol 17:821, 1985
39. Winegrad S: Regulation of cardiac contractile proteins: correlation between physiology and biochemistry. Circ Res 55:565, 1984
40. Wang J, Morgan JP: Endocardial endothelium modulates myofilament Ca^{2+} responsiveness in ferret myocardium. Circ Res 69:582, 1991
41. De Hert SG, Gillebert TC, Andries LJ, Brutsaert DL: Role of the endocardial endothelium in the regulation of myocardial function: Physiologic and pathophysiologic implications. Anesthesiology 79:1354, 1993
42. Clementi F, Palace GE: Intestinal capillaries: Structural effects of EDTA and histamine. J Cell Biol 42:706, 1969
43. Nagy Z, Goehlert UG, Wolfe LS, Hüttner I: Ca^{2+} depletion-induced disconnection of right junctions in isolated rat brain microvessels. Acta Neuropathol (Berl) 68:48, 1985
44. De Hert SG, Brutsaert DL: Modulation of left ventricular performance by endocardial endothelium is sensitized by cyclooxygenase inhibitors. Circulation 4:II-308, 1991
45. De Hert SG: Role of the Endocardial Endothelium in the Modulation of Myocardial Performance in Vivo. PhD thesis. Antwerp, Belgium, University of Antwerp, 1992
46. Colden-Stanfield M, Schilling WP, Ritchie AK, Eskin SG, Navarro LT, Kunze DL: Bradykinin-induced increases in cytosolic calcium and ionic currents in cultured bovine aortic endothelial cells. Circ Res 61:632, 1987
47. Smith JA, Shah AM, Lewis MJ: Factors released from endocardium of the ferret and pig modulate myocardial contraction. J Physiol (Lond) 439:1, 1991
48. Palmer RMJ, Ferrige AG, Moncada S: Nitric oxide releases accounts for the biological activity of endothelium-derived relaxing factor. Nature 327:524, 1987
49. Ku DD, Nelson JM, Caulfield JB, Winn MJ: Release of endothelium-derived relaxing factors from canine cardiac valves. J Cardiovasc Pharmacol 16:212, 1990

50. Schulz R, Smith JA, Lewis MJ, Moncada S: Nitric oxide synthase in cultured endothelial cells of the pig. Br J Pharmacol 104:21, 1991
51. Henderson AH, Lewis MJ, Shah AM, Smith JA: Endothelium, endocardium, and cardiac contraction. Cardiovasc Res 26:305, 1992
52. Holtz J, Forstermann U, Pohl U, Giesler M, Bassenge E: Flow-dependent endothelium-mediated dilatation of epiocardial coronary arteries in conscious dogs: Effect of cyclooxygenase inhibition. J Cardiovas Pharmacol 6:1161, 1984
53. Hutcheson IR, Griffith TM: Release of endothelium-derived relaxing factor is modulated both by frequency and amplitude of pulsatile flow. Am J Physiol 261:H257, 1991
54. Blumenthal DK, Stull JT, Gill JN: Phosphorylation of cardiac troponin by guanosine 3',5' monophosphate-dependent kinase. J Biol Chem 253:334, 1978
55. Clement O, Puceat M, Vassort G: Protein kinase modulate Ca sensitivity of cardiac myofilaments in rat skinned cells. J Physiol (Lond) 438:96P, 1991
56. McClellan GB, Winegrad S: Cyclic nucleotide regulation of the contractile proteins in mammalian cardiac muscle. J Gen Physiol 75:283, 1980
57. Mohan P, Brutsaert DL, Paulus WJ, Sys SU. Nitric oxide potentiates endothelium-denuded myocardium. Circ Res, in press, 1995
58. Beavo JA, Reifsnyder DH: Primary sequence of cyclic nucleotide phosphodiesterase isoenzymes and the design of selective inhibitors. Trends Pharmacol Sci 11:150, 1990
59. Walter U: Physiological role of cGMP and cGMP-dependent protein kinase in the cardiovascular system. Rev Physiol Biochem Pharmacol 113:42, 1989
60. Levi RC, Alloatti G, Fischmeister R: Cyclic GMP regulates the Ca-channel current in guinea pig ventricular myocytes. Pflugers Arch 413:685, 1989
61. Méry P.F., Lohmann SM, Walter U, Fischmeister R: Ca^{2+} current is regulated by cyclic GMP-dependent protein kinase in mammalian cardiac myocytes. Proc Natl Acad Sci USA 88:1197, 1991
62. Finkel MS, Oddis CV, Jacob TD, Watkins SC, Hattler BG, Simmons RL: Negative inotropic effects of cytokines on the heart mediated by nitric oxide. Science 257:387, 1992
63. Shah AM, Shattock MJ, Lewis MJ: Action potential duration and endocardial modulation of myocardial contraction. Cardiovasc Res 26:376, 1992
64. Takanashi M, Endoh M: Characterization of positive inotropic effect of endothelin on mammalian ventricular myocardium. Am J Physiol 261:H611, 1991
65. Moody CJ, Dashwood MR, Sykes RM, Chester M, Jones SM, Yacoub MH, Harding SE: Functional and autoradiographic evidence for endothelin-1 receptors on human and rat cardiac myocytes. Circ Res 67:764, 1990
66. Mebazaa A, Mayoux E, Maeda K, Martin LD, Lakatta EG, Robotham JL, Shah AJ: Paracrine effects of endocardial endothelial cells on myocyte contraction mediated via endothelin. Am J Physiol 265:H1841, 1993
67. Shah AM, Lewis MJ, Henderson AH: Inotropic effects of endothelin in ferret ventricular myocardium. Eur J Pharmacol 163:365, 1989
68. Brandt R, Nowak J, Sonnenfeld T: Prostaglandin formation from exogenous precursor in homogenates of human cardiac tissue. Basic Res Cardiol 79:135, 1984
69. Manduteanu I, Popov D, Radu A, Simionescu M: Calf cardiac valvular endothelial cells in culture: Production of glycosaminoglycans, prostacyclin and fibronectin. J Mol Cell Cardiol 20:103, 1988
70. Mebazaa A, Martin LD, Robotham JL, Maeda K, Gabrielson EW, Wetzel RC: Right and left ventricular cultured endocardial endothelium produces prostacyclin and PGE_2. J Mol Cell Biol 25:245, 1993

71. Brutsaert DL: Endocardial and coronary endothelial control of cardiac performance. NIPS 8:82, 1993
72. Li K, Rouleau JL, Andries JL, Brutsaert DL: Effects of dysfunctional vascular endothelium on myocardial performance in isolated papillary muscles. Circ Res 72:768, 1993
73. McClellan G, Weisberg A, Kato NS, Ramaciotti R, Sharkey A, Winegrad S: Contractile proteins in myocardial cells are regulated by factor(s) released by blood vessels. Circ Res 70:787, 1992
74. Ramaciotti C, McClellan G, Sharkey A, Rose D, Weisberg A, Winegrad S: Cardiac endothelial cells modulate contracility of rat heart in response to oxygen tension and coronary flow. Circ Res 72:1044, 1993
75. Sonnenblick EH: The mechanisms of myocardial contraction. In Briller SA, Conn HL Jr (eds): The Myocardial Cell: Structure, Function and Modification by Cardiac Drugs, p. 173. Philadelphia, University of Pennsylvania Press, 1966
76. Furlong B, Henderson AH, Lewis MJ, Smith JA: Endothelium-derived relaxing factor inhibits in vitro platelet aggregation. Br J Pharmacol 90:687, 1987
77. Radomski MW, Palmer RMJ, Moncada S: The role of nitric oxide and cGMP in platelet adhesion to vascular endothelium. Biochem Biophys Res Commun II:1057, 1987
78. Brutsaert DL: Role of endocardium in cardiac overloading and failure. Eur Heart J 11:G8, 1991
79. Lecarpentier YC, Martin JL, Gastineau P, Hatt PY: Load dependence of mammalian heart relaxation during cardiac hypertrophy and heart failure. Am J Physiol 242:H855, 1982
80. Lecarpentier YC, Waldenström A, Clerque M: Major alterations in relaxation during cardiac hypertrophy induced by aortic stenosis in guinea pig. Circ Res 61:107, 1987
81. Rouleau JL, Juneau C, Stephens H, Shenasa H, Parmley WW, Brutsaert DL: Mechanical properties of papillary muscle in cardiac failure: Importance of pathogenesis and of ventricle of origin. J Mol Cell Cardiol 21:817, 1989
82. Curtiss C, Cohn JN, Vrobel T, Franciosa JA: Role of the renin-angiotensin system in the systemic vasoconstriction of chronic congestive heart failure. Circulation 58:763, 1978
83. Levine TB, Francis GS, Goldsmith SR, Simon AB, Cohn JN: Activity of the sympathetic nervous system and renin-angiotensin system assessed by plasma hormone levels and their relation to hemodynamic abnormalities in congestive heart failure. Am J Cardiol 49:1659, 1982
84. Swedberg K, Viquerat C, Rouleau JL, Roizen M, Atherton B, Parmley WW, Chatterjee K: Comparison of myocardial catecholamine balance in chronic congestive heart failure and in angina pectoris without failure. Am J Cardiol 54:783, 1984
85. Goldsmith SR, Francis GS, Cowley AW Jr, Levine TB, Cohn JN: Increased plasma arginin vasopressin in patients with congestive heart failure. J Am Coll Cardiol 1:1385, 1983
86. Gotlieb SS, Kuhin MC, Ahern D, Packer M: Prognostic importance of atrial natriuretic peptide in patients with chronic heart failure. J Am Coll Cardiol 13:1534, 1989
87. Hochman JS, Platia EB, Bulkley BH: Endocardfial abnormalities in left ventricular aneurysms. Ann Intern Med 100:29, 1984
88. Johnson RC, Crissman RS, Didio LJA: Endocardial alterations in myocardial infarction. Lab Invest 40:183, 1979

89. Li K, Calderone A, Rouleau JL: Reduced myocardial alpha-adrenergic contractile responsiveness in pacing-overdrive model of heart failure in the dog: Potential role of the endocardial endothelium. Eur Heart J 11:S79, 1990

90. Blaise G, Sill JC, Nugent M, Van Dyke RA, Vanhoutte PM: Isoflurane causes endothelium-dependent inhibitio of contractile responses of canine coronary arteries. Anesthesiology 67:513–517, 1987

91. Muldoon SM, Hart JL, Bowen KA, Freas W: Attenuation of endothelium-mediated vasodilation by halothane. Anesthesiology. 68:31, 1988

92. Stone DJ, Johns RA: Endothelium-dependent effects of halothane, enflurane and isoflurane on isolated rat aortic vascular rings. Anesthesiology 71:126, 1989

93. Toda H, Nakamura K, Hatano Y, Nishiwada M, Kakuyama M, Mori K: Halothane and isoflurane inhibit endothelium-dependent relaxation by acetylcholine. Anesth Analg 75:198, 1992

94. Uggeri MJ, Proctor GJ, Johns RA: Halothane, enflurane and isoflurane attenuate both receptor and non-receptor mediated EDRF production in rat throacic aorta. Anesthesiology 76:1012, 1992

95. Johns RA: Endothelium, anesthetics, and vascular control. Anesthesiology 79:1381, 1993

96. Lechlecter J, Greuner R: Halothane shortens acetylcholine receptor channel kinetics without affecting conductance. Proc Natl Acad Sci USA 81:2929, 1989

97. Forstermann U, Pollock JS, Schmidt HHHW, Heller M, Murad F: Calmodulin-dependent endothelium-derived relaxing factor/nitric oxide synthase activity is present in the particulate and cytosolic fractions of bovine aortic endothelial cells. Proc Natl Acad Sci USA 88:1788, 1991

98. Pollock JS, Forstermann U, Mitchell JA, Warner TD, Schmidt HHHW, Nakane M, Murad F: Purification and characterization of particulate endothelium-derived relaxing factor synthase from cultured and native bovine aortic endothelial cells. Proc Natl Acad Sci USA 88:10480, 1991

99. Yoshida KI, Okahe E. Selective impairment of endothelium-dependent relaxation by sevoflurane: Oxygen free radical participation. Anesthesiology 76:440, 1992

100. Hart JL, Jing M, Bina S, Freas W, Van Dyke RA, Muldoon SM: Effects of halothane on EDRF/cGMP-mediated vascular smooth muscle relaxations. Anesthesiology 79:323, 1993

101. Petros AJ, Bogle RG, Pearson JD: Propofol stimulates nitric oxide release from cultured porcine aortic endothelial cells. Br J Pharmacol 109:6, 1993

102. Chang KSK, Davis RF: Propofol produces endothelium-independent vasodilation and may act as a Ca^{2+} channel blocker. Anesth Analg 76:24, 1993

103. Coughlan MG, Flynn NM, Kenny D, Warltier DC, Kampine JP: Differential relaxant effect of high concentrations of intravenous anesthetics on endothelin-constricted proximal and distal canine coronary arteries. Anesth Analg 74:378, 1992

104. Terasako K, Nakamura K, Toda H, Kakuyama M, Hatano Y, Mori K: Barbiturates inhibit endothelium-dependent and independent relaxations mediated by cGMP. Anesth Analg 78:823, 1994

105. Johns RA: Local anesthetics inhibit endothelium-dependent vasodilation. Anesthesiology 70:805, 1989

William C. Little
Che-Ping Cheng

3 | Left Ventricular Systolic and Diastolic Performance

SYSTOLIC PERFORMANCE

Indices of Left Ventricular Systolic Function

The evaluation of left ventricular systolic performance is an important problem in clinical practice and physiological investigation. Conventional measures of left ventricular performance, such as ejection fraction and maximum rate of change of left ventricular pressure (dP/dt_{max}), are influenced not only by myocardial contractile state but also by loading conditions.[1,2] Left ventricular performance has been analyzed in the pressure-volume plane to help overcome these limitations (Fig. 3–1).[1–7] Most attention was initially focused on the left ventricular end-systolic pressure-volume relation (ESPVR). The slope of a linear approximation of this relation (E_{es}) responds to the contractile state and is relatively insensitive to loading conditions. However, recent observations suggest that the ESPVR may be quite variable, nonlinear, and shifted by alterations in arterial loading.[2,6,8–11]

Two other measures of left ventricular performance derived from variably loaded left ventricular pressure-volume diagrams have been proposed[2,12]: linear relations between dP/dt_{max} and the end-diastolic volume and between left ventricular stroke work and end-diastolic volume (Fig. 3–2). Both the dP/dt_{max}-end-diastolic volume relation and

Ventricular Function, edited by David C. Warltier. Williams & Wilkins, Baltimore © 1995.

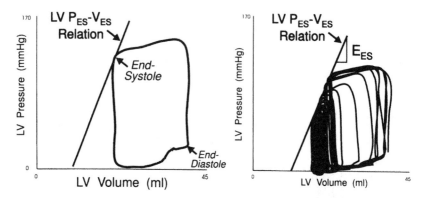

FIGURE 3-1. The *left panel* contains a steady-state pressure-volume loop recorded in a conscious dog. End-systole occurs at the *upper lefthand corner* of the loop, on the left ventricular end-systolic pressure-volume (P_{es}-V_{es}) relation. The *righthand panel* shows variably loaded beats produced by caval occlusion. The *upper left hand corners* fall along the left ventricular end-systolic pressure-volume relation whose slope is E_{es}. LV, left ventricular. (*Adapted from Little WC, Cheng CP. Am J Physiol 261:H70–H76, 1991*)

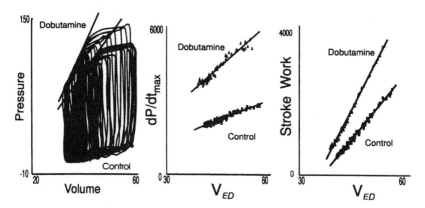

FIGURE 3-2. The *lefthand panel* contains variably loaded pressure-volume loops produced by caval occlusion recorded from a conscious dog before and after increasing contractile state with dobutamine. The *upper lefthand corners* of the loops denote the left ventricular end-systolic pressure-volume relation. The relation is shifted to the left with an increased slope in response to dobutamine. In the other panels of dP/dt$_{max}$-end-diastolic volume (V_{ED}) relation and stroke work end-diastolic volume relation derived from these loops are shown. In both instances the relations shifted toward the left with an increase in slope in response to an increase of contractile state produced by dobutamine. (*Adapted from Little WC et al. Circulation 80:1378–1387, 1989*)

ESPVR can be derived from the time-varying elastance model of the left ventricle.[2] The stroke work-end-diastolic volume relation also called preload recruitable stroke work (PRSW) is a modification of the traditional Frank-Starling cardiac function curve in which left ventricular end-diastolic pressure is replaced by end-diastolic volume.[12] This substitution linearizes the Frank-Starling relation. The slopes of the dP/dt_{max}-end-diastolic volume and PRSW relations have been reported to respond to changes in contractile state but not to load alterations.[2,12]

The PRSW relation integrates data obtained throughout the cardiac cycle, thus potentially damping out noise and beat-to-beat variations (see Chapter 4). Following inferior vena caval occlusion (a sudden decrease in preload), both determinants of stroke work, left ventricular pressure, and stroke volume fall. Thus, a larger range of stroke work is generated as compared to end systolic pressure or dP/dt_{max}.[13,14] In addition, the PRSW relation is the only relation that displayed no statistically significant deviation from linearity. These factors contribute to the marked stability and reproducibility of this relationship. The PRSW relation depends on the position of both the end-systolic and end-diastolic pressure-volume relations. The PRSW relation does not change as much as the ESPVR in response to the positive inotropic agent, dobutamine because the diastolic pressure-volume relation is not altered in response to the enhanced contractile state.

In contrast to the PRSW relation, which integrates data obtained throughout the cardiac cycle, the dP/dt_{max}-end-diastolic volume relation is derived from the period of isovolumic contraction, when the left ventricle is undergoing a rapid transition from a passive diastolic to an active systolic state. Differentiation increases the magnitude of any noise in the left ventricular pressure signal. Although at steady-state, dP/dt_{max} does not significantly vary more from beat-to-beat than stroke work, it appears that dP/dt_{max} does not significantly vary more from beat-to-beat than stroke work, it appears that dP/dt_{max} may be subject to greater potential beat-to-beat variation following inferior vena caval occlusion. Furthermore, because the range of dP/dt_{max} produced following a decrease in preload is less than the range of stroke work, the dP/dt_{max}-end-diastolic volume relationship cannot be as accurately defined as the PRSW relation. The dP/dt_{max}-end-diastolic volume relation is well approximated by a straight line, but it is somewhat concave toward the volume axis.[15] Thus, linear approximations of this relation over different ranges may also produce variations in the calculated slope. These factors are reflected in the observation that the slope of the dP/dt_{max}-end-diastolic volume relation is subject to almost an 11% variation between repeated determinations.[14]

The ESPVR uses data obtained at a single time in the cardiac cycle, end-systole, when left ventricular pressure and volume are not rapidly changing.[3-5] Furthermore, at end-systole, the potentially varying effects of the time course of ejection and contraction may tend to cancel.[3,7,16] Thus, it is not surprising that the stability of repeat determinations of the ESPVR is intermediate between the PRSW and dP/dt_{max}-end-diastolic volume relations. Our observation[14] of an 8% variation in repeated determinations of E_{es} is similar to that reported by Lee et al.[17] in conscious dogs. We also found that E_{es} responds to alterations in the contractile state in contrast to observations by Crottogini et al.

The variability of repeated determinations of the three relations should be considered when interpreting changes resulting from an intervention. Small changes (especially of the dP/dt_{max}-end-diastolic volume relation) may well be due to spontaneous variability, but averaging repeated determinations provides a method of improving the precision with which the parameters are defined.[14] Moreover, the position of the relations (in the middle of the range from which the data are collected) shows less variation than the slopes and is less dependent on the choice of the model (linear or quadratic) used to fit the data. The accuracy with which the position of the relations in the physiological range can be determined and the consistent shift of the relations with inotropic stimulation make the positions of these relations ideal measures of pump function. Thus, it is important to assess the positions of the relations and not simply the slopes.[5]

The response of these relations to a marked increase in afterload (i.e., end-systolic pressure increased by approximately 50 mm Hg has also been investigated.[14] The slopes did not change by more than 10%. Although all three slopes of the relations decreased, only the change in the slope of the dP/dt_{max}-end-diastolic volume relation approached statistical significance. These changes, although relatively small, may reflect an underlying curvilinearity in the relations, in which the slopes decrease at the higher ranges.[2,17,19-21] This shift of the ESPVR is consistent with previous investigations using other methods of producing arterial vasoconstriction in intact animals, open-chest preparations, and isolated hearts. The lack of shift of the dP/dt_{max}-end-diastolic volume and PRSW relations with arterial loading is also consistent with previous reports in intact animals.[2,12] In contrast, Baan and Vander Velde[11] found that arterial constriction shifted both the ESPVR and dP/dt_{max}-end-diastolic volume relation. These conflicting results may be due to differences in the loading protocols used in these two studies. The position of the dP/dt_{max}-end-diastolic volume relation and the PRSW relation do not consistently shift with the increase in arterial load, but the ESPVR shifts to the left.[2,6,9-11] More marked increases in arterial load must influence the PRSW relation because an isovolumic beat produces zero stroke work.[22]

Interaction between Ventricular and Arterial Systems

The function of the cardiovascular system is to provide for the perfusion of the tissues. This requires that the left ventricle produces both flow (stroke volume) and perfusion pressure (arterial pressure). Left ventricular stroke work integrates both these parameters, and thus it provides a simple means of quantitating the performance of the cardiovascular system.[23] The interaction of the left ventricle and the arterial system, in addition to determining stroke work, also importantly influences the determinants of myocardial oxygen demand.[24] Accordingly, alterations of the coupling between the left ventricle and arterial system on stroke work and pressure-volume area in conscious animals have been studied (see Chapter 5).[22]

In our investigation, we studied stroke work at a constant end-diastolic volume and contractile state. We found that stroke work is maximized when left ventricular end-systolic elastance, E_{es}, and arterial elastance (E_a) are equal (i.e., $E_{es}/E_a = 1$). However, there is a broad plateau to the relation of stroke work to E_{es}/E_a. Stroke work was within 95% of its maximum value when E_{es}/E_a was between 0.74 and 1.20. When E_{es} exceeded E_a further, stroke work remained high, still being approximately 83% of its maximum with an E_{es}/E_a equal to 2.2. Only when E_a markedly exceeded E_{es} (i.e., $E_{es}/E_a<0.56$) was stroke work substantially (>20%) reduced. Our data indicate the cardiovascular system of the resting, conscious dog with intact autonomic reflexes operates near the center of the plateau with nearly equal E_{es} and E_a. Thus, during most physiological perturbations in E_{es} and E_a, it appears that the left ventricle operates on the plateau of the stroke work E_{es}/E_a relation, where the left ventricle and arterial system interact to produce nearly maximal stroke work.

The relation between stroke work and E_{es}/E_a which we observed is similar to that predicted by Sunagawa et al.[23] and Burkhoff and Sagawa.[24] These investigators modeled ventriculoarterial coupling in the pressure-volume plane, using linear ESPVR and end-systolic pressure-stroke volume relations to describe the left ventricle and the arterial system (see Chapter 5). Their analysis includes several assumptions that are not completely correct. For example, the ESPVR is not perfectly linear, but instead it is concave toward the volume axis when evaluated over a wide range of pressures.[5,19,21] However, over a 30 to 60 mm Hg range, as evaluated in this study, the ESPVR is closely approximated by a straight line.[21] The theoretical analysis assumed that the left ventricular ESPVR is independent of the mode of ejection. In contrast, we found that arterial vasoconstriction tended to shift the ESPVR to the left while vasodilation tended to shift the ESPVR toward the right. This is consistent with previous observations in isolated dog hearts[10] and intact animals.[6,25,26] However, despite marked changes in the arterial system, the slope of the ESPVR remains relatively unchanged. The afterload-dependent shifts of the ESPVR help to preserve stroke work as E_a increases.[27] The theoretical analysis of Sunagawa et al.[23] and Burkhoff and Sagawa[24] assumed that mean ejection pressure was closely approximated by end-systolic pressure and left ventricular-diastolic pressures were zero. Despite some inaccuracy in these simplifying assumptions, we found that the shape of the stroke work-E_{es}/E_a relation (Fig. 3–3) directly determined in the intact cardiovascular system of conscious animals was very similar to that predicted by the model. However, the stroke work at each E_{es}/E_a was consistently less than predicted by the theoretical pressure-volume analysis. This lower than predicted stroke work may at least partially be due to the nonzero diastolic pressures and deviation of mean ejection pressure from end-systolic pressure. Our results are consistent with the predictions of pressure-volume analysis with this quantitatively small exception and suggest it provides an accurate approximation of left ventricle arterial coupling in conscious animals.

Thus, stroke work is insensitive to changes in E_a in the normal operating range. This is reflected in the lack of effect of changes in afterload within the physiogical range on the PRSW relation.[1,12,28] This is not

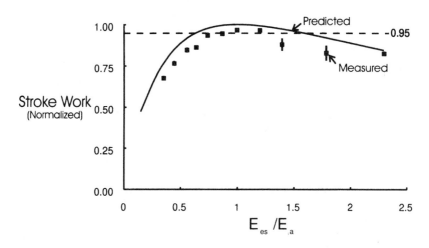

FIGURE 3-3. Plot of stroke work (SW) occurring at constant end-diastolic volume normalized by maximum SW produced at each contractile state vs ratio (E_{es}/E_a) of slopes of left ventricular end-systolic pressure-volume and arterial end-systolic pressure-stroke volume relation. Maximum SW occurs when $E_{es}/E_a = 1$. SW predicted by theoretical model proposed by Sunagawa et al.[23] and Burkhoff and Sagawa[24] is also shown. Data are shown as group means ± SE. (*Adapted from Little WC, Cheng CP. Am J Physiol 261:H70–H76, 1991*)

the case when E_a greatly exceeds E_{es}, as may occur in many patients with heart failure in which E_{es} is reduced and E_a increased. In this situation, stroke work is very sensitive to changes in E_a and both stroke work and the ratio of stroke work to pressure-volume area would be improved by a reduction in E_a, as would be produced by a vasodilator drug.

Conclusions

The PRSW relation, which integrates data obtained throughout the cardiac cycle, is the most stable but also the least sensitive to alterations in the contractile state. It has the widest range of values following inferior vena caval occlusion, shows no deviation from linearity, and is the only relation with a reproducible volume-axis intercept that is not altered by enhanced contractile state or arterial vasconstriction. Thus, it has advantages over the other relations to serially evaluate left ventricular performance. It also has an advantage over the other relations if the volume-axis intercept cannot be repeatedly determined or if pressure-volume loops are only available over a limited range. The dP/dt_{max}-end-diastolic volume relation is the least reproducible but most sensitive to changes in the contractile state. Thus, it may be of greatest value in excluding small changes in the contractile state. Using data obtained from inferior vena caval occlusions, the positions of these three relations in the physiological range respond consistently to inotropic stimulation and can be determined more reproducibly than their slopes. Therefore, it is also important to assess the position of each relation and not merely the slope. Arterial vasoconstriction shifts the ESPVR toward the left, and the position of this relation should not be used in situations in which arterial properties are markedly altered. The ESPVR, dP/dt_{max}-end-diastolic and PRSW relations have somewhat different characteristics, and in many situations, they can provide complementary means of evaluating left ventricular performance from variably loaded pressure-volume loops.

DIASTOLIC PERFORMANCE

The importance of left ventricular systolic function has traditionally been emphasized in cardiac evaluation, while left ventricular diastolic function has received less attention. However, abnormal diastolic function may result in congestive heart failure despite a normal systolic contractile state.[29–32] A single measure of left ventricular diastolic function is not available, and a confusing array of measures of diastolic function has been proposed.[33,34] The basis for this is straight forward. Diastole represents a complex sequence of interrelated events.

Definition of Normal Left Ventricular Diastolic Performance

Normal left ventricular diastolic performance can be defined as filling of the left ventricle that is sufficient to produce a cardiac output commensurate with the needs of the body at a mean pulmonary venous pressure of less than 12 mm Hg.[33–36] When defined in such a manner, left ventricular diastolic dysfunction is present when the mean pulmonary venous pressure is elevated. This simple definition of diastolic dysfunction avoids the ambiguity and confusion inherent in characterizing diastolic dysfunction in terms of the multiple determinants of left ventricular filling. The most common cause of left ventricular diastolic dysfunction (using our definition) is reduced systolic performance. However, primary diastolic dysfunction in the absence of systolic dysfunction is an important, increasingly recognized condition. Abnormalities of left ventricular filling that would not produce an adequate cardiac output with a mean pulmonary venous pressure below 12 mm Hg activate compensatory mechanisms which ultimately elevate pulmonary venous pressure. As such, abnormalities of left ventricular diastolic filling do not usually produce a reduction of cardiac output at rest. Instead, pulmonary venous congestion is the most common result of diastolic dysfunction. Patients with abnormalities of diastolic filling caused by left ventricular hypertrophy, restrictive cardiomyopathy, ischemia, or pericardial disease may have symptoms of pulmonary congestion despite normal or even enhanced left ventricular systolic performance. Accordingly, normal left ventricular systolic function does not rule out the possibility of a cardiac cause of dyspnea.[29,33,36]

Determinants of Left Ventricular Diastolic Performance

Diastole can be divided into four phases: 1) isovolumic relaxation, 2) early rapid filling, 3) diastasis, and 4) atrial systole.[30] These phases are illustrated in Figure 3–4.The timing, rate, and amount of ventricular filling and the relative importance of each of the phases of diastole are determined by four major factors: 1) myocardial relaxation; 2) the passive filling characteristics of the left ventricle; 3) the characteristics of the left atrium, pulmonary veins, and mitral valve; and 4) the heart rate.[33,34] Each of these determinants of diastolic performance can be influenced by different physiological stimuli and can be altered by dis-

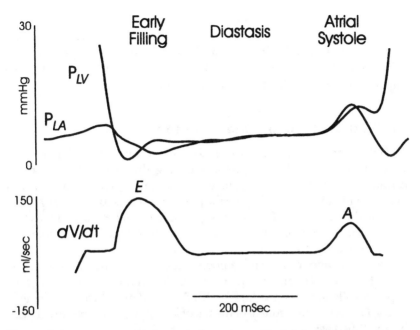

FIGURE 3-4.   Recording of left ventricular pressure (P_{LV}), left atrial pressure (P_{LA}), and the rate of change of left ventricular volume (dV/dt) in a conscious animal. The left ventricular filling rate is indicated by dV/dt. Filling of the ventricle occurs at two times: during the first 100 msec of diastole during the early filling phase and during the last 100 msec of diastole during atrial systole. During mid-diastole, the period of diastasis, there is very little filling. The early filling occurs in response to a pressure gradient generated as left ventricular pressure falls below left atrial pressure. Late filling during atrial systole occurs in response to the pressure gradient generated as left atrial pressure increases above left ventricular pressure during atrial contraction. (*Adapted from Cheng CP et al. Circ Res 66:814–823, 1990*)

ease states.[30,33] These factors are closely interrelated in that alterations in one may ultimately result in changes in the others.

Evaluation of Diastolic Performance

Complete assessment of diastolic function requires measurement of both left atrial and left ventricular pressures and the left ventricular volume throughout diastole. Analysis of the passive properties of the left ventricle requires evaluation of the left ventricular diastolic pressure-volume relation over a wide range of volumes. Ideally, this should also include determination of the ventricular stress-strain relation. With the development of current interest in diastolic function, there has been a tremendous increase in the number of indices proposed to analyze diastolic performance. Most of these are based on a noninvasive evaluation of the pattern of left ventricular filling. These methods provide useful information about diastolic filling, but they fail to provide evaluation of important determinants of filling.

Evaluation of Isovolumic Relaxation

The left ventricle is normally a closed chamber during isovolumic relaxation. Thus, the decline of pressure during this period reflects myocardial relaxation. The time course of isovolumic pressure decline has been quantitatively described by the peak rate of pressure fall (dP/dt_{min}) and the time constant of isovolumic pressure decline τ. Each of these require measurement of left ventricular pressure with a micromanometer. Left ventricular dP/dt_{min} is strongly influenced by the pressure at aortic valve closure and, thus, is not a good measure of the rate of isovolumic relaxation. Weiss et al. demonstrated that left ventricular pressure falls exponentially between the time of dP/dt_{min} and mitral valve opening.[37] Accordingly, the time course of the fall of left ventricular pressure (P) can be quantified as:

$$P(t) = P_0 e^{-t/\tau}$$

where P_0 is the left ventricular pressure at the time of aortic valve closure or peak negative dP/dt, t is the time after the onset of relaxation, and τ is the time constant of isovolumic relaxation. τ is usually calculated using the linear least squares technique after a logarithmic transformation. The exponential fall in left ventricular pressure can be described by τ which represents the time for the pressure to fall to $1/e$ of its initial value. The smaller the value of τ, the faster the rate of relaxation. This simple exponential model has been quite valuable in describing the rate of left ventricular relaxation.

Several limitations of the simple exponential model, however, need to be considered.[38] First, this simple model assumes that the pressure in the ventricle will be equal to 0 when relaxation is complete. This assumption is not correct because in the absence of filling and following complete relaxation, left ventricular pressure is subatmospheric. This indicates that the ventricle normally ejects beyond its equilibrium volume.[39-42] The pressure after total relaxation may also be influenced by an external pressure (the pericardial pressure).[41,43,44] These factors can be partially overcome by the addition of an intercept (P_B) to the exponential relation:

$$P(t) = (P_0 - P_B)e^{-t/\tau} + P_B.$$

This technique is quite helpful in accounting for changes in external pressure.[43] However, it does not accurately describe left ventricular pressure beyond the time of mitral valve opening. There is some indication that in the absence of changes in external pressure, the simple exponential equation, though not completely accurate, may provide a closer estimation of the true rate of left ventricular relaxation.[41,43,44] In addition, the exponential equation with the intercept cannot be fit using a simple logarithmic transformation.

The time constant of isovolumic relaxation is strongly influenced by active myocardial relaxation, but it is also sensitive to alterations in loading conditions and heart rate.[45–47] An increase in arterial systolic pressure slows relaxation while an increase in heart rate accelerates relaxation. The load sensitivity of isovolumic relaxation has important practical implications in the clinical and experimental use of this variable. The time constant of isovolumic relaxation is normally in the range of 20 to 40 msec. However, evaluation of relaxation usually consists of comparing time constants before and after an intervention. Care must be exercised in ascribing the change in this time constant to alterations in active myocardial relaxation, since it may have resulted from changes in arterial pressure. It is also important to recognize that τ represents the speed of relaxation, not the completeness of relaxation.[44]

Evaluation of the Passive Diastolic Characteristics of the Left Ventricle

The passive chamber properties of the left ventricle can be evaluated by plotting the relation between left ventricular diastolic pressure and volume. Optimally, this curve should be constructed from points obtained after relaxation is complete and when ventricular filling is slow, so that it represents only the passive characteristics of the left ventricle.[38,48] One approach is to examine the diastolic portion of a steady-state pressure-volume diagram. This technique is commonly used in clinical studies. However, most of the diastolic portion of the left ventricular pressure-volume loop is actually generated early in diastole while the ventricle is relaxing and mitral flow is high.[49] Thus, a diastolic pressure-volume relation obtained in this manner does not simply represent the passive properties of the left ventricle. Apparent shifts of the diastolic portion of the left ventricular pressure-volume loop during an intervention may occur secondary to altered relaxation, viscous properties, external constraints, or passive myocardial properties (see also Chapter 4). Another approach is to use points obtained from a single beat during diastasis and atrial systole.[50,51] This approach avoids the problems of incomplete relaxation, but the range of volumes is very limited.

The passive left ventricular pressure-volume relationship can be determined from the end-diastolic points obtained from several variably loaded beats. Under most circumstances, relaxation is complete at end-diastole, so the end-diastolic pressure-volume relation provides information about the passive properties of the left ventricle. The use of variably loaded beats, however, may introduce other confounding factors. For example, the right ventricular and pericardial pressures may be altered, causing a shift in the left ventricular pressure-volume relation.[52] Furthermore, it is frequently difficult to obtain a wide range of ventricular volumes.

The slope of the pressure-volume curve is the chamber stiffness.[38,53] The reciprocal is the compliance. The normal passive pressure-volume relation of the left ventricle is exponential in shape. Because of this exponential relationship, the chamber stiffness (or compliance) is not a constant, but changes with pressure and volume. This indicates that the left ventricle becomes stiffer at higher diastolic pressures. The position of the pressure-volume curve may be even more important than the slope in determining the passive diastolic properties of the left ventricle.[48,54] A shift upward and to the left, regardless of the chamber stiffness, indicates that a higher pressure will be required to fill the ventricle to the same volume. If the myocardium is abnormal, as may occur with amyloid infiltration, a higher pressure will be required to distend the left ventricular chamber. A higher pressure will also be required to fill the left ventricle if its walls are abnormally thick, even if the myocardial tissue characteristics are normal.

Chamber stiffness (or compliance) depends on the point on the diastolic pressure-volume curve in which it is measured.[38,48,53] Several techniques have been proposed to correct for this effect by normalizing chamber stiffness. One approach is to approximate the pressure-volume relation by an exponential function.[55] Another technique is to compare the chamber stiffness at a common pressure or volume. Analysis of chamber stiffness, however, does not account for the importance of shifts of the pressure-volume relation that can occur with alteration of load, diseases, or pharmacological agents.[38,48,54]

As discussed above, the end-diastolic pressure-volume relation represents the net passive characteristics of the left ventricular chamber. The effects of wall thickness, ventricular configuration, size, and external pressure must be removed in order to derive information concerning the properties of the myocardium alone.[38] The usual method to accomplish this is to derive the myocardial stress-strain relation from the chamber pressure-volume relation. In contrast to the pressure-volume relation, which assesses the ability of the ventricular chamber to distend under pressure, the stress-strain relation represents the resistance of the myocardium itself to stretching when it is subjected to a stress. It should not be influenced by the configuration of the left ventricle.

The calculation of stress involves measurement of left ventricular wall thickness and configuration. Stress is directly proportional to radius (r) and pressure (p) and inversely proportional to wall thickness (h) for a thin walled sphere.

$$\text{Stress} = p \cdot r / h.$$

Clearly, the left ventricle is not a thin-walled sphere. However, the simple equation does provide an approximation indicating that the effect of increased pressure and chamber size to increase wall stress can be offset by increased wall thickness (e.g., the compensatory nature of left ventricular hypertrophy to pressure overload). More accurate calculation of wall stress requires assumptions concerning left ventricular configuration. Recent reviews[38,56] consider this in more detail.

Calculation of strain requires some assumptions concerning unstressed left ventricular volume. Determination of the left ventricular stress-strain relation requires accurate measurements over a wide range of ventricular pressures and volumes. Since stress-strain analysis can most simply be applied to the determination of purely passive or mechanical properties, measurements made during rapid filling will be inappropriately influenced by active myocardial relaxation and viscoelastic effects. Measurements made in diastasis and atrial systole will not encounter this problem but may not supply a wide enough range of points. The theoretical problems and the technical difficulties in determining myocardial stress-strain relations have limited their clinical usefulness.

Evaluation of the Pattern of Left Ventricular Diastolic Filling

There has been considerable recent interest in quantifying left ventricular diastolic performance by analysis of the pattern of ventricular filling. Such information can be obtained from measurement of left ventricular volume or dimension throughout the cardiac cycle using contrast or radionuclide angiography, the conductance catheter, M-mode or 2D echocardiography, or by measurement of left ventricular inflow using Doppler determination of mitral valve flow velocities. The most widely used methods at present are radionuclide angiography[57-61] and Doppler mitral valve flow velocity determination.[62-69] These methods quantify various aspects of early rapid filling, diastasis, and atrial systole. Early rapid filling can be estimated by determining the peak filling rate. Other indices compare the degree of filling during the early rapid filling phase to that during atrial systole, and the rate and time for deceleration of early filling.

The pattern of left ventricular filling determined by Doppler echocardiography or radionuclide angiography, is used to noninvasively evaluate diastolic performance (see also Chapter 8). Interpretation of these observations requires an understanding of the mechanism of both the normal and abnormal patterns of left ventricular filling. The left ventricle fills in diastole in response to the pressure gradient between the left atrium and ventricle.[33,49,70-72] This occurs at two times during a single cardiac cycle: early in diastole following mitral valve opening and late in diastole during atrial systole. Normally, the majority of filling occurs early in diastole as left ventricular pressure falls below that in the left atrium. The magnitude of early filling is influenced by the rate of relaxation and elastic recoil of the left ventricle, the left atrial pressure, and the pressure-volume characteristics of the left ventricle and atrium.[33,49,71-73] Atrial contraction late in diastole again produces a gradient to propel blood from the atrium to the ventricle.

The normal pattern of left ventricular filling is altered in congestive heart failure (Fig. 3–5).[74-79] Early in the course of ventricular failure

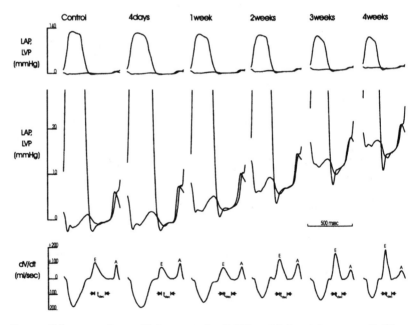

FIGURE 3-5. Recordings of left ventricular (*LVP*) and left atrial pressure (*LAP*) and the rate of change of left ventricular pressure volume (*dV/dt*) in conscious dogs serially during the development of pacing-induced heart failure. The early filling (E) and the atrial filling (A) are indicated. After 4 days the rate of left ventricular relaxation is reduced and the E to A ratio falls below 1. With increasing left atrial pressure the E to A ratio returns to its normal level by 2 weeks and becomes elevated by 4 weeks. The increased E to A ratio at 4 weeks is distinguished from the normal by the much shorter time for filling deceleration (t_{dec}). (*Reproduced with permission from Ohno M et al. Circulation 89:2241–2250, 1994*)

the amount and rate of early filling are reduced, and the relative importance of filling during atrial contraction is enhanced. The normal ratio of degree of early to late ventricular filling is reversed. This is due to a slowing of the rate of left ventricular relaxation.[75,77,79] Later in the course of congestive failure, the rate of early filling returns to its normal level. This "pseudonormalization" is due to the effect of increasing left atrial pressure.[75,79,80] The peak early filling rate may be higher than normal even later in the course of ventricular failure. The enhanced rate of early filling observed in advanced congestive failure is distinguished from normal by a faster rate of deceleration of the early flow and a shortened early filling deceleration time (t_{dec}). This more rapid deceleration of early filling in heart failure is due to an increase in the net stiffness of the left atrium and ventricle.[79,81–83] Our preliminary observations suggest that left ventricular chamber stiffness can be calculated from t_{dec}.

References

1. Kass A, Maughan WL, Guo AM, Kona A, Sunagawa K, Sagawa K: Comparative influence of load versus inotropic states on indexes of ventricular contractility: Experimental and theoretical analysis based on pressure-volume relationships. Circulation 76:1422–1436, 1987
2. Little WC: The left ventricular dP/dt$_{max}$-end-diastolic volume relation in closed chest dogs. Circ Res 56:808–815, 1985
3. Sagawa K: End-systolic pressure-volume relationship in retrospect and prospect. Fed Proc 43:2399–2400, 1984
4. Sagawa K: The left ventricular pressure-volume diagram revisited. Circ Res 43:677–678, 1978
5. Kass DA, Maughan WL: From "Emax" to pressure-volume relations: A broader view. Circulation 77:1203–1212, 1988
6. Sodums MT, Badke FR, Starling MR, Little WC, O'Rourke RA: Evaluation of ventricular contractile performance utilizing end-systolic pressure-volume relationships in conscious dogs. Circ Res 54:731–739, 1984
7. Weber KT, Janicki JS, Hunter WC, Shroff S, Pearlman ES, Fishman AP: The contractile behavior of the heart and its functional coupling to the circulation. Prog Cardiovasc Dis 24:375–400, 1982
8. Spratt JA, Tyson GS, Glower DD, Davis JW, Muhlbaier LH, Olsen CO, Rankin JS: The end-systolic pressure-volume relationship in conscious dogs. Circulation 75(6):1295–1309, 1987
9. Freeman GL, Little WC, O'Rourke RA: The effect of vasoactive agents on the left ventricular end-systolic pressure-volume relation in closed-chest dogs. Circulation 74:1107–1113, 1986
10. Maughan WL, Sunagawa K, Burkhoff D, Sagawa K: Effect of arterial impedance changes on the end-systolic pressure-volume relation. Circ Res 54:595, 1984
11. Baan J, Van der Velde ET: Sensitivity of left ventricular end-systolic pressure-volume relation to type of loading intervention in dogs. Circ Res 62:1247–1258, 1988
12. Glower DD, Spratt JA, Snow ND, Kabas JS, Davis JW, Olsen CO, Tyson GS, Sabiston DC, Rankin JS: Linearity of the Frank-Starling relationship in the

intact heart: The concept of preload recruitable stroke work. Circulation 71:994–1009, 1985

13. Fenely MP, Skelton TN, Kisslo KB, Rankin JS, Bashore TM: Comparison of preload recruitable stroke work and end-systolic pressure-volume relationships in man (abstr). Circulation 75:IV–163, 1987

14. Little WC, Cheng CP, Mumma M, Igarashi Y, Vinten-Johansen J, Johnston WE: Comparison of measures of left ventricular contractile performance from pressure-volume loops in conscious dogs. Circulation 80:1378–1387, 1989

15. Little WC, Rassi A, Freeman GL: Effect of dobutamine and ouabain on left ventricular contraction and relaxation in closed-chest dogs. J Clin Invest 80:613–620, 1987

16. Little WC, Freeman GL: Description of LV pressure-volume relations by time-varying elastance and source resistance. Am J Physiol 253:H83–H90, 1987

17. Lee J, Tajimi T, Widmann T, Ross J: Application of end-systolic pressure-volume and pressure-wall thickness relations in conscious dogs. J Am Coll Cardiol 9:136–146, 1987

18. Crottogini AJ, Willshaw P, Barra JG, Armentano R, Caberera, Fisher El, Pichel RH: Inconsistency of the slope and the volume intercept of the end-systolic pressure-volume relationship as individual indexes of inotropic state in conscious dogs: Presentation of an index combining both variables. Circulation 76(5):1115–1126, 1987

19. Burkhoff D, Sugawa S, Yue DT, Sagawa K: Contractility-dependent curvilinearity of end-systolic pressure-volume relations. Am J Physiol 252: H1218–1227, 1987

20. Kass DA, Beyar R, Lankford E, Heard M, Maughan WL, Sagawa K: Influence of contractile state on curvilinearity of in situ end-systolic pressure-volume relations. Circulation 79:167–178, 1989

21. Little WC, Cheng CP, Peterson T, Vinten-Johansen J: Response of the left ventricular end-systolic pressure-volume relation in conscious dogs to a wide range of contractile states. Circulation 78:736–745, 1988

22. Little WC, Cheng CP: Left ventricular-arterial coupling in conscious dogs. Am J Physiol 261:H70–H76, 1991

23. Sunagawa K, Maughan WL, Sagawa K: Optimal arterial resistance for the maximal stroke work studied in isolated canine left ventricle. Circ Res 56:586, 1985

24. Burkhoff D, Sagawa K: Ventricular efficiency predicted an analytical model. Am J Physiol 250:R1021–R1027, 1986

25. Freeman GL, Little WC, O'Rourke RA: Influence of heart rate on the left ventricular performance in conscious dogs. Circ Res 61:455–464, 1987

26. Little WC, O'Rourke RA: Effect of regional ischemia on the left ventricular end-systolic pressure-volume relationship in chronically instrumented dogs. J Am Coll Cardiol 5:297–302, 1985

27. Freeman G: Effects of increased afterload on left ventricular function in-closed-chest dogs. Am J Physiol 259:H619–H625, 1990

28. Little WC, Park RC, Freeman GL: Effect of alterations on the left ventricular activation sequence on left ventricular systolic performance. In Sideman S, Beyar R, (eds): Activation, Metabolism and Perfusion of the Heart: Simulation and Experimental Models. The Hague, Martinus Nijhoff, 1987

29. Dougherty AH, Nacarelli GV, Gray EL, Hicks CH, Goldstein RA: Congestive heart failure with normal systolic function. Am J Cardiol 54:778–782, 1984

30. Santamore WP, Little WC: Left ventricular diastolic performance. Cardiology 3:43–46, 1986
31. Soufer R, Wohlgelernter D, Vita NA, Amuchestegui M, Sostman D, Berger HJ, Zaret BL: Intact systolic left ventricular function in clinical congestive heart failure. Am J Cardiol 55:1032–1036, 1985
32. Topol EJ, Traill TA, Fortuin NJ: Hypertensive hypertrophic cardiomyopathy of the elderly. N Engl J Med 312:277–283, 1985
33. Little WC, Downes TR: Clinical evaluation of left ventricular diastolic performance. Prog Cardiovasc Dis 32:273–290, 1990
34. Little WC, Downes TR, Applegate RJ: Invasive evaluation of left ventricular diastolic performance. Herz 15:362–376, 1990
35. Little RC, Little WC: Physiology of the Heart and Circulation, 4th ed. pp. 1–377. Boston, Yearbook Publishers, 1988
36. Applegate RJ, Little WC: Left ventricular systolic and diastolic function in heart failure. Cardiology 4/2:63–77, 1991
37. Weiss JL, Frederiksen JW, Weisfeldt ML: Hemodynamic determinants of the time-course of fall in canine left ventricular pressure. J Clin Invest 58:751–760, 1976
38. Mirsky I: Assessment of diastolic function: Suggested methods and future considerations. Circulation 69:836–841, 1984
39. Suga H, Goto Y, Igarashi Y, Yamada O, Nozawa T, Yasumura Y: Ventricular suction under zero source pressure for filling. Am J Physiol 251:H47–H55, 1986
40. Suga H, Yasumura Y, Nozawa T, Futaki S, Tanaka N: Pressure-volume relation around zero transmural pressure in excised cross-circulated dog left ventricle. Circ Res 63:361–372, 1988
41. Yellin EL, Hori M, Yoran C. Sonnenblick EH, Gabbay S, Frater RWM: Left ventricular relaxation in the filling and nonfilling intact canine heart. Am J Physiol 250:H620–H629, 1986
42. Nikolic S, Yellin EL, Tamura K, Vetter H, Tamura T, Meisner JS, Frater RW: Passive properties of canine left ventricle: Diastolic stiffness and restoring forces. Circ Res 62:1210–1222, 1988
43. Frais MA, Bergman DW, Kingma I, Smiseth OA, Smith ER, Tyberg JV: The dependence of the time constant of left ventricular isovolumic relaxation (Tau) on pericardial pressure. Circulation 81:1071–1080, 1990
44. Gilbert JC, Glantz SA: Determinants of left ventricular filling and of the diastolic pressure-volume relations. Circ Res 64:827–852, 1989
45. Brutsaert DL, Housmans PR, Geothals MA: Dual control of relaxation. It's role in the ventricular function in the mammalian heart. Circ Res 47:637–652, 1980
46. Brutsaert DL, Rademakers FE, Sys SU: Triple control of relaxation: Implications in cardiac disease. Circulation 69:190–196, 1984
47. Brutsaert DL, Rademakers FE, Sys SU, Gillebert TC, Housmans PR: Analysis and relaxation in the evaluation of ventricular function of the heart. Prog Cardiovasc Dis 28:143–163, 1985
48. Glantz SA. Computing indices of diastolic stiffness has been counterproductive. Fed Proc 39:162–168, 1980
49. Cheng CP, Freeman GL, Santamore WP, Constantinescu MS, Little WC: Effect of loading conditions, contractile state, and heart rate on early diastolic left ventricular filling in conscious dogs. Circ Res 66:814–823, 1990
50. Ludbrook PA, Byrne JD, Kurnik PB, McKnight RC: Influence of reduction of preload and afterload by nitroglycerin on left ventricular diastolic pressure-volume relations and relaxation in man. Circulation 56:937–943, 1977

51. Ludbrook PA, Byrne JD, Reed RC, McKnight RC: Modification of left ventricular diastolic behavior by isometric handgrip exercise. Circulation 62:357–370, 1980

52. Little WC, Badke FR, O'Rourke RA: Effect of right ventricular pressure on the end-diastolic left ventricular pressure-volume relationship before and after chronic right ventricular overload. Circ Res 54:719–730, 1984

53. Grossman W, McLaurin LP: Diastolic properties of the left ventricle. Ann Intern Med 84:316–326, 1976

54. Glantz SA, Parmley WW: Factors which affect the diastolic pressure-volume curve. Circ Res 42:171, 1978

55. Kennish A, Yellin E, Frater RW: Dynamic stiffness profiles in the left ventricle. J Appl Physiol 39:665–671, 1975

56. Regen DM: Calculation of left ventricular wall stress. Circ Res 67:245–252, 1990

57. Bacharach SL, Green MV, Borer JS, Hyde JE, Farkas SP, Johnston GS: Left ventricular peak ejection rate, filling rate, and ejection fraction-frame rate requirements at rest and exercise: Concise communication. J Nucl Med Res 20:189–193, 1978

58. Bonow RO, Bacharach SL, Green MV, Kent KM, Rosing DR. Lipson LC, Leon MB, Epstein SE: Impaired left ventricular diastolic filling in patients with coronary artery disease: Assessment with radionuclide angiography. Circulation 64:315–323, 1981

59. Reduto LA, Wickemeyer WJ, Young JB, Del Ventura LA, Reid JW, Glaeser DH, Quinones MA, Miller RR: Left ventricular diastolic performance at rest and during exercise in patients with coronary artery disease: Assessment with first-pass radionuclide angiography. Circulation 63:1228–1237, 1981

60. Polak JF, Kemper AJ, Bianco JA, Parisi AF, Tow DE: Resting early peak diastolic filling rate: A sensitive index of myocardial dysfunction in patients with coronary artery disease. J Nucl Med 23:471–478, 1982

61. Magorien DJ, Shaffer P, Bush C,Magorien RD, Kolibash AJ, Vaverferth DV, Bushore TM: Hemodynamic correlation for timing intervals, ejection rate and filling rate derived from the radionuclide angiographic volume curve. Am J Cardiol 53:567–571, 1984

62. Traill TA, Gibson DG: Left ventricular relaxation and filling: Study by echocardiography. Br Heart J 40:596–601, 1978

63. Upton MT, Gibson DG: The study of left ventricular function from digitized echocardiograms. Prog Cardiovasc Dis 20:359–384, 1978

64. Lewis JF, Kuo LC, Nelson JG, Limacher MC, Quinones MA: Pulsed Doppler echocardiographic determination of stroke volume and cardiac output: Clinical validation of two new methods using the apical window. Circulation 70:425–431, 1984

65. Rokey R, Kuo LC, Zoghbi WA, Limacher MC, Quinones MA: Determination of parameters of left ventricular diastolic filling with pulsed Doppler echocardiography: Comparison with cineangiography. Circulation 71:543–550, 1985

66. Spirito P, Maron BJ, Bonow RO: Noninvasive assessment of left ventricular diastolic function: Comparative analysis of Doppler echocardiographic and radionuclide angiographic techniques. J Am Coll Cardiol 7:518–526, 1986

67. Friedman BJ, Drinkovic N, Miles H, Shih WJ: Assessment of left ventricular diastolic function: Comparison of Doppler echocardiography and gated blood pool scintigraphy. J Am Coll Cardiol 8:1348–1354, 1986

68. Spirito P, Maron BJ: Doppler echocardiography for assessing left ventricular diastolic function. Ann Intern Med 109:122–126, 1988
69. Plehn JHF: Noninvasive assessment of diastolic function. Cardiology 5:89, 1987
70. Courtois M, Kovacs SJ, Ludbrook PA: Transmitral pressure-flow velocity relation: Important of regional pressure gradients in the left ventricle during diastole. Circulation 78:661–671, 1988
71. Ishida Y, Meisner JS, Tjujioka K, Gallo JI, Yoran, C, Frater RWM, Yellin EL: Left ventricular filling dynamics: Influence of left ventricular relaxation and left atrial pressure. Circulation 74:187–196, 1986
72. Yellin EL, Nikolic S. Frater RWM: Left ventricular filling dynamics and diastolic function. Prog Cardiovasc Dis 32/4:247–271, 1990
73. Yamamoto K, Masuyama T, Tanouchi J, Uematsu M, Doi Y, Naito J, Hori M, Tada M, Kamada T: Importance of left ventricular minimal pressure as a determinant of transmitral flow velocity pattern in the presence of left ventricular systolic dysfunction. J Am Coll Cardiol 21:662–672, 1993
74. Appleton CP, Hatle LK, Popp RL: Relation of transmitral flow velocity patterns to left ventricular diastolic function: New insights from a combined hemodynamic and Doppler echocardiographic study. J Am Coll Cardiol 12:426–440, 1988
75. Appleton CP: Doppler assessment of left ventricular diastolic function: The refinements continue. J Am Coll Cardiol 21:1697–1700, 1993
76. Kono T, Sabbah HN, Rosman H, Alam M, Stein PD, Goldstein S: Left atrial contribution to ventricular filling during the course of evolving heart failure. Circulation 86:1317–1322, 1992
77. Nishimura RA, Abel MD, Hatle LK, Holmes DR Jr, Housmans PR, Ritman EL, Tajik AJ: Significance of Doppler indices of diastolic filling of the left ventricle: Comparison with invasive hemodynamics in a canine model. Am Heart J 118:1248–1258, 1989
78. Vanoverschelde JLJ, Raphael DA, Robert AR, Cosyns JR: Left ventricular filling in dilated cardiomyopathy: Relation to functional class and hemodynamics. J Am Coll Cardiol 15:1288–1295, 1990
79. Ohno M, Cheng CP, Little WC: Mechanism of altered patterns of left ventricular filling during the development of congestive heart failure. Circulation 89:2241–2250, 1994
80. Appleton CP, Hatle LK: The natural history of left ventricular filling abnormalities: Assessment by two-dimensional and Doppler echocardiography. Echocardiography 9/4:437–457, 1992
81. Thomas JD, Weyman AE: Echocardiographic Doppler evaluation of left ventricular diastolic function: Physics and physiology. Circulation 84:977–990, 1991
82. Thomas JD, Newell JB, Choong CYP, Weyman AE: Physical and physiological determinants of transmitral velocity: Numerical analysis. Am J Physiol 260(Hrt Circ Phys23):H1718–H1730, 1991
83. Flachskampf FA, Weyman AE, Guerrero JL, Thomas JD: Calculation of atrioventricular compliance from the mitral flow profile: Analytic and in vitro study. J Am Coll Cardiol 19:998–1004, 1992

David A. Kass

4 | Clinical Ventricular Pathophysiology: A Pressure-Volume View

The latter half of the twentieth century has witnessed extraordinary changes in how heart disease is diagnosed, characterized, and treated. Recent advances in biochemistry and molecular biology are providing novel views of cardiac pathophysiology with truly revolutionary potential. Advances in imaging methodologies, including echodoppler cardiography, nuclear magnetic resonance, radionuclide scintigraphy, etc. continue to expand our ability to define what goes wrong with the human heart and focus on new approaches toward correcting it.

Even the way in which the heart is characterized as a pump has evolved. A major goal has been development of methods to describe cardiac function that separately identify the importance of its principal determinants: preload, afterload, contractility, relaxation, diastolic stiffness, and heart rate. As pioneered by the work of Suga, Sagawa, and colleagues in the early 1970s,[1,2] pressure-volume relations have come the closest to achieving this goal. The initial focus of these relations was on the end-systolic pressure-volume relation as a *"load-independent"* index of cardiac contractility,[3] but the value of the pressure-volume approach is far more powerful and broad.[4] One advantage of the representation, well known to Carnot and other 19th century engineers,[5] is that in one diagram, both active and passive filling properties of the pump, its efficiency, and coupling with external loads, are *all* quantifiable. As to whether the end-systolic elastance is indeed a load-

Ventricular Function, edited by David C. Warltier. Williams & Wilkins, Baltimore © 1995.

independent index of contractility, research has shown that it falls short of these claims.[6-9] This can complicate simple interpretations of data under some circumstances, but it has not reduced the utility of the pressure-volume approach for characterizing cardiac function.

One limitation to the clinical application of pressure-volume relations has been the difficulty of measuring continuous chamber volumes. Many investigations have used image-contouring methods, varying cardiac load by use of vasodilators or constrictors.[10,11] These approaches are unfortunately cumbersome because of the requirement for extensive off-line image analysis. Furthermore, one does not actually visualize the pressure-volume data during the study, which is a great impediment to assessing changes in left ventricular function during various interventions. Finally, analysis is typically limited to a few cardiac cycles or interventions. This prevents examination of continuous changes during ischemia or following acute drug administration, or beat-to-beat variations induced by varying cycle length.

New catheter-based instrumentation has been developed over the past decade that for the first time has enabled the essential measurements of instantaneous pressure, volume, and variable cardiac loading to be made in intact patients.[12-14] The invasive measurements employ an intracardiac conductance (or impedance) catheter that provides a continuous signal proportional to chamber blood volume. In the mid-1980s, we first demonstrated how the conductance catheter method could be combined with transient obstruction of inferior vena cava blood inflow to determine pressure-volume relations. Since then, we and others have employed this approach to examine mechanisms of human disease and the efficacy of drug and nonpharmacological therapies.[15-18] In this chapter, several of these studies are reviewed with specific examples selected to highlight major issues regarding the interpretation of pressure-volume relations in human cardiac disease.

PRESSURE-VOLUME DIAGRAM: METHODS AND PRINCIPLES OF ANALYSIS

Figure 4–1*A* displays time plots of pressure-volume data in a human subject. The four tracings shown (from the top down) are right atrial pressure, left ventricular volume, left ventricular pressure, and electrocardiogram. Continuous volumes (*second tracing from top*) were measured by a conductance catheter and demonstrate both early rapid and late atrial systolic filling phases. To generate pressure-volume relations, the loading conditions of the heart must be varied. As noted above, this is achieved by temporarily obstructing inflow to the heart with a balloon-typed catheter placed in the inferior vena cava. The on-

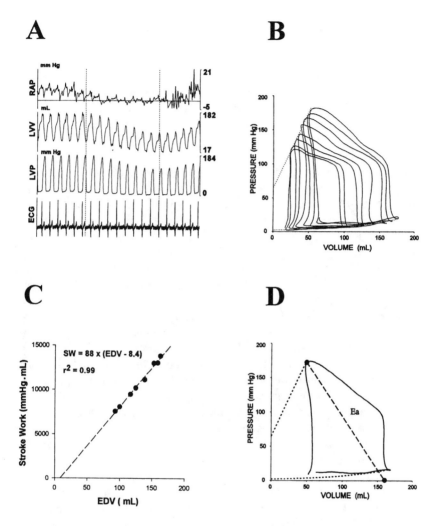

FIGURE 4-1. (A) Time plot of simultaneous right atrial pressures (*RAP*), left ventricular volume (*LVV*), left ventricular pressure (*LVP*) and electrocardiogram (*ECG*) before and during transient preload reduction by acute obstruction of inferior vena caval inflow. There is an early rapid decline in RAP, followed within 1 to 2 beats by a gradual decline in left heart filling and pressures (*dotted vertical line*). These data are used to derive pressure volume relations. (B) Pressure-volume (PV) loops plot from the same data shown in panel A. The set of successive cardiac cycles is taken from between the two cursors in the previous panel. End-systolic and diastolic PV relations (*dashed lines*) form the boundaries of cardiac performance. (C) Plot of stroke work versus end-diastolic volume determined from each of the multiple cardiac cycles displayed in panel B. Although this function relation indexes integrated cardiac performance, it is primarily influenced by systolic properties. (D) Afterload calculation from PV loop. The effective arterial elastance (E_a) is the ratio of end-systolic pressure/stroke volume, and is depicted by the line connecting the end-systolic PV point to zero pressure and ED (bold dashed line).

set of inferior vena caval inflation is clearly identified by the sudden decline in right atrial pressure (top tracing), about 1 to 2 beats prior to the vertical dotted line. Right atrial pressure declines to near zero over the ensuing three cardiac cycles. Importantly, there is minimal change in left ventricular filling or systolic pressure for these same beats. Thereafter, both left ventricular volume and pressure gradually decline, generating a set of pressure-volume loops. Consecutive cycles are selected from this sequence from the onset of loading change to peak effect (usually occurring over a period of 10 seconds or less), and this is delineated between the vertical dotted lines in Figure 4–1A. Because of the decline in preload is quick, it often occurs with minimal change in heart rate, as indicated by the electrocardiogram tracing (*bottom panel*). This is an important advantage of this type of mechanical unloading maneuver. It is not necessarily the case when pharmacological loading interventions are used to determine pressure-volume relations, as recently reported by Crottogini et al.[19]

Figure 4–1B displays the pressure-volume loops and relations that are determined by this maneuver. There are two boundaries that are delineated by the set of beats, the diastolic and end-systolic pressure-volume relationships. To a great extent, cardiac pump function and dysfunction are characterized by changes in these two critical boundaries of pressure-volume data. Changes in the slope and/or position of each boundary define alterations in systolic pump function, diastolic chamber stiffness, geometric remodeling. etc.

The systolic boundary to the upper left is the end-systolic pressure-volume relation and defines the systolic pump performance capacity of the heart. Points of maximal pressure/volume are first determined for each cardiac cycle. These are then fit to linear (or nonlinear if required) analyses to estimate a volume axis intercept (V_0). This is then used to determine points of maximal $[P/(V - V_0)]$ ratio for each beat, and the process of fitting is repeated. This is iterated until there is minimal change in V_0 estimates. An additional feature of the analysis routinely employed is the use of perpendicular rather than the more conventional linear regression analysis. Perpendicular regression minimizes the perpendicular distance of each point to the regression line. Unlike standard least-squares linear regression, this method does not make assumptions that the x-axis coordinate is the highly controlled "independent" variable and the y-axis coordinate is the dependent variable. Instead, both variables receive equal weighing about the regression line. The advantage of perpendicular regression is that it always yields a relation that passes through the actual outer envelope of the pressure-volume data, with less influence of one or two outliers.

The slope of the end-systolic pressure-volume relation (ESPVR) termed the end-systolic elastance (E_{es}), can provide an index of contractile function under many but certainly not all circumstances. For example, if a drug is administered acutely, shifts in this relation provide reasonable assessments of contractile change. As described in more detail below, position shifts in the ESPVR also occur, and these convey information regarding changes in the systolic pump function of the heart as well. More importantly, for the intact chamber, the slope of the ESPVR is reflective of myocyte contractile properties as well as structural and geometric wall properties of the heart. Thus, in chronic disease conditions, E_{es} can be markedly influenced without necessarily indicating contractile change.

In addition to the end-systolic pressure-volume relation, the same set of pressure-volume diagrams measured at varying preloads can be used to derive other valuable pump function relations. One such relation is a linear correspondence between the stroke work for each beat and the end-diastolic volume for the same cycle.[20] (Fig 4–1C) This latter relation, often termed preload recruitable stroke work (PRSW) is a modification of the classic Sarnoff curve, which itself is a modification of the original Frank-Starling relationship. This is a pump function relation. Since stroke work combines information regarding systolic and diastolic function, it can in fact be altered purely by abnormalities in diastole.[17] However, this is not typically the case, and generally this relationship reflects changes in systolic pump performance. In clinical studies, the stroke work-end diastolic volume relation or PRSW has some advantages. The slope of this relation has units of mm Hg, because the ratio of work to volume is a pressure. Thus, the absolute value of PRSW is less dependent upon chamber size than is for example E_{es}, which has units of mm Hg/milliliter. The slope of the PRSW has proven to be remarkably consistent in normal hearts, both from humans and small and large animals. It normally ranges about 75 to 90 mm Hg ($\sim 10^5$ n/m^2).

The PRSW is also more statistically robust than the ESPVR, and this can be useful for the purpose of quantifying "contractile change." This is because the ESPVR is obtained from a collection of single points extracted from the pressure volume loops. Stroke work, on the other hand, is the integral of the area within the loop and is therefore less subject to signal noise than is a single pressure-volume point. Secondly, the range of change in stroke work is greater during inferior vena caval inflow obstruction inasmuch as both stroke volume and pressure are declining simultaneously. Therefore, regression relations derived from stroke work and end-diastolic volume span a broader range and provide improved statistical certainty regarding the zero-pressure axis intercept. The important concept is not that one version of pump function index is "better" than another, but that from the set of data displayed in Figure 4–1B one can derive many of these indices, all of which have strengths and weaknesses but, when combined, provide a more complete view of the systolic contractile performance of the cardiac chamber.

Ventricular preload and afterload can also be obtained from the pressure-volume diagram. Cardiac preload is defined by end-diastolic volume. The utility of volume as opposed to pressure is clear from the example in Figure 4–1B. Diastolic pressure-volume relations in humans are often very flat. As a consequence, a considerable degree of ventricular filling can occur with only minimal alteration in chamber diastolic pressure. These variations in pressure may fall into a noise range despite substantial and often physiologically significant changes in ventricular preload volume. Also, ventricular diastolic pressures do not uniquely vary with filling volume but are also influenced by external forces such as those applied by ventricular interaction and pericardial constraint. Alterations in these forces directly influence diastolic pressure without changing preload volume and similarly without changing cardiac output.

Cardiac afterload is also measurable from the pressure-volume diagram. One fairly widespread notion is that ventricular afterload is represented by arterial systolic pressure. This stems from isolated muscle experiments in which contracting muscle initiates shortening only after developed force equals that of a fixed suspended weight. In the intact circulation, however, the arterial pressure is not a fixed weight but varies considerably throughout cardiac ejection. Furthermore, the volume of ejected blood itself alters this pressure. This is clearly demonstrated by the set of pressure-volume loops shown in Figure 4–1B which were constructed by simply reducing ventricular preload volume. Defining "afterload" by the arterial pressure automatically establishes an ambiguity in that "afterload" must change with altered preload.

If, however, afterload is defined as the impedance properties of the arterial tree (see Chapter 5), then this characterization is far more independent of preload. Furthermore, this assessment of vascular load can also be determined from the pressure-volume loop. Sunagawa et al.[22] first proposed that the ratio of end-systolic pressure to stroke volume (effective arterial elastance or E_a) provides a measure of arterial impedance. Kelly et al.[23] later validated this measurement in patients. These investigators used simultaneous central aortic pressure and flow data to obtain vascular impedance spectra, and from these spectra, an elastance index of total vascular load was derived. This parameter was then compared to the ratio of end-systolic pressure and stroke volume ($P_{es}/SV = E_a$) obtained from simultaneously measured pressure-volume loop data. The results demonstrated near complete agreement, showing that this simple E_a parameter indeed embodied the major vascular loading features.

E_a is graphically depicted in Figure 4–1D. The long dashed diagonal line connects the end-systolic pressure-volume point with a point at an end-diastolic volume of zero (EDV, 0). The absolute value of the slope of this line is $(P_{es} - 0)/(EDV\text{-}ESV)$, or P_{es}/SV, which is E_a. Vasodilators or constrictors alter the slope of this line, and the magnitude of vascular afterload change can be easily measured from pressure-volume relations. The capacity of simultaneously displaying loading, diastolic, and systolic elements of cardiac contraction and performance is one of the unique and powerful features of the pressure-volume diagram.

The method of measuring pressure-volume data continuously during rapid preload reduction, as shown in Figure 4–1A and B, has also proven very valuable for the study of human diastolic chamber function. Figure 4–2 shows diastolic pressure-volume data from single beats at resting steady-state cardiac cycles (SS) and the diastolic pressure-volume relation (DPVR) determined after inferior vena caval inflow obstruction. For the DPVR, only late diastolic points (preatrial systole) are used from multiple beats to measure passive chamber properties. There is a clear difference between data obtained from steady-state pressure-volume loops and those obtained during preload reduction. This has provided several important insights into human pathophysiology. Diastolic pressure-volume data for the steady-state cycle are elevated relative to the DPVR. This is primarily due to the influence of external pressures from the pericardium and right heart on the resting diastolic pressures of the left ventricle. As previously described (Fig. 4–1A), right heart filling pressures decline rapidly after inferior vena caval inflow obstruction, generally preceding the decline in *left* heart preload. This leads to a downshift of the diastolic pressure-volume curve. The difference between the resting diastolic pressure-

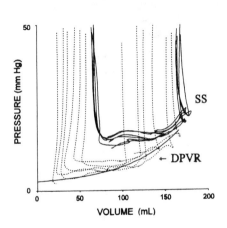

FIGURE 4-2. Disparity between resting steady state (SS) cardiac diastolic pressure-volume data and the diastolic PV relation (*DPVR*) derived only from late diastolic points taken from multiple beats at varying preloads. The latter is measured once inferior vena caval occlusion has been initiated and is displaced downward from the steady-state data. This reflects removal of most external constraints (i.e., pericardium, right heart filling) that influence the diastolic PV data at rest.

volume data and the DPVR reflects influences of early filling, ongoing relaxation, and external constraining forces. By minimizing these factors, the DPVR represents the closest measure of passive chamber properties yet obtainable in the intact human.

METHODOLOGICAL ISSUES OF VENTRICULAR VOLUME MEASUREMENT BY INTRACARDIAC CONDUCTANCE

The conductance catheter technique used to measure left ventricular volume is an evolution of an older concept for measuring cardiac stroke volume by thoracic impedance. In the case of the catheter technique, the alternating current field is applied locally to electrodes positioned at the apex of the heart and above the aortic valve. The local field application has major advantages, since the signal to noise ratio is vastly improved, and the signal itself derived primarily from changes in blood volume. In contrast, total thoracic impedance measurements derive their signal primarily from changes in blood flow.

The conductance catheter has intervening electrodes between point source electrodes, and these measure voltages which are inversely *proportional* to segmental blood volume signals. The segmental volumes (for each electrode pair) are combined in real time to generate a time-varying signal for total volume. The word proportional is emphasized, because the relation between the conductance catheter signal and real chamber blood volume is influenced by several factors. Conductivity into the left ventricular muscle wall and surrounding structures adds a signal offset to what is measured. Deviation of the real current field from an assumed idealized homogeneous field contributes to a nonunity proportionality constant. Furthermore, over a very broad range of volumes, these two "constants" are actually variables, so that the correspondence between real volume and catheter signal can be complex.

Fortunately, the correspondence between catheter signal and chamber blood volume is fairly linear over the range of volumes typically measured in a given experiment or in a given patient. This indicates that the calibration factors are for, practical purposes, reasonably constant. Calibration of the signal can be performed in several ways. One method is to simply match end-systolic and end-diastolic volumes to those measured by some external standard. This can stem from ventriculographic or other image data or might be derived by combining ejection fraction and mean cardiac flow estimates. An alternative method involves direct estimation of the signal offset by injection of hypertonic saline into the pulmonary artery.[12,13] This mixes with blood, increasing its conductivity but not total volume. As a consequence, the volume signal from the catheter will increase (proportional with net blood conductivity), yet actual volumes are unchanged. The component due to muscle wall and other external structure conductances can be calculated by a regression algorithm.

Once the catheter is calibrated, the signal generally remains stable unless blood conductivity changes (e.g., during hemodilution associated with cardiopulmonary bypass) or the catheter is moved within the left ventricular chamber. In either instance, recalibration is essential in order to generate meaningful comparisons to other data. In summary, this catheter approach is very useful for applying pressure-volume analysis to patients. However, like any methodology, the value of the data obtained depends upon careful and consistent procedures employed in using this method and an understanding and regard for potential sources of artifact and error.

PRESSURE-VOLUME RELATIONS AND CARDIAC DISEASE

In the classification of cardiac dysfunction, abnormalities are typically divided into dilated cardiomyopathy, restrictive cardiomyopathy, and hypertrophic cardiomyopathy. Figure 4–3 displays an example from each type of disease, as viewed by pressure-volume relations. Data from a normal patient are shown at the upper left, and this subject's (ESPVR) data are reproduced in each disease panel for comparison.

Dilated cardiomyopathy is associated with a decline in the slope of the ESPVR, and a marked rightward shift of the systolic and diastolic pressure-volume relations and of the loops themselves. In this patient with chronic compensated failure, stroke volume was similar to that of the normal comparison subject. In decompensated heart failure, stroke volume is limited, and the ESPVR volume axis intercept shifts rightward (e.g., Fig. 4–6A).

Restrictive cardiomyopathy is associated with a rightward shift of the ESPVR, often with a normal or steep slope and a steep DPVR. Thus, both systolic and diastolic chamber stiffness is increased. The data shown in Figure 4–3C were obtained from a patient with cardiac amyloidosis and demonstrate how restrictive disease narrows the pressure-volume space between diastolic and systolic boundaries. The ESPVR slope does not necessarily deviate from normal but may reflect stiffening influences of the amyloid protein deposited within the myocardial interstitium. This points to an important aspect of ESPVR interpretation in human disease. Unlike the simple interpretation based on experiments conducted in normal, isolated canine ventricles that equates a low slope with cardiodepression and a high slope with increased contractility, chronic dis-

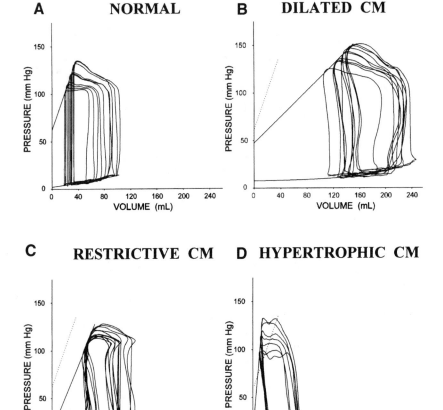

FIGURE 4-3. Examples of PV relations in four patients representing class cardiac disease conditions. (A) Normal ventricle. (B) Dilated cardiomyopathy (CM). (C) Restrictive heart disease. (D) Hypertrophic cardiomyopathy. See text for details.

eases influence the ESPVR in a more complex manner. Myocyte function is important, but the geometry of the ventricular chamber, the presence or absence of fibrosis or increased collagen content, edema, or interstitial protein deposition, and other factors can all contribute to the ESPVR. Interpretations of changes in the ESPVR measured over long time courses following therapies that chronically alter cardiac constitutive and geometric properties must therefore be made cautiously.

The second feature of the restrictive pressure-volume relation example shown in Figure 4–3 is the rightward shift of the ESPVR. This may result from an inability of the myocytes to contract to shorter sarcomere lengths when they are imbedded within the amyloid matrix. Alternatively, amyloid which pathologically aggregates around the muscle fibers, may act as a diffuse scar within the myocardium, limiting the extent of chamber shortening. This rightward shift (compared to the position of a normal control) bears many similarities to that which is observed with chronic infarction or acute ischemia. (c.f. Fig. 4.5. below)

Unlike the prior two examples, hypertrophic cardiomyopathy is most often associated with a leftward shift and steep slope of the ESPVR and reduced chamber volumes. The steepness of the ESPVR may not be due to improved myocardial contractility but, instead, to small-chamber volumes, muscle hypertrophy, interstitial fibrosis, or a combination of these changes. Abnormalities of the DPVR are often less dramatic than might be anticipated, even in the presence of profound left ventricular hypertrophy. This is demonstrated in this patient example, (Fig. 4–3D), for which the DPVR appears quite flat despite marked hypertrophy and substantially higher end-systolic stiffness as compared to control.

While it can be difficult to translate the resting ESPVR slope (E_{max} or E_{es}) into a measure of "contractility," this slope does provide useful and relevant information about the way in which the cardiovascular system is likely to respond to changes in blood volume or arterial tone. For example, in restrictive and hypertrophic heart disease, changes in circulating blood volume often result in rapid and dramatic changes in arterial pressures. This can be directly related to the steepness of the ESPVR, which defines the sensitivity of systolic pressure generation to changes in end-diastolic volume. As shown in the example of a patient with left ventricular hypertrophy (Fig. 4–3D), fairly small changes in preload filling volume result in nearly twice the decline in systolic pressure as observed in a normal subject. A patient with a very steep ESPVR will also have limited contractile reserve capacity. Increasing ESPVR slope 10-fold may not actually amount to much leftward shift of the relation and, thus, not increase stroke volume or work capacity. In contrast, a 10-fold rise in slope in the patient with dilated cardiomyopathy (Fig. 4–3B) would markedly increase pump function and result in enhanced cardiac output. Similarly, if vascular tone is altered, ventricles with steeper ESPVRs will experience greater changes in systolic pressure and relatively less change in cardiac output than those with shallower ESPVRs.

ACUTE INOTROPIC INTERVENTION AND ESPVR

Chronic cardiac diseases and associated changes in the composition and geometry of the heart can complicate interpretations of pressure-volume relation contractile indices, but acute changes in these indices due to an intervention are more easily interpreted. An example is the assessment of inotropic change due to intravenous verapamil in patients with left ventricular hypertrophy. As shown in Figure 4–4*A*, verapamil (10 mg IV bolus) does not alter ejection fraction or cardiac output, and reduces systolic pressure only slightly. However, E_{es} declines by nearly 30%. The example in Figure 4–4*B* depicts pressure-volume diagrams before and after verapamil and demonstrates this marked change in contractility. The lack of change in conventional ejection indices results from simultaneous peripheral vasodilation, offsetting the negative inotropic effect of verapamil. Similar analysis of acute inotropic changes have proven valuable for studies of inotropic agents, such as amrinone,[24] and novel clinical heart failure drugs with simultaneous effects on venous, arterial, and cardiac chamber properties[25] (see Chapter 6).

The acute decrease in ESPVR slope with minimal alteration in the

A

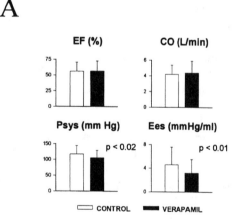

FIGURE 4-4. Influence of verapamil on hemodynamics and pressure-volume relations in hypertrophied human hearts. (A) Resting ejection fraction (*EF*) and cardiac output (*CO*) not altered due to vasodilating properties of verapamil (end-systolic pressure [*Psys*] declined slightly). However, the end-systolic elastance (*Ees*) was reduced by nearly 30%. (B) Pressure-volume loops from one patient displays a marked reduction in the ES-PVR slope (*dotted line*) compared to control (*solid line*). LV, left ventricular.

B

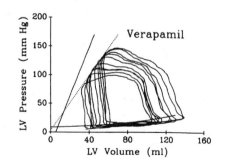

volume axis intercept (V_0) (Fig. 4–4B) is a classic example of negative inotropic change as first observed in the isolated canine heart studies of Suga and colleagues.[2] However, this is not the only manifestation of reduced chamber systolic function. Figure 4–5 displays data from a study performed in humans undergoing acute coronary occlusion by balloon inflation during angioplasty.[16] Regional ischemia produces heterogeneous cardiac dysfunction, with a portion of the wall generating normal contraction and another portion essentially bulging passively, as if arrested in diastole. The result, as predicted by Sunagawa et al.[26] is a rightward shift of the ESPVR. These investigators first demonstrated both theoretically and experimentally that the extent of shift correlated with the magnitude of ischemic myocardium. The greater the ischemic zone size, the greater the regional bulging, and the more the end-systolic volume increases. Regional ischemia can also influence the slope (E_{es}) of the net chamber ESPVR. The elastance of the eschemic region is assumed to remain similar to diastolic muscle throughout cardiac ejection. Adding this elastance to the stiffer elastance of the residual nonischemic myocardium results in a change in the net stiffness, and the magnitude of this change is very dependent upon the initial elastance of the intact chamber. For example, in a heart which has a high baseline E_{es}, adding even a fairly small region with much reduced stiffness (low regional E_{es}) will have a profound effect on the net elastance of the combined chamber. Alternatively, if the initial chamber end-systolic stiffness is low, then regional ischemia will not alter this stiffness. This result has been confirmed in animal studies[27] and in a human study of patients undergoing coronary angioplasty.[16]

The interpretation of the E_{es} in regional ischemia is not straightforward because it does not simply reflect "contractile" properties of remote normal myocardium. Rather, it is the sum of remote viable and regionally ischemic systolic stiffness coupled together. The ESPVR still

FIGURE 4-5. Influence of acute coronary occlusion and regional ischemia on pressure-volume relations in humans. Patient example shows a rightward parallel shift of the ES-PVR (*solid* to *dashed line*). In contrast, there was minimal change in the diastolic PV relation. See text for details.

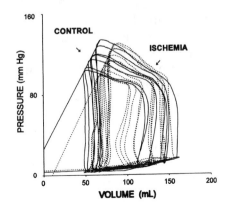

provides a measure of the net systolic performance of the whole ventricle and conveys useful information regarding loading sensitivities of systolic pressure or stroke volume.

The example in Figure 4–5 raises another important interpretive point concerning the ESPVR. Both reductions in slope or rightward parallel shifts of the relation represent a decline in systolic chamber performance, and only by measuring the actual data can statements about these changes be made. Studies that focus solely upon a slope estimate (maximal pressure/end-systolic volume ratio) can overlook the true underlying pathophysiology and fail to properly characterize the real change in left ventricular systolic function.

ESPVR AND CHRONIC INTERVENTIONS

In chronic disease states, changes in pressure-volume loop position and corresponding shifts in systolic and diastolic relations are often the most dramatic alterations. Figure 4–6A displays data from a patient with chronic idiopathic dilated cardiomyopathy. The most striking feature is a rightward shift of the pressure-volume diagram, similar to that observed during acute coronary artery occlusion (see Fig. 4–5). Ventricular volumes are markedly increased as a result of chronic chamber remodeling in dilated cardiomyopathy. Interestingly, the slope of the ESPVR is normal, although this does not necessarily mean that the heart has "normal" systolic function. In fact, this is highly unlikely. Chronic dilated cardiomyopathy associated with ventricular fibrosis and increases in wall mass, and these nonmyocyte changes will also influence the ESPVR.

Chronic chamber remodeling can also be the major consequence of heart failure therapy. Figure 4–6B and C show data from the another patient with dilated cardiomyopathy before (B) and 1 year after (C) undergoing cardiomyoplasty.[28,29,30] Cardiomyoplasty is a novel surgical procedure in which the latissimus dorsi muscle is wrapped around the heart and chronically stimulated to contract synchronously with left ventricular systole. The most striking effect of this procedure was a shift in the position of the pressure-volume loops and ESPVR. Both shifted *leftward* toward normal. In contrast, there was only a minimal change in ESPVR slope. Interpreting the lack of change in slope in this case is just as difficult as it was in the patient with chronic congestive heart failure shown in panel A. The myoplasty procedure altered the fundamental geometry of the heart, shifting the ESPVR leftward, just as chronic dilation from cardiomyopathy had initially resulted in a rightward shift. This leftward translation of the ESPVR clearly represents an improvement in systolic pump function, regardless of any

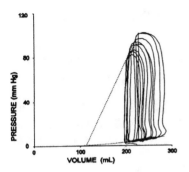

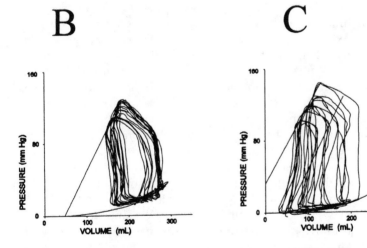

FIGURE 4-6. Influence of chronic disease and therapy on PV relations. (A) Patient with chronic dilated cardiomyopathy displaying marked chamber remodeling. The result is a large rightward shift of the systolic and diastolic PV relations to a very positive volume axis intercept (compare to normal subject in Fig. 4–3). (B) Another similar patient shown at baseline. Again there is a right shift of the PV data, with very high baseline diastolic pressures. (C) The same patient 1 year after undergoing cardiomyoplasty. The procedure has resulted in a left shift of the data—moving the ESPVR back to a more normal position. This is an example of chronic therapy inducing reversal of chamber remodeling.[30]

change in slope. However, it is impossible to discern how much of this change reflects alterations in the contractile properties of the myocytes vs geometric remodeling.

DISEASES OF DIASTOLIC FUNCTION

Assessment of ventricular function from pressure-volume relationships is not only restricted to evaluations of systolic performance. Well before investigators explored the ESPVR and other derived indices of systolic function, the diastolic pressure-volume relation was widely used to assess chamber compliance. Evolution of methods combining continuous volume measurements with rapid preload reduction has yielded DPVRs relatively free from influences of external pressures or constraints and has led to new pathophysiological insights.

One example of how this approach has produced new information about cardiac disease was reported in a recent study of patients with rheumatic mitral stenosis.[17] This disorder is primarily one in which left ventricular filling is limited by a narrowed valve orifice. However, there is also extensive endocardial scarring and thickening of the chordae tendineae, and this has been suggested to alter both systolic and diastolic properties of the chamber. These changes are difficult to study, because most measurements of left ventricular function are themselves influenced by abnormal filling due to valvular stenosis. Liu et al.[17] studied 10 such patients and compared them to normal controls. These investigators found that chamber compliance was reduced in patients with mitral stenosis by more than 50% of that in normal patients, while the ESPVR remained essentially unchanged. This decrease in compliance indicated that independent of the actual amount of chamber filling, the left ventricle in mitral stenosis was intrinsically stiffer. When many of these same patients with mitral stenosis underwent balloon mitral valvuloplasty, chamber compliance increased within 1 hour after the procedure to near normal values, and this change persisted at 3 month follow-up. This result suggested that the influence of mitral stenosis on diastolic passive stiffness could be acutely reversed by a procedure that simply altered the mobility of the mitral valve apparatus. This raised the hypothesis that mitral stenosis causes an internal mechanical tethering of the valve to the left ventricular myocardium, much like a "pericardial constraint" on the inside of the heart. Balloon valvuloplasty by freeing the valve leaflets was able to acutely release this tethering and increase chamber compliance. This is the first evidence for such an effect and suggests an alternative mechanism by which valvuloplasty or for that matter commissurotomy or valve surgery, can improve left ventricular diastolic function.

Another example of how pressure-volume analysis has resulted in a new perspective of the pathophysiology of cardiac disease comes from a study of the acute influence of coronary occlusion on diastolic chamber stiffness.[16] Ischemia has long been thought to stiffen myocardium secondary to mechanical influences of discoordinate wall motion, abnormal calcium handling, edema, and other factors. Studies performed in patients undergoing coronary angioplasty have revealed that the diastolic pressure-volume data shifts upward during coronary occlusion, consistent with such reduced distensibility.[31] To more carefully examine this behavior, we studied 10 patients by continuous pressure-volume analysis before, during, and after angioplasty for single vessel coronary artery disease.[16] The most striking results pertained to the diastolic pressure-volume data. As with prior studies, resting cardiac cycles measured before and during coronary artery occlusion shifted upward (solid to dashed lines in Fig. 4–7A). However, when DPVRs were measured, using only late diastolic pressure-volume data from multiple cardiac cycles measured during transient inferior vena caval obstruction, a very different result was found. Rather than shifting upward, these DPVRs were virtually superimposable (diamond symbols, Fig. 4–7A). This strongly suggested that the apparent lowered distensibility observed in resting cardiac cycles was due to forces extrinsic to the left ventricle, i.e., those that could be simply removed by obstructing right heart inflow. Similar results were subsequently demonstrated in an animal study, in which the upward shift during coronary artery occlusion could be eliminated if the pericardium was first removed.[32] This similarity of DPVR data during acute severe ischemia is also displayed in Figure 4–5. Despite the rightward shift of the ESPVR and reduction in cardiac output, the diastolic pressure-volume relations are virtually superimposable.

Analogous disparities between the effects of acute interventions on resting diastolic pressure-volume data (derived from steady-state beats) vs DPVRs (derived from postinferior vena caval occlusion loop data) have been presented in a study of the effects of calcium channel blocking agents in hypertrophied human hearts.[15] Verapamil has been reported to shift the steady-state diastolic pressure-volume diagram downward, and this has been interpreted to reflect an *improvement* in chamber distensibility induced by calcium channel blockade. Figure 4–7B shows an example of this response, with the steady-state loop shifting downward after verapamil with even an increase in diastolic volume despite the lowered diastolic pressures. It has been assumed that improved relaxation and calcium handling produced by verapamil result in an enchantment of chamber distensibility. However, as also shown in Figure 4–7B, DPVR data derived from the same two conditions (same hearts) are virtually superimposable. This again indicates

A

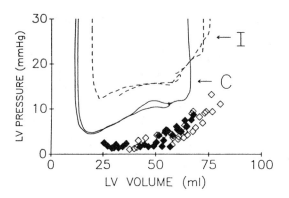

B

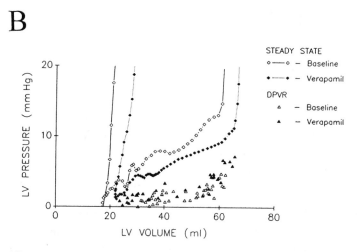

FIGURE 4-7. Interventions that may alter the resting diastolic pressure-volume data do not necessarily change passive left ventricular (*LV*) chamber properties. (*A*) Data are from a patient undergoing coronary balloon angioplasty. During coronary occlusion, the loops shifted upward (*C*, control *I*; ischemia), suggesting a decline in chamber diastolic distensibility. However, when DPVR data are obtained by the inferior vena caval inflow occlusion method, the diastolic curves (◆- control, ◇ - ischemia) were superimposable. This indicates that real passive chamber properties were not altered. (*B*) Similar concept, but in this instance the data were in a patient with LV hypertrophy receiving IV verapamil. The resting (steady state) data displayed a downward shift, suggesting improved distensibility from the drug. However, the DPVR data (*triangle symbols*) were again virtually superimposable.

that the downward shift of the pressure-volume loop at steady-state does not reflect a change in intrinsic myocardial stiffness but rather the removal of external constraints (venous and pericardial unloading).[15]

The relative constancy of the diastolic pressure-volume relation in humans following a host of acute interventions has led to the strong suspicion that this relation is rarely changed acutely. This is likely because the DPVR primarily reflects structural properties of the heart, rather than being influenced by actively controlled cellular processes. Certainly, in settings in which profound global ischemia, reperfusion, cardiac edema, or other major insults occur, the DPVR can be altered. However, in many settings in which drugs are being provided to improve "diastolic function," the DPVR is minimally changed.

SUMMARY

Pressure-volume analysis provides an ideal window through which to view cardiac function. If continuous pressure-volume loops could be monitored in the patient undergoing surgery or in the intensive care unit, there is little doubt that the interpretation of changes in cardiovascular function would be greatly facilitated. Indeed, this has been our experience in nearly 30 years of animal research in isolated and intact hearts and now in the catheterization laboratory in humans. As molecular biology advances our understanding of human cardiac disease at a very basic level, there still remains much to be discovered by pressure-volume analysis of ventricular systolic and diastolic function effects of novel therapies. New advances in imaging technology are making this approach ever more practical,[33] and these will hopefully pave the way for future insights.

Acknowledgment

I gratefully thank the late Dr. Sagawa and Drs. Maughan, Suga, and Sunagawa for their support and inspiration. I would also like to acknowledge Dr. Chung Pen Liu, Mathew Wolff, Raymond P. Kelly, Chih-Tai Ting, and Peter H. Pak from among the many who have contributed to our studies of human pressure-volume relations.

References

1. Sagawa K, Maughan WL, Suga H, Sunagawa K: Cardiac Contraction and the Pressure-Volume Relationship. New York, Oxford University Press, 1988

2. Suga H, Sagawa K, Shoukas AA: Load independence of the instantaneous pressure-volume ratio of the canine left ventricle and effects of epinephrine and heart on the ratio. Circ Res 32:314, 1973

3. Sagawa K, Suga H, Shoukas AA, Bakalar KM: End-systolic pressure-volume ratio: A new index of ventricular contractility. Am J Cardiol 40:748, 1979

4. Kass DA, Maughan WL: From "Emax" to pressure-volume relations: A broader view. Circulation 77:1203–1212, 1988

5. Wilson SS: Sadi Carnot. Sci Am 245:134–145, 1981

6. Freeman GL, Little WC, O'Rourke RA: The effect of vasoactive agents on the left ventricular end-systolic pressure-volume relation in closed-chest dogs. Circulation 74:1107–1113, 1986

7. Freeman GL: Effects of increased afterload on left ventricular function in closed-chest dogs. Am J Physiol 259:H619–H625, 1990

8. Suga H, Hisano R, Goto Y, Hamada O: Normalization of end-systolic pressure-volume relation and Emax of different sized hearts. Jpn Circ J 48:136–143, 1984

9. Zile MR, Izzi G, Gaasch WH: Left ventricle diastolic dysfunction limits use of maximum systolic elastance as an index of contractile function. Circulation 83:674–680, 1991

10. McKay RG, Aroesty JM, Heller GV, Royal HD, Warren WE, Grossman W: Assessment of the end-systolic pressure-volume relationship in human beings with the use of a time varying elastance model. Circulation 74:97–104, 1986

11. Kronenberg MW, Parrish MD, Jenkins DW Jr, Sandler MP, Friesinger GC: Accuracy of radionuclide ventriculography for estimation of left ventricular volume changes and end-systolic pressure-volume relations. J Am Coll Cardiol 6:1064–1072, 1985

12. Baan J, Van der Velde ET, de Brun HG, Smeenk GJ, Koops J, van Dijk AD, Temmerman D, Senden J, Buis B: Continuous measurement of left ventricular volume in animals and humans by conductance catheter. Circulation 70:812–823, 1984

13. Kass DA, Yamazaki T, Burkhoff D, Maughan WL, Sagawa K: Determination of left ventricular end-systolic pressure-volume relationships by the conductance (volume) catheter technique. Circulation 73:586–595, 1986

14. Kass DA, Midei M, Graves W, Brinker JA, Maughan WL: Use of a conductance (volume) catheter and transient inferior vena caval occlusion for rapid determination of pressure-volume relationships in man. Cathet Cardiovasc Diagn 15:192–202, 1988

15. Kass DA, Wolff MR, Ting CT, Liu CP, Lawrence W, Chang MS, Maughan WL: Diastolic compliance of hypertrophied ventricle is not acutely altered by pharmacologic agents influencing active processes. Ann Intern Med 119:466–473, 1993

16. Kass DA, Midei M, Brinker J, Maughan WL: Influence of coronary occlusion during PTCA on end-systolic and end-diastolic pressure-volume relations in humans. Circulation 81:447–460, 1990

17. Liu CP, Ting CT, Yang TM, Chen JW, Chang MS, Maughan WL, Lawrence W, Kass DA: Reduced left ventricular compliance in human mitral stenosis. Role of reversible internal constraint. Circulation 85:1447–1456, 1992

18. Liu CP, Ting CT, Lawrence W, Maughan WL, Chang MS, Kass DA: Diminished contractile response to increased heart rate in intact human left ventricular hypertrophy: Systolic versus diastolic determinants. Circulation 88(Pt 1):1893–1906, 1993

19. Crottogini AJ, Willshaw P, Barra JG, Pichel RH: Left ventricular end-systolic elastance is incorrectly estimated by the use of stepwise afterload variations in conscious, unsedated, autonomically intact dogs. Circulation 90:1431–1440, 1994
20. Glower DD, Spratt JA, Snow ND, Kabas JS, Davis JW, Olsen CO, Tyson GS, Sabiston DC, Rankin JS: Linearity of the Frank-Starling relationship in the intact heart: The concept of preload recruitable stroke work. Circulation 71:994–1009, 1985
21. Kass DA, Kelly RP: Ventriculo-arterial coupling: Concepts, assumptions, and applications. Ann Biomed Eng 20:41–62, 1992
22. Sunagawa K, Maughan WL, Burkhoff D, Sagawa K: Left ventricular interaction with arterial load studied in isolated canine ventricle. Am J Physiol 245:H773–H780, 1983
23. Kelly RP, Ting CT, Yang TM, Maughan WL, Chang MS, Kass DA: Effective arterial elastance as index of arterial vascular load in humans. Circulation 86:513–521, 1992
24. Kass DA, Grayson R, Marino P: Pressure-volume analysis as a method for quantifying simultaneous drug (amrinone) effects on arterial load and contractile state. J Am Coll Cardiol 16:726–732, 1990
25. Feldman MD, Haber HL, Wu CC, Tedesco CL, Carnivale M, Pak PH, Feldman AM, Bergin JD, Cowart TD, Powers ER, Kass DA: Clinical determination of myocardial versus load effects of OPC-18790: A novel intravenous agent for the treatment of patients with congestive heart failure. Circulation 88:(abstr):I–301, 1993
26. Sunagawa K, Maughan WL, Sagawa K: Effect of regional ischemia on the left ventricular end-systolic pressure-volume relationship of isolated canine hearts. Circ Res 52:170–178, 1983
27. Kass DA, Marino P, Maughan WL, Sagawa K: Determinants of end-systolic pressure-volume relations during acute regional ischemia in situ Circulation 80:1783–1794, 1989
28. Carpentier A, Chachques JC: Clinical dynamic cardiomyoplasty: Method and outcome. Semin Thorac Cardiovasc Surg 3:136–139, 1991
29. Jatene AD, Moreira LF, Stolf NA, Bocchi EA, Seferian P, Fernandes MP, Abensur H: Left ventricular function changes after cardiomyoplasty in patients with dilated cardiomyopathy. J Thorac Cardiovasc Surg 102:132–139, 1991
30. Kass DA, Baughman KL, Pak PH, Cho PW, Levin HR, Gardner TJ, Halperin HR, Tsitlik JE, Acker MA: Reverse remodeling from cardiomyoplasty in human heart failure: External constraint versus active assist. Circulation (In Press, 1995).
31. Serruys PW, Wijns W, van den Brand M, Meji S, Slager C, Schuubiers JCH, Hugenholtz PG, Brower RW: Left ventricular performance, regional blood flow, wall motion, and lactate metabolism during transluminal angioplasty. Circulation 70:25–36, 1984
32. Applegate RJ: Load dependence of left ventricular diastolic pressure-volume relations during short-term coronary artery occlusion. Circulation 83:661–673, 1991
33. Gorcsan JI, Romand JA, Mandarino WA, Deneault LG, Pinsky MR: Assessment of left ventricular performance by on-line pressure-area relations using echocardiographic automated border detection. J Am Coll Cardiol 23:242–252, 1994

Douglas A. Hettrick
David C. Warltier

5 Ventriculoarterial Coupling

A great deal of focus is rightfully placed on ventricular function in the determination of the effect of disease state or pharmacological intervention on cardiovascular performance. However, ventricular performance may also be markedly altered by afterload in systole.[1] Furthermore, the function of the arterial system itself may also be affected by the disease state or pharmacological intervention under study. In order to fully appreciate alterations in cardiovascular function, the main concern should not be for the individual properties of the ventricle or the arterial system, but rather their combined effects in tandem.

Capillaries of various tissues require a steady flow of blood which is provided for by the intermittently pumping heart. The role of the arterial system is to transform (rectify) the discrete motion of blood supplied by the ventricle into the constant flow needed by the capillaries. Evolutionary pressure would favor the development of an arterial system with mechanical properties sufficient to perform this task with minimal loss of energy produced by the ventricle. The amount of energy required by the ventricle for any given cardiac output and heart rate is determined by the relationship between the combined mechanical properties (resistance and elastance) of the ventricle and the arterial system. The challenge to physiologists over the past 20 years has been to devise a framework for comparing these properties between chambers.

Ventricular Function, edited by David C. Warltier. Williams & Wilkins, Baltimore © 1995.

This chapter will describe the important mechanical properties of the ventricular and arterial systems, some of the modeling frameworks developed to relate these properties, and the effects of pathological (age and cardiovascular disease) and pharmacological (including anesthetic agents) interventions on ventriculoarterial coupling. Two excellent reviews emphasizing the limitations and applications of ventricloarterial coupling have recently been published.[2,3]

MECHANICAL PROPERTIES OF THE VENTRICLE

The mechanical properties of the ventricle may be most easily interpreted through the left ventricular pressure-volume relationship (see Chapters 3 and 4). The ventricle may be considered as an elastic chamber, the elasticity of which varies with time throughout the cardiac cycle. Elasticity is defined as the ratio of a change in pressure to change in volume ($\Delta P / \Delta V$). The ventricle is maximally compliant (compliance is defined as the inverse of elastance) during diastole in order to facilitate filling. Elastance then begins to dramatically increase as tension develops in the myocardium during isovolumic contraction. Elastance continues to rise throughout systole, peaking at end ejection (E_{max}). Elastance finally declines during isovolumic relaxation. This time-varying elastance model of the left ventricle originally proposed by Suga and Sagawa[4-6] has proven useful for determining inotropic state (Chapters 3 and 4). The E_{max} curve, which represents ventricular systolic stress-strain relationships, may be determined by linear regression of the end-systolic points of differently loaded pressure-volume loops. E_{max} has been demonstrated to be a reasonably load-independent index of contractility.[6,7] Left ventricular end-systolic pressure (P_{es}) may be related to E_{max} from this model by the equation

$$P_{es} = E_{max} (V_{ed} - SV - V_o) \tag{1}$$

where V_{ed} is left ventricular end-diastolic volume, SV is stroke volume, and V_0 is the theoretical chamber volume at zero pressure. This equation defines a linear relationship between ventricular end-systolic pressure and stroke volume.

ARTERIAL SYSTEM MECHANICS

The elastic nature of the aorta and peripheral arteries allows these vessels to store part of the energy supplied by the left ventricle during ejection and return it during diastole. Arterial blood pressure would decline to zero during diastole (and coronary perfusion would cease) if the aorta and peripheral arteries were rigid tubes. The higher the arterial compliance, the closer are the absolute values of diastolic and mean blood pressure due to the rectifying qualities of the compliance. Aging or disease states which decrease arterial compliance lower diastolic pressure and increase pulse pressure (the absolute difference between systolic and diastolic pressures).

Total peripheral resistance, defined as mean arterial pressure divided by mean arterial flow, would completely describe the hydraulic resistance of the arteries if the heart were a steady flow pump ejecting into a rigid tube. The actual arterial wall is not rigid but possesses viscoelastic properties. A viscoelastic material is one which demonstrates stress relaxation (a decrease in stress in response to a sudden strain), creep (an increase in strain in response to a sudden stress), and hysteresis (differential stress-strain relationships during cyclic loading and unloading).[8] This implies that the change in pressure that occurs in response to a change in blood flow in the arterial system will not be instantaneous. The phase difference (time lag) between pressure and flow waves is frequency-dependent. Thus, the simplistic calculation of phasic hydraulic resistance obtained by dividing instantaneous aortic pressure by instantaneous aortic flow is incorrect. Analysis has focused on the aortic input impedance (Z_{in}) as a tool for interpreting the mechanical function of the arterial system while taking into account its viscoelastic, frequency-dependent, and time-invariant nature. Z_{in} is determined by performing Fourier analysis (or the fast Fourier transform) on pressure and flow waveforms to obtain transformation from the time domain into the frequency domain.

AORTIC INPUT IMPEDANCE

Z_{in} is the complex ratio of pressure (the forces acting on the blood) to flow (the resultant motion of the blood) at the aortic root.[9,10] From a control systems standpoint, if aortic flow is considered the input to the system and pressure the output, then Z_{in} is the transfer ($Z_{in} = P/F$). From an electrical engineering standpoint, this relation is analogous to Ohm's law for AC circuits where pressure and flow are analogous to voltage and current, respectively, and hence the term inpedance. Z_{in} is most commonly displayed by plotting its magnitude and phase as a function of frequency (Fig. 5–1). This is known as the aortic input impedance spectrum.

The magnitude of Z_{in} ($|Z_{in}|$ expressed in dyn $\cdot$ sec/cm^5) is defined as the magnitude of the pressure divided by the magnitude of the flow at each point in the frequency domain. The phase is determined by subtracting the phase angle of the flow from the phase angle of the pressure at each frequency. Note in Figure 5–1 that the phase angles are usually negative especially at low frequencies. This implies that at low frequencies flow actually leads pressure. The zero frequency intercept (Y intercept) of the aortic impedance spectrum is the steady state (mean) ratio of pressure to flow which is equivalent to total peripheral resistance by definition.

Z_{in} can be calculated by determining the Fourier series of measured aortic pressure and flow waves or by spectral analysis.[11,12] Spectral analysis (via the fast Fourier transform) may provide a more continuous spectrum if the input data used consists of varying heart rates. Most of the spectral energy of Z_{in} is concentrated at low frequencies. Plots of Z_{in} rarely extend further than 15 to 20 Hz because of the low energy at higher frequencies. A range of 0 to 15 Hz usually encompasses 5 to 15 harmonics depending on the heart rate. Figure 5–1 shows raw pressure and flow waveforms (approximately 20 sec of data sampled at 200 Hz) and the corresponding Z_{in} spectrum. Z_{in} depends on the physical properties of the arterial wall including diameter and visoelasticity (which determine the characteristic impedance), as well as reflected waves.[13] Vasoactive substances or disease states which alter the mechanical properties of the arterial wall will change Z_{in} (Fig. 5–2).[14] Alterations in Z_{in} may be difficult to quantify, and, thus, Z_{in} is often interpreted through an analytical model known as the three-element Windkessel.

WINDKESSEL APPROXIMATION

The three-element Windkessel model (Fig. 5–3) is an electrical analog of Z_{in} which displays most of its general characteristics in the frequency domain.[15] In this model, Z_c represents the characteristic impedance of the aorta. Characteristic impedance may be defined as the input impedance of an individual length of vessel minus the effects of reflected waves. It is a property of the vessel itself and is not affected by proximal or distal vessels.[10] Z_c is referred to as an impedance (rather than a resistance) because its value is influenced not only by the Pouiseullian resistance of the aorta but also (inversely) by the aortic compliance. Pressure-induced distension of a vessel will cause a decrease in Pouiseullian resistance and thereby decrease impedance. Distension will simultaneously cause the arterial wall to stiffen, reducing compliance and thereby increasing impedance. The net change in Z_c depends on the elastic properties of the wall, vessel dimension, and intravascular pressure.[10,16]

Total arterial resistance (R) is equivalent to total peripheral resis-

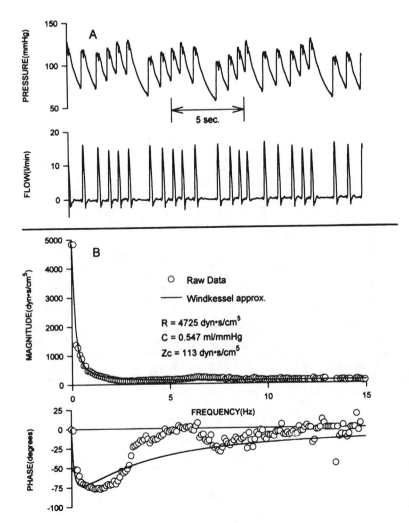

FIGURE 5-1. Calculation of aortic input impedance spectrum (A) Raw pressure and flow waves consisting of 4096 data points sampled at 200 Hz from a conscious dog. (B) Corresponding aortic input impedance spectrum (*open circles*) calculated *via* spectral analysis. Because the dog was experiencing sinus arrhythmia, a multitude of heart rates are present creating a continuous spectrum. Data points with magnitude squared coherence less than 0.8 were omitted. *Solid lines* represent frequency response of calculated Windkessel parameters.

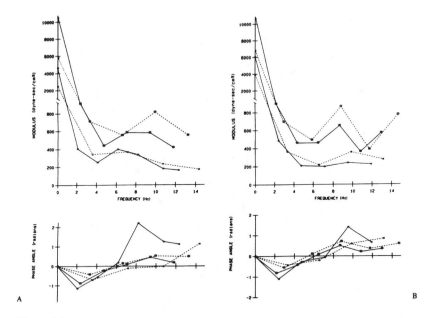

Figure 5-2. Changes in the magnitude and phase of the aortic input impedance spectrum with exercise, age, and pharmacological intervention. (A) *Circles* and *squares* represent young and senescent dogs at rest (*solid lines*) and during exercise (*dashed lines*), respectively. (B) Same as A in the presence of propranolol. (Reproduced with permission from Yin FCP. In Yin FCP (ed): *Ventricular/Vascular Coupling*. New York, Springer-Verlag, 1987.)

Figure 5-3. Three-element Windkessel. Zc represents characteristic aortic impedance. R represents total arterial resistance. C represents total arterial compliance. A represents the aortic valve. *F(t)* is aortic flow. *P(t)* is aortic root pressure. Z(ω ± represents the combined impedance of the three elements (Z$_c$, R, and C).

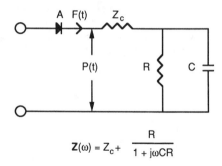

3 ELEMENT WINDKESSEL

$$\mathbf{Z}(\omega) = Z_c + \frac{R}{1 + j\omega CR}$$

tance minus Z_c. R is generally an order of magnitude greater than Z_c. This is consistent with the physiological concepts of the aorta as a low-resistance, high-compliance conduit and the arterioles as the primary resistance vessels. C is the total arterial compliance (the energy storage element). The majority of C (>90%) is contained in the aorta.[17,18] The values of the three elements of the Windkessel model may be estimated from Z_{in} determined experimentally. The zero frequency magnitude intercept of Z_{in} is equal to the sum of R and Z_c (total peripheral resistance). The electrical impedance of a capacitor (Z_{cap}) is inversely proportional to frequency [$Z_{cap} = 1/j\omega C$ where $j = (-1)^{0.5}$]. At low frequencies, the impedance of the capacitor (total arterial compliance) is high, causing most of the current (blood flow) to pass through Z_c and R. As frequency increases, the impedance of the capacitor decreases, and it draws more of the total flow away from R. At even higher frequencies, C behaves as a short circuit (zero impedance) leaving Z_c as the only impedance to flow (see the formula in Fig. 5–3). The rate of decay of the magnitude of Z_{in} as it decreases from R + Z_c to Z_c is proportional to C. C may be estimated by a number of techniques in both the time and frequency domain,[19–22] perhaps the most common being the method of Liu et al.[23] This method is also based on the Windkessel model and does not assume exponential decay of the pressure wave during diastole, thus allowing for the influence of reflected waves.

R and the resistive component of Z_c are primarily Pouiseullian resistances and may be affected by changes in blood viscosity or vessel diameter. Since the radius of the vessel varies during the cardiac cycle, R and the resistive component of Z_c may be thought of as mean hydraulic resistances. The value C is not directly related to diameter but is rather a mechanical property of the arterial wall. It is primarily determined by the interrelation between collagen, elastin, and smooth muscle.[24,25] C is nonlinearly related to pressure. An increase in pressure causes an increase in diameter (distension) which alters the interrelationship between elastin, collagen, and smooth muscle, resulting in reduced compliance. C has also been shown to vary during the cardiac cycle.[26] The Windkessel approximation of C represents a mean value for all vessels of the arterial system over the cardiac cycle.

Interpretation of Z_{in} through the three-element Windkessel model allows quantification of the mechanical properties of the aorta and distal arterial system. It should be emphasized that Z_{in} as well as R, Z_c, and C are properties of the arterial system alone and are not affected by the ventricle. More elaborate models of the arterial system such as the t-tube (transmission line)[27–30] or more detailed lumped parameter models[31,32] offer alternatives to the Windkessel. Some of these models may account for reflected waves and more faithfully reproduce details of Z_{in} but all are considerably more complex. Burkhoff et al.[12] suggested that from a coupling standpoint, the fine details in Z_{in} not accounted for by the three-element Windkessel model may not have significant impact on its interpretation.

WAVE REFLECTION

One aspect of Z_{in} that is not accounted for in the three-element Windkessel model is reflected waves. When a vessel branches, the characteristic impedance (input impedance minus the effects of wave reflection) of the proximal trunk may not be equivalent to the combined characteristic impedances of the distal branches. This hydraulic impedance mismatch causes some of the forward energy to be reflected back toward the heart. From an intuitive standpoint, it might be expected that the morphology (if not the phase) of the pressure wave should be similar to that of the flow wave. In fact, if the forward traveling component is separated from the reflected component, the waves indeed look identical (Fig. 5–4). However, since the reflected wave adds to the pressure wave and subtracts from the flow wave, the result is the familiar nonisomorphic relation between pressure and flow waves.

Wave reflections may be beneficial for the cardiovascular system. Diastolic pressure is augmented if the reflected pressure is phasically related to the aortic root pressure in such a manner that the peak of the reflected wave occurs during diastole. This may improve coronary perfusion. If the reflection occurs during systole, the result is an increased systolic load on the ventricle. Fig. 5–5 demonstrates the effects of reflected waves on measured aortic root pressure waveforms. The wave-

Figure 5-4. Effects of wave reflections on aortic pressure and flow wave morphology. Reflected pressure and flow waves are identical in form but 180° out of phase. The forward pressure and flow waves are also identical in form. When the forward and reverse waves are summed to create the measured waveforms, the familiar nonisomorphism is apparent. (Reproduced with permission from Nichols WW et al. In Yin FCP (ed): *Ventricular/Vascular Coupling.* New York, Springer-Verlag, 1987.)

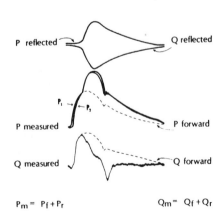

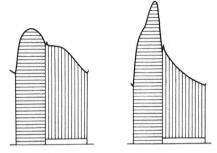

Figure 5-5. Effect of wave reflections on aortic root pressure. Reflected waves create an increase in diastolic pressure in the waveform on the *left,* while causing an increase in systolic pressure in the waveform on the *right. Hatched areas* demonstrate a greater discrepancy between mean systolic and diastolic pressure when the reflected wave occurs during systole. Thus, the increased systolic loading and decreased diastolic pressure augmentation impair the efficient transfer of the stroke volume from the ventricle to the arterial system (*Reproduced with permission from O'Rourke MF, et al. Physiol Rev 62:570–623, 1982*)

form on the left shows an increase in pressure during diastole due to wave reflection. The mean pressure (hatched areas) is similar during both systole and diastole. In contrast, the waveform on the right shows a late increase in pressure during ejection due to wave reflection. End-diastolic pressure is much lower. The difference between mean systolic and diastolic pressure (hatched areas) is more pronounced, implying a decrease in the efficiency of the arterial system to accept pulsatile flow from the heart.[33] Pressure waveform morphology is dependent on the site where the measurement is made because the phase relation of the reflected wave to the incident wave is different in various regions of the arterial system. Radial artery systolic and diastolic pressures do not match aortic root pressures for this reason.

Wave reflections are manifested in aortic input impedance spectra as oscillations of $|Z_{in}|$ at higher frequencies. The magnitude of the oscillations of $|Z_{in}|$ is directly proportional to the magnitude of the reflections.[10] The frequency of the first minimum of $|Z_{in}|$ resulting from these oscillations and the frequency of the first zero crossing of the phase have been shown to be correlated with the distance to the major reflecting site.[10] The major reflecting site is not a true anatomical branching point but is a mean distance that describes the average sum of all reflecting sites in relation to the aortic root. Another factor which affects the phase relation of the incident to reflected wave is pulse wave velocity. A faster moving wave will reach the aortic root more quickly. An increase in pulse wave velocity may also be quantified via the aortic input impedance spectrum as an increase in the frequency of the first minimum of $|Z_{in}|$.[14,25] Both pulse wave velocity and distance to reflection sites must be considered as possible causes for a change in the first minimum of $|Z_{in}|$. Pulsatile flow delivered at a frequency with low $|Z_{in}|$ (such as the first minimum of $|Z_{in}|$) would encounter the least impedance. In fact, under normal conditions, the highest energy flow harmonics are associated with the first minimum of $|Z_{in}|$. Thus, reflected waves may contribute to decreased afterload.[9,25,34,35]

Because wave reflections originate at a multitude of sites, their phase relations differ. Reflected waves may be additive or algebraically cancel each other out. The net result as "seen" from the ascending aorta is two discrete reflecting sites, one arising from the proximal superior arterial vasculature and the other from the inferior distal vasculature. Occluding the descending aorta eliminates the effect of reflections arising from the lower body. This results in the Z_{in} spectrum becoming dominated by reflections arising from the upper body, thereby eliminating the minimum of Z_{in}.[9,36] This implies that aortic cross-clamping during surgery could alter wave reflection possibly to the detriment of the ventricle, but this remains unstudied.

AFTERLOAD

Afterload may be defined as the external forces opposing ventricular ejection. It is commonly interpreted as being equal to total peripheral resistance, systolic myocardial wall stress, or ventricular pressure. These interpretations have been criticized as less than adequate for various reasons.[13] Minor proposed Z_{in} as an operational definition of afterload.[13] This viewpoint has gained wide, albeit nonuniversal, acceptance. Although it provides a complete and somewhat quantifiable method of interpreting afterload, it is difficult to adapt Z_{in} into a coupling framework with the ventricle because it is calculated in the frequency domain.[2]

TIME DOMAIN

The inverse Fourier transform of Z_{in} is known as the impulse response function. This is a time domain representation of the resultant aortic pressure wave which would occur from a hypothetical flow pulse of unit volume and of infinitely small duration.[12,37,38] The impulse response is more easily applied to coupling comparisons with ventricular properties because it is expressed in the time domain. Determination of the impulse response, however, may require extrapolation of Z_{in} beyond the actual frequency range measured.[12]

COUPLING FRAMEWORKS

Once the mechanical properties of the ventricle and arterial system have been established, the next challenge is to combine them within a coupling framework in order to determine the quality (optimality) of their interaction. Guyton's well-known cardiac output-venous return diagrams represented the earliest attempt to quantify ventriculovascular interaction as a determinant of cardiac output.[39] This framework, however, does not emphasize the individual contributions of the cardiac chambers and vascular divisions.[40] Van den Horn et al.[41] introduced a framework involving mean ventricular pressure plotted against mean ventricular outflow. The slope of this function curve is ventricular internal source resistance. Total peripheral resistance obtained from mean arterial pressure and flow data (assuming a linear relationship) could be represented on the same plot. The intersection of the two curves defines the coupling point of the system. This approach provides a useful framework from routinely measured hemodynamic variables, but it ignores the pulsatile component of the system as well as ventricular diastolic function and energetics.[2]

Sunagawa and his associates[42] described a coupling framework that links the preload system to the three-element Windkessel model.

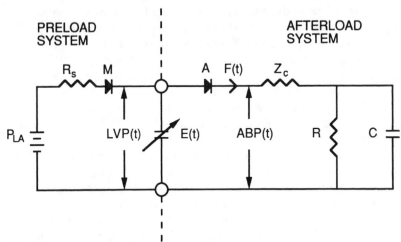

Figure 5-6. Electrical analog model for coupling the preload system and the afterload system. P_{LA} is left atrial pressure. R_s is the internal resistance to filling of the left ventricle. Diodes M and A represent the mitral and aortic valve, respectively. $E(t)$ is the time-varying elastance of the left ventricle. $LVP(t)$ and $ABP(t)$ are left ventricular and ascending aortic pressure, respectively. $E(t)$ is the time-varying elastance of the left ventricle. $LVP(t)$ and $ABP(t)$ are left ventricular and ascending aortic pressure, respectively. $F(t)$ is aortic flow. Z_c, R, and C are the three elements of the Windkessel comprising afterload. (*Modified with permission from Sunagawa K, et al. Ann Biomed Eng 12:163–189, 1984*)

Fig. 5–6 depicts an electrical analog of this framework. P_{LA} is a constant voltage source representing left atrial pressure. R_s is an internal ventricular source resistance that opposes filling. E(t) is the time-varying elastance of the left ventricular chamber. M and A are diodes analogous to the mitral and aortic valves, respectively. Z_c, C and R are the three components of the Windkessel as previously described. Left ventricular and aortic blood pressures are represented as voltages as shown in the figure.

When left ventricular pressure is lower than P_{LA}, current (flow) will fill the capacitor (ventricle) with charge (blood) through diode M (mitral valve). The ventricle then begins to develop tension (increase elastance), and as left ventricular pressure exceeds P_{LA}, diode M shuts off (filling ceases). As E(t) continues to increase, pressure in the left ventricle exceeds that in the aorta, diode A (aortic valve) opens, and E(t) begins to discharge (eject) into the Windkessel. Some of the current (blood flow) is dissipated through the load (R), while some of the current charges C (total arterial compliance) during ejection. E(t) decreases as the ventricle begins to relax. Left ventricular pressure decreases to levels below that in the aorta, and diode A closes while C begins to simultaneously discharge across the load (R) (total arterial resistance), thereby maintaining diastolic aortic pressure at relatively high values. Aortic blood pressure would fall to zero when diode A (aortic valve) closes in the absence of C. Note that during diastole, P_{LA} is charging E(t) while C is simultaneously discharging (elastically recoiling) across R. The key to the performance of the entire system is the time variance of E(t).

Sunagawa et al. estimated ventricular parameters from arterial mechanical properties and stroke volume by applying this model to a servo-controlled afterload system in an isolated heart preparation.[43] These investigators were able to individually assess the effects of changing each of the afterload parameters (R, C, or Z_c) on ventricular pressure-volume relationships while maintaining all other model parameters (including E_{es} and end-diastolic volume) constant. Their results are shown in Figure 5–7. This figure demonstrates that the main effect of a pure increase in total arterial resistance is a decrease in stroke volume for a given E_{es}. The effect of increasing C is more subtle, being primarily characterized by a decrease in left ventricular pressure during ejection (Fig. 5–7). The concept that increased C unloads the ventricule during ejection has been supported by other investigators.[19,44–47] An increase in C also causes an increase in diastolic arterial pressure which is accompanied by a decrease in pulse pressure (resulting in the same mean pressure). Left ventricular end-systolic pressure is lower with an increased compliance, but left ventricular pressure at the beginning of ejection is higher. Thus, stroke work for a given stroke vol-

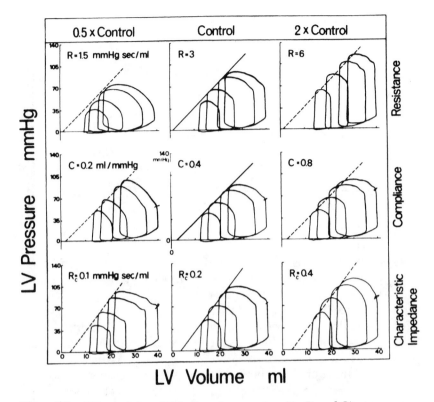

Figure 5-7. Effects of altered Windkessel parameters (Z_c, R, and C) on pressure-volume relations in the isolated canine ventricle. E_{es} was held relatively constant, and end-diastolic volume was adjusted to four different levels for nine computer-simulated combinations of Z_c, R, and C. See text for further explanation. (*Reproduced with permission from Maughan WL, et al. Circ Res 54:595–602, 1984*)

ume remains approximately the same. The effects of a change in C on left ventricular pressure-volume relations are not as dramatic as those observed with a change in R, but both variables must be considered when assessing the effects of a change in afterload on cardiac performance.

Characteristic aortic impedance (Z_c) may be increased through an increase in aortic resistance and/or a decrease in aortic compliance. The results are similar to those observed when changing both R and C. An increase in Z_c causes stroke volume to decrease slightly and left ventricular pressure to increase during ejection.

Sunagawa et al. developed a coupling framework based on pres-

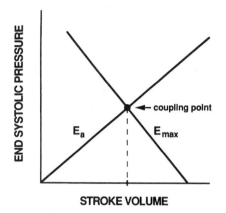

Figure 5-8. End-systolic pressure-stroke volume plane representation of ventriculoarterial coupling framework. E_{max} represents ventricular properties according to equation 1. E_a represents arterial mechanical properties ($E_a = P_{es}/SV$). The intersection of these two curves (*coupling point*) determines stroke volume. (*Adapted from Sunagawa K, et al. Am J Physiol 265:H773–H780, 1983*)

sure-volume relations from this model linking the preload and afterload systems.[47] Figure 5–8 depicts a schematic diagram of this framework. E_{max} is the maximal elastance curve of the ventricle. Effective arterial elastance (E_a) was defined as the slope of the arterial end-systolic pressure vs stroke volume curve ($E_a = P_{es}/SV$). Recall that E_{max} (E_{es}) could also be plotted on the end-systolic pressure-stroke volume plane by equation[1]. The intersection of the E_{max} (E_{es}) curve (which represents ventricular function) and the E_a curve (which represents arterial mechanical properties) is the coupling point and occurs at the stroke volume intercept. This coupling point determines end-systolic pressure (Fig. 5–8). E_a may also be expressed in terms of the Windkessel afterload components by the equation

$$E_a = \frac{Z_c + R}{t_s + R \cdot C(1 - e^{td/R \cdot C})} \tag{2}$$

where t_s and t_d are the elapsed times of systole and diastole, respectively.

E_a does not include high-frequency components of Z_{in} and does not specifically describe the actual elastance of any part of the arterial system, but it was chosen as a coupling parameter for several reasons. E_a incorporates the mechanical properties of arterial load (including heart rate), is easily derived from the pressure-volume plane, and has the same units as E_{es} for comparison.[48–50] In the pressure-volume plane, E_a is the negative of the slope of a line drawn through the end-ejection and end-diastolic corners of the pressure-volume diagram (Fig. 5–9). This approach for estimating E_a has been shown to agree with E_a determined by equation 2 in humans.[48] It can be shown that for any E_{es} and end-diastolic volume, stroke work (estimated as the product of

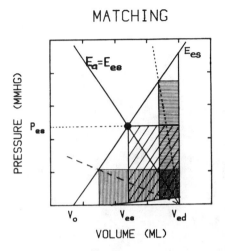

MATCHING

Figure 5-9. Pressure-volume plane representation of coupling framework. For any given ventricular elastance (E_{es}) and end-diastolic volume the value of E_a which will maximize stroke work (*shaded area*) will be equal to E_{es}. E_a is represented on this plane as the magnitude of the slope of the line connecting the end-ejection and end-filling points of the pressure-volume loop (*Reproduced with permission from Sunagawa K, et al. Ann Biomed Eng 12:163–189, 1984*)

end-systolic pressure and stroke volume) will be maximal when E_a is equal to E_{es} (Fig. 5–9).[42,51,52]

EFFICIENCY

Stroke work is that work accomplished by the ventricle that contributes to ejection but is not necessarily all the work performed by the ventricle. The total work performed may be depicted in the pressure-volume plane as the area bounded by the E_{es} curve on the left, end-systolic pressure on the top, end-diastolic volume on the right, and the diastolic pressure-volume curve on the bottom (Fig. 5–10). Efficiency is defined as the ratio of stroke work to total work (pressure-volume area). It can be shown from equations 1 and 2 that this ratio is maximized when E_{es} is equal to twice the E_a. The question that arises from this information is: does the cardiovascular system operate optimally in terms of maximum efficiency or maximum stroke work?

OPTIMIZATION

Criteria describing optimization must be defined before it can be determined if a pharmacological agent or pathological state creates a more or less optimal relationship between the ventricle and the arterial system. It can be shown that for any electric circuit such as that depicted in Figure 5–6 with a voltage source (P_{LA}) and source impedance (R_s plus E_{es}), there is a specific combination of afterload values (Z_c, R, and C)

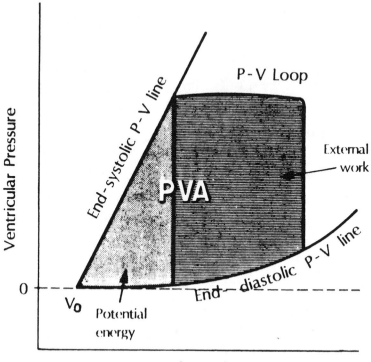

Figure 5-10. Stroke work area vs pressure volume area. The *shaded region* represents pressure volume area (the total work performed by the ventricle). The *darker shaded region* inside the pressure volume loop is stroke work representing the external work performed by the ventricle. The *lighter shaded region* represents potential energy (still stored in the myocardium at end-systole). The ratio of stroke work to pressure volume area is a measure of ventricular efficiency. (*Reproduced with permission from Sagawa K, et al. Cardiac Contraction and the Pressure-Volume Relationship. New York, Oxford University Press, 1988*)

which will maximize the power across the load (R). In physiological terms, for any given hemodynamic state (inotropy, end-diastolic volume, and heart rate), there is a unique combination of arterial properties which will allow stroke work to be maximized. Likewise, at any given afterload, there is a unique combination of ventricular properties that will fulfill the demands of the systemic circulation with minimal energy expenditure (oxygen consumption). A great deal of research has been conducted to establish criteria for optimization.[3,42,53–55] These studies have determined that under normal conditions the cardiovascular system operates at nearly optimal values.

Sunagawa's coupling framework of two elastic chambers theoretically implies that the maximal transfer of potential energy from one chamber to another occurs when E_{es} is equal to E_a.[42] Sunagawa and his associates determined a formula based on the equations for arterial elastance and ventricular elastance to calculate the maximal external work [stroke work (SW)] for a given set of ventricular properties:

$$SW_{max} = E_{es}/4 \bullet (V_{ed} - V_o)^2. \qquad (3)$$

These investigators defined optimization criteria including an arterial quality factor (Q_{load}), i.e., the ratio of actual SW to SW_{max}. Likewise, they determined a ventricular quality factor (Q_{heart}) as the ratio of the minimum myocardial oxygen consumption possible to the actual oxygen consumption. Figure 5–11 shows the relation of Q_{heart} and Q_{load} to E_a/E_{es}. The load (SW) is optimized at $E_a/E_{es} = 1$, and the heart (efficiency in terms of MVO_2) is optimized when $E_a/E_{es} = 0.5$. Note, however, that there is a relatively wide range of E_a/E_{es} ratios where Q_{load} and Q_{heart} are nearly maximal. Figure 5–11 also demonstrates the effects of exercise, volume loading, volume depletion, and reduced left ventricular function on E_a/E_{es}. Volume depletion and decreased left ventricular function adversely affect coupling by increasing E_a/E_{es} so that neither the ventricle nor the load is optimized. In contrast, exercise and volume loading maintain nearly optimal coupling. The finding that ventriculoarterial coupling is maintained during exercise is supported by results obtained in chronically instrumented dogs.[56] Exercise-in-

Figure 5-11. Heart and load optimization as a function of E_a/E_{es} ratio. The "heart" is optimized at an E_a/E_{es} ratio of 0.5 while the E_a/E_{es} is optimized at an E_a/E_{es} ratio of 1.0. Note the range of $E_a E_{es}$ ratios which will nearly optimize both curves. Exercise (EX) and volume loading (VOL) create E_a/E_{es} ratios in the nearly optimal range. Volume depletion (HEM) or ventricular dysfunction (D) shift E_a/E_{es} ratios into a range of neither optimal load nor heart (ventriculoarterial mismatch). (*Reproduced with permission from Sunagawa K, et al. Basic Res Cardiol* 88:75–90, 1993)

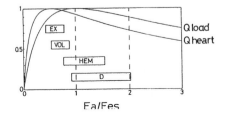

duced increases in both E_{es} and E_a maintain E_a/E_{es} ratios near resting values.

ALTERATIONS IN VENTRICULOARTERIAL COUPLING RELATIONS

Many studies have examined the effects of pharmacological agents on ventriculoarterial coupling. Vasoactive substances primarily affect ventriculoarterial coupling by changing aortic input impedance (arterial wall mechanics) through alterations in smooth muscle activity.[10] Vasoconstriction or vasodilation alters both the resistance and the compliance of individual vessels. Most vasoactive substances act through receptors which are not evenly distributed between larger and smaller arteries. Therefore, a change in characteristic impedance produced by a vasoactive substance can vary from vessel to vessel. This may disturb impedance matching relations between vessels and thereby alter wave reflections. Aside from the obvious change in R, most vasoactive substances have little effect on Z_c and primarily affect Z_{in} by increasing wave reflections.[10]

Several investigations[16,34,57] have documented age-related changes in aortic input impedance due to impaired distensibility caused by arterial wall thickening, increases in collagen, and decreases in elastin content. Alterations with aging include increased Z_c and R, decreased C, and increased wave reflection magnitude and pulse wave velocity. Such changes in afterload cause the ventricle and arterial system to become uncoupled and, thus, reduce cardiac performance. Other investigators[24,34,58] have suggested that vasodilator therapy in hypertension should focus on agents that can restore the normal arterial system properties in order to reduce wave reflections, not merely on drugs that decrease mean arterial pressure.

Watanabe et al.[59] found that dogs with chronically decreased aortic compliance in addition to coronary artery stenosis (similar to that observed in humans with atherosclerosis) had reduced subendocardial blood flow. In the same model but in the absence of a coronary artery stenosis, dogs with decreased aortic compliance also demonstrated subendocardial ischemia during the administration of a positive inotropic agent, isoproternol.[60] This study also showed evidence of increased "backwards" coronary blood flow during systole. These findings emphasize the importance of aortic compliance in maintaining the aortic to intramyocardial pressure gradient in order to facilitate coronary perfusion.

Increases in E_a/E_{es} have been reported in patients with long-term mitral regurgitation.[61] This was a result of decreased E_{es} without a corresponding change in E_a. The increase in E_a/E_{es} was associated with a decrease in left ventricular pump efficiency. Ventricular failure also has detrimental effects on aortic input impedance parameters,[62-65] including increases in aortic characteristic impedance and total arterial resistance, as well as decreases in total arterial compliance. These changes in afterload may contribute to the progression of failure. One of the earliest hemodynamic changes occurring in ventricular failure may be an increase in aortic characteristic impedance preceding changes in systemic vascular resistance.[62]

In humans, increased afterload (*via* methoxamine) caused E_a/E_{es} to increase toward optimal loading (and away from optimal efficiency) due to increases in stroke work and decreased efficiency. Decreases in afterload (*via* sodium nitroprusside) decreased E_a/E_{es} towards optimal ventricular properties (efficiency) by increasing efficiency and decreasing stroke work. Positive inotropy (*via* dobutamine) caused a similar decrease in E_a/E_{es} secondary to an increase in stroke work without a change in efficiency.[52]

Maruyama et al.[45] recently demonstrated that a reduction in aortic compliance can cause a decrease in stroke volume due to increased end-ejection pressure. If E_{es} is held constant, the decrease in stroke volume is magnified in ventricles with impaired systolic function. Hypoxia increases E_a/E_{es} (toward optimal load) in anesthetized dogs by increasing E_a and decreasing E_{es}.[66] Oshita et al.[67] showed that nicardipine decreases E_a/E_{es} in humans. Both these studies calculated E_{es} without altering load by using a single beat method proposed by Takeuchi et al.[69] This method employs a sinusoidal curve fit to estimate maximal isovolumic ventricular pressure (P_{max}) and then extrapolates E_{es} from P_{es}, P_{max}, and stroke volume.

The only published report of the effects of volatile anesthetics on ventriculoarterial coupling also used this single beat estimation technique in dogs with a baseline anesthesia consisting of pentobarbital and α-chloralose.[69] Halothane but not isoflurane was demonstrated to increase (uncouple) E_a/E_{es} (Fig. 5–12). Isoflurane anesthesia equally decreased both E_{es} and E_a while halothane depressed left ventricular function to a greater extent than arterial system function.

Recently, we measured aortic input impedance spectra of chronically instrumented dogs during the conscious and anesthetized (halothane or isoflurane) states. Aortic input impedance spectra were quantified by estimating the Windkessel parameters. The results (Fig. 5–13) demonstrated that halothane caused no change in R, while isoflurane and sodium nitroprusside administered in the conscious state decreased R. All agents increased C, but the increase in C produced by halothane and isoflurane was considerably smaller than that caused by sodium nitroprusside. Isoflurane and halothane but not nitroprusside

Ea/Ees

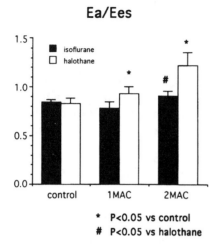

Figure 5-12. Effects of halothane and isoflurane on E_a/E_{es} ratios in acutely instrumented dogs with single beat estimation of E_{es}. Both anesthetics equally depressed arterial function. Halothane, however, decreased ventricular function more than isoflurane, resulting in an increased E_a/E_{es} (*Reproduced with permission from Kawasaki T, et al. Anesth Analg 79:681–686, 1994*)

increased Z_c. The increase in aortic characteristic impedance was probably due to pressure-induced decreases in aortic diameter. Sodium nitroprusside but not halothane or isoflurane reduced the frequency of the first minimum of $|Z_{in}|$, indicating an alteration of arterial wave reflections. These results emphasized that the major actions of halothane and isoflurane on afterload are secondary to effects on total arterial re-

Figure 5-13. Effects of halothane, isoflurane, and sodium nitroprusside (*SNP*) on Windkessel parameters in chronically instrumented dogs. Low, medium, and high doses of anesthetic are 1.25, 1.5, and 1.75, respectively. SNP doses were chosen to create comparable changes in mean arterial pressure. All data are mean ± SEM, °significantly different (*P* < 0.05) from control; † significantly different (*P* < 0.05) than low dose; §, significantly different (< 0.05) than medium dose; ‡ , significantly different (*P* < 0.05) than halothane at the same dose.

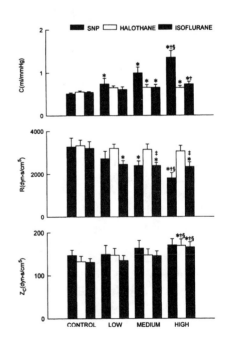

sistance, a property of arterioles and not the aorta. Thus, the primary difference in effects of halothane and isoflurane may be occurring at the arteriolar level. The increase in C observed during halothane and isoflurane anesthesia may have been solely a nonspecific result of a decline in pressure. Figure 5–14 demonstrates the concept of aortic compliance increasing during a reduction of arterial pressure. A higher compliance at any decreased level of mean arterial pressure is observed in the presence of sodium nitroprusside in comparison to the volatile anesthetics.

PULMONARY VASCULATURE

The pulmonary artery input impedance spectrum resembles that of the aorta with only a few differences. Pulmonary artery characteristic impedance is much lower than aortic characteristic impedance despite the fact that both vessels have similar diameters (indicating similar hydraulic resistances). The difference results from the greater compliance of the pulmonary artery which decreases impedance.[10,25] Pulmonary vascular resistance (mean pressure/mean flow) is lower than total peripheral resistance due in part to the shorter distance the blood must travel through the pulmonary circulation. Pulmonary artery input impedance is also affected by wave reflections. Because of the symmetry of the lungs, the reflections appear to arise from a single reflecting site rather than from two discrete sites (head and body) as in the systemic circulation.[25]

Piene and Sund[70,71] used a coupling framework consisting of mean hydraulic power vs pulmonary load resistance to evaluate the optimization of right ventriculopulmonary arterial coupling. Hydraulic power (W) may be interpreted through the three-element Windkessel as the product of mean flow (F_m) through load (R) and mean pressure (P_m) across the load ($W = P_m \bullet F_m$). If pressure is interpreted to be the

Figure 5-14. Relationship of mean arterial pressure to total arterial compliance. Halothane (*squares*) and isoflurane (*circles*) create similar increases in compliance with decreasing pressure. Sodium nitroprusside (*triangles*) steepens the relationship. Halothane and isoflurane may be following the normal pressure compliance relationship, but SNP steepens this relation.

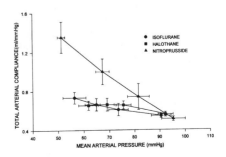

product of flow and resistance ($P_m = F_m \cdot R$), then power can be expressed in two forms by substitution

$$W = F_m^2 \cdot R \qquad (4a)$$
$$W = P_m^2 \cdot R . \qquad (4b)$$

A diagram of these two relations in the mean hydraulic power vs load resistance plane reveals a coupling point (intersection) as seen in Figure 5–15. Actual plots of R vs W constructed by Piene and Sund from isolated cat heart preparations revealed that under the normal pressure range the right heart-pulmonary vascular system operated very near this coupling point, thereby maximizing delivery of hydraulic power from the ventricle to the vasculature.[70–72] Decreasing pulmonary artery compliance shifted the curve to the left, causing peak power to occur outside the normal pressure range (Fig. 5–15). A reduced compliance also lowered the magnitude of the peak indicative of a decrease in power available for the load (impedance mismatch). The curve steepens at higher resistances, indicating a smaller range of load resistances which provide nearly optimal power delivery. These effects emphasize the importance of compliance for maintaining favorable ventriculoarterial coupling relations.

Serotonin has been demonstrated to increase pulmonary vascular resistance without altering characteristic impedance.[73] The minimal

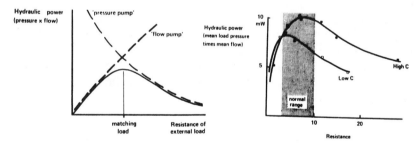

Figure 5-15. Right ventricular-pulmonary artery coupling framework (*left side of figure*). *Dashed curves* represent hydraulic power as a function of resistance from a pressure or flow source (equations 4a and 4b). The *solid line* represents the experimentally determined power-load relation. The "matching load" point represents the optimum coupling point. Shifting the operating point to the left or right of the optimal point implies that the ventricle is acting primarily as a flow or pressure pump, respectively. Right ventricular power-load function curves at high and low pulmonary compliance levels in the cat (*right side of figure*). Decreased compliance lowers the maximum power available and shifts this optimal coupling point to the edge of the normal resistance range. (*Reproduced with permission from Piene H. In Yin FCP (ed): Ventricular/Vascular Coupling. New York, Springer-Verlag, 1987*)

frequency of pulmonary input impedance increased due to reduced distance to wave reflection sites and increased pulse wave velocity. Both changes occurred secondary to alterations in the elastic properties of the arterial wall, resulting in characteristic impedance mismatches between adjacent vessels. Zuckerman et al.[74] studied the effects of physiological changes in arterial mechanics due to pulmonary hypertension in a high altitude calf model. These investigators concluded that the increases in characteristic impedance and decreases in total arterial compliance resulted only from an elevated pressure despite the observed thickening of the pulmonary arterioles.

FUTURE WORK

Compliance is, by definition, the ratio of a change in volume to a change in pressure ($\Delta V / \Delta P$). Total arterial compliance is usually derived from a model (such as the Windkessel) applied to direct measurements of pressure and flow (not volume) data. Effective arterial elastance has been shown to be insensitive to dynamic coupling during ventricular ejection because it ignores the higher frequency components of afterload.[49,50] Its usefulness as a coupling variable stems from its ease of measurement and compatibility with ventricular function parameters (E_{es}) despite the fact that it is not a true measure of the elastance of any specific portion of the arterial system. A measure of aortic compliance derived from directly measured aortic volume and pressure might provide more meaningful insights into coupling relationships. Ferguson et al.[18] used the conductance catheter technique for chamber volume measurement to track changes in aortic segment volume (not absolute volume) with simultaneous pressure measurement. The conductance catheter has already proven to be an essential tool for determining ventricular pressure-volume relations[75-78] (see Chapter 4). As coupling models and techniques for experimentally determining modeling parameters improve, a much greater understanding of the effects of drugs on ventriculoarterial coupling can be expected. At present, the role of ventriculoarterial coupling in the effects of anesthetic agents on overall cardiac performance remains speculative.

References

1. Sagawa K, Maughn L, Suga H, Sunagawa K: Cardiac Contraction and the Pressure-Volume Relationship. New York, Oxford University Press, 1988
2. Kass DA, Kelly RP: Ventriculo-arterial coupling: Concepts, assumptions, and applications. Ann Biomed Eng 20:41–62, 1992
3. Sunagawa K, Sugimachi M, Todaka K, Kobota T, Hayashida K, Itaya R,

Chishaki A, Takeshita A: Optimal coupling of the left ventricle with the arterial system. Basic Res Cardiol 88:75–90, 1993

4. Suga H. Time course of left ventricular pressure-volume relationship under various end-diastolic volume. Jpn Heart 10:509–51, 1969
5. Suga H. Left ventricular pressure-volume ratio in systole as an index of myocardial inotropism. Jpn Heart J 12:153–160, 1971
6. Suga H, Sagawa K, Shoukas AA. Load independence of the instantaneous pressure-volume ratio of the canine left ventricle and effects of epinephrine on the ratio. Circ Res 32:314–322, 1973
7. Sagawa K. The end-systolic pressure-volume relation of the ventricle: Definition, modifications and clinical use. Circulation 63:1223–1227, 1981
8. Fung YC. Biomechanics: Mechanical Properties of Living Tissues, 2nd ed. New York, Springer Verlag, 1993
9. O'Rourke MF, Taylor MG: Input impedance of the systemic circulation. Circ Res 4:365–380, 1967
10. Minor WR: Hemodynamics. Baltimore, Williams & Wilkins, 1989
11. Taylor MG: Use of random excitation and spectral analysis in the study of parameters of the cardiovascular system. Circ Res 18:585–595, 1966
12. Burkhoff D, Alexander J Jr, Schipke J: Assessment of Windkessel as a model of aortic input impedance. Am J Physiol 255:H742–H753, 1988
13. Minor WR: Arterial impedance as ventricular afterload. Circ Res 36:565–570, 1975
14. Nichols WW, O'Rourke MF, Avolio AB, Yaginuma T, Murgo JP, Pepine CJ, Conti ER: Age related changes in left ventricular/arterial coupling. In Yin FCP (ed): Ventricular/Vascular Coupling. New York, Spinger Verlag, 1987
15. Elzinga G, Westerhof N: Pressure and flow generated by the left ventricle against different impedances. Circ Res 32:178–186, 1973
16. Yin FCP: Aging and vascular impedance. In Yin FCP (ed): Ventricular/Vascular Coupling. New York, Springer-Verlag, 1987
17. Westerhof N, Bosman F, De Vries CJ, Noordergraaf A: Analog studies of the human systemic arterial tree. J Biomech 2:121–143, 1969
18. Ferguson JJ III, Miller MJ, Sahagian P, Aroesty JM, McKay RG: Assessment of aortic pressure-volume relationships with an impedance catheter. Cathet Cardiovasc Diagn 15:27–36, 1988
19. Vrettos AM, Gross DR: Instantaneous changes in arterial compliance reduce energetic load on left ventricle during systole. Am J Physiol 267:H24–H32, 1994
20. Toorop GP, Westerhof N, Elzinga G: Beat-to-beat estimation of peripheral resistance and arterial compliance during pressure transients. Am J Physiol 252:H1275–H1283, 1987
21. Shim Y, Pasipoularides A, Straley GA, Hampton TG, Soto PF, Owen CH, Davis JW, Glower DD: Arterial Windkessel parameter estimation: A new time-domain method. Ann Biomed Eng 22:66–77, 1994
22. Laskey WK, Parker HG, Ferrari VA, Kussmaul WG, Noodergraaf A: Estimation of total systemic arterial compliance in humans. J Appl Physiol 69:112–119, 1990
23. Liu Z, Brin KP, Yin FCP: Estimation of total arterial compliance: An improved method and evaluation of current methods. Am J Physiol 251: H588–H600, 1986
24. Pepine CJ, Nicols WW, Curry RC Jr, Conti CR: Aortic input impedance during nitroprusside infusion: A reconsideration of afterload reduction and beneficial action. J Clin Invest 64:643–654, 1979

25. Nichols WW, O'Rourke MF: McDonald's blood flow in arteries: Theoretic, experimental and clinical principles. Philadelphia, Lea & Febiger, 1990
26. Li JKJ, Cui T, Drzewiecki GM: A nonlinear model of the arterial system incorporating a pressure-dependent compliance. IEEE Trans Biomed Eng 37:674–676, 1990
27. Burattini R, Campbell KB: Modified asymmetric T-tube model to infer arterial wave reflection at the aortic root. IEEE Trans Biomed Eng 36:805–814, 1989
28. Burattini R, Knowlen GG, Campbell KB. Two arterial effective reflecting sites may appear as one to the heart. Circ Res 68:85–99, 1991
29. Burattini R, Campbell KB. Effective distributed compliance of the canine descending aorta estimated by modified T-tube model. Am J Physiol 264:H1977–H1987, 1993.
30. Campbell KB, Burattini R, Bell DL, Kirkpatrick RD, Knowlen GG: Time-domain formulation of asymmetric T-tube model of arterial system. Am J Physiol 258:H1761–H1774, 1990.
31. Burattini R, Fogliardi R, Campbell KB: Lumped model of terminal aortic impedance in the dog. Ann Biomed Eng 1994:381–391, 1994
32. Grant BJB, Paradowski LJ: Characterization of pulmonary arterial input impedance with lumped parameter models. Am J Physiol 252:H585–H593, 1987
33. O'Rourke MF: Vascular impedance in studies of arterial and cardiac function. Physiol Ref 62:570–623, 1982
34. O'Rourke M: Coupling between the left ventricle and arterial system in hypertension. Eur Heart J 11:24–28, 1990
35. O'Rourke M: Arterial compliance and wave reflection. Arch Mal Coeur 84:45–48, 1991
36. Van Den Bos GC: Reflection in the systemic arterial system: Effects of aortic and carotid occlusion. Cardiovasc Res 10:565–573, 1976
37. Latson TW, Yin FCP, Hunter WC: The effects of finite wave velocity and discrete reflections on ventricular loading. In Yin FCP (ed): Ventricular/Vascular Coupling. New York, Springer-Verlag, 1987
38. Laxminarayan S, Sipkema P, Westerhof N: Characterization of the arterial system in the time domain. IEEE Trans Biomed Eng BME-25:177–183, 1978
39. Guyton AC: Textbook of Medical Physiology, 8th ed. Philadelphia, WB Saunders, 1991
40. Sunagawa K, Sagawa K, Maughan WL: Vantricular interaction with the loading system. Ann Biomed Eng 12:163–189, 1984
41. Van den Horn GJ, Westerhof N, Elzinga G: Interaction of the heart and arterial system. Ann Biomed Eng 12:151–162, 1984
42. Sunagawa K, Maughan WL, Sagawa K: Optimal arterial resistance for the maximal stroke work studied in isolated canine left ventricle. Circ Res 56:586–595, 1985
43. Maughan WL, Sunagawa K, Burkhoff D, Sagawa K: Effect of arterial impedance changes on the end-systolic pressure-volume relation. Circ Res 54:595–602, 1984
44. Urschel CW, Covell JW, Sonnenblick EH, Ross J Jr, Braunwald E: Effects of decreased aortic compliance on performance of the left ventricle. Am J Physiol 214:298–304, 1968
45. Maruyama Y, Nishioka O, Nozaki E, Kinoshita H, Kyono H, Koiwa Y, Takishima T: Effects of arterial distensility on left ventricular ejection in the depressed contractile state. Cardiovasc Res 27:182–187, 1993

46. Kelly RP, Tunin R, Kass DA: Effect of reduced aortic compliance on cardiac efficiency and contractile function of *in situ* canine left ventricle. Circ Res 71:490–502, 1992
47. Sunagawa K, Maughan WL, Burkhoff D, Sagawa K: Left ventricular interaction with arterial load studied in isolated canine ventricle. Am J Physiol 265:H773–H780, 1983
48. Kelly RP, Ting C-T, Yang T-M, Liu C-P, Maughan WL, Chang M-S, Kass DA: Effective arterial elastance as index of arterial vascular load in humans. Circulation 86:513–521, 1992
49. Little WC, Cheng C-P: Left ventricular-arterial coupling in conscious dogs. Am J Physiol 261:H70–H76, 1991
50. Little WC, Cheng C-P: Coupling of the left ventricular and arterial system. Med Biol Eng Comput 32:205–209, 1994
51. Burkhoff D, Sagawa K: Ventricular efficiency predicted by an analytical model. Am J Physiol 250:R1021–R1027, 1986
52. Starling MR: Left ventricular-arterial coupling relations in the normal human heart. Am Heart J 125:1659, 1993
53. Myhre ESP, Johansen A, Piene H: Optimal matching between canine left ventricle and afterload. Am J Physiol 254:H1051–H1058, 1988
54. Piene H, Sund T. Does normal pulmonary impedance constitute the optimum load for the right ventricle? Am J Physiol 242:H154–H160, 1982
55. Hamalainen JJ: Optimal stroke volume in left-ventricular ejection. IEEE Trans Biomed Eng 36:172–182, 1989
56. Hayashida K, Sunagawa K, Noma M, Sugimachi M, Ando H, Nakamura M: Mechanical matching of the left ventricle with the arterial system in exercising dogs. Circ Res 71:481–489, 1992
57. Murgo JP, Westerhof N, Giolma JP, Altobelli SA: Aortic input impedance in normal man: Relationship to pressure wave forms. Circulation 62:105–116, 1980
58. Carroll JD, Shroff S, Wirth P, Halsted M, Rajfer SI: Arterial mechanical properties in dilated cardiomyopathy. J Clin Invest 87:1002–1009, 1991
59. Watanabe H, Ohtsuka S, Kakihana M, Sugishita Y: Coronary circulation in dogs with an experimental decrease in aortic compliance. J Am Coll Cardiol 21:1497–1506, 1993
60. Ohtsuka S, Kahihana M, Watanabe H, Sugishita Y: Chronically decreased aortic distensibility causes deterioration of coronary perfusion during increased left ventricular contraction. J Am Coll Cardiol 24:1406–1414, 1994
61. Starling MR: Left ventricular pump efficiency in long-term mitral regurgitation assessed by means of left ventricular-arterial coupling relations. Am Heart J 127:1324–1335, 1994
62. Eaton GM, Cody RJ, Binkley PF: Increased aortic impedance precedes peripheral vasoconstriction at the early state of ventricular failure in the paced canine model. Circulation 88:2714–2721, 1993
63. Finkelstein SM, Cohn JN, Collins R, Carlyle PF, Shelley WJ: Vascular hemodynamic impedance in congestive heart failure. Am J Cardiol 55:423–427, 1985
64. Merillon JP, Fontenier G, Lerallut JF, Jaffrin MY, Chastre J, Assayag P, Motte G, Gourgon R: Aortic input impedance in heart failure: Comparison with normal subjects and its changes during vasodilator therapy. Am Heart J 5:447–455, 1984
65. Asanoi H, Sasayama S, Kameyama T: Ventriculoarterial coupling in normal and failing heart in humans. Circ Res 65:483–493, 1989
66. Kawasaki T, Hoka S, Okamoto H, Okuyama T, Takahashi S: The effects of

hypoxia on ventriculo-arterial coupling in dogs. Anesthesiology 81:A719, 1995

67. Oshita S, Kaieda R, Murakawa T, Masuda N, Funatsu N, Sakabe T: Effects of nicardipine on ventriculo-arterial coupling in humans. Anesthesiology 81:A128, 1995

68. Takeuchi M, Igarashi Y, Tomimoto S, Odake M, Hayashi T, Tsukamoto T, Hata K, Takaoka H, Fukuzaki H: Single-beat estimation of the slope of the end-systolic pressure-volume relation in the human left ventricle. Circulation 83:202–212, 1991

69. Kawasaki T, Hoka S, Okamoto H, Okuyama T, Takahashi S: The difference of isoflurane and halothane in ventricular-arterial coupling in dogs. Anesth Analg 79:681–686, 1994

70. Piene H: Impedance matching between ventricle and load. Ann Biomed Eng 12:191–207, 1984

71. Piene H, Sund T: Flow and power output of right ventricle facing load with variable input impedance. Am J Physiol 237:H125–H130, 1979

72. Piene H: Matching between right ventricle and pulmonary bed. In Yin FCP (ed): Ventricular/Vascular Coupling. New York, Springer-Verlag, 1987

73. Yin FCP, Guzman PA, Brin KP, Maughan WL, Brinker JA, Traill TA, Weiss JL, Weisfeldt ML: Effect of nitroprusside on hydraulic vascular loads on the right and left ventricle of patients with heart failure. Circulation 67:1330–1359, 1983

74. Zuckerman BD, Orton EC, Stenmark KR, Trapp JA, Murphy JR, Coffeen PR, Reeves JT: Alteration of the pulsatile load in the high-altitude calf model of pulmonary hypertension. J Appl Physiol 70:859–868, 1991

75. Burkhoff D: The conductance method of left ventricular volume estimation: Methodologic limitations put into perspective. Circulation 81:703–706, 1990

76. Kass DA, Yamazaki T, Burkhoff D, Maughan WL, Sagawa K: Determination of left ventricular end-systolic pressure-volume relationships by the conductance (volume) catheter technique. Circulation 73:586–595, 1986

77. Kass DA, Midei M, Graves W, Brinker JA, Maughan WL: Use of a conductance (volume) catheter and transient inferior vena caval occlusion for rapid determination of pressure-volume relationships in man. Cathet Cardiovasc Diagn 15:192–202, 1988

78. Baan J, Van Der Velde ET, De Bruin HG, Smeenk GJ, Koops J, Van Duk AD, Temmerman D, Senden J, Buis B: Continuous measurement of left ventricular volume in animals and humans by conductance catheter. Circulation 70:812–823, 1984

Robert G. Merin

Positive Inotropic Drugs
6 and Ventricular Function

Inotropic is defined as "effecting the force or energy of muscular contractions" and positive inotropic as "increasing the strength of muscular contraction."[1] For the purpose of this chapter, the inotropic response will be that of cardiac muscle. Although the basic physiology and pharmacology of cardiac muscle have been investigated primarily in isolated papillary or muscle strips (and even the nomenclature has been derived from these experiments, e.g. preload and afterload), the emphasis in this chapter will be predominately on humans with failing hearts because that is the major indication for these drugs. Results of animal experimentation will also be reviewed when information is lacking from human studies. Notice that my definition of "inotropic" does not simply refer to left ventricular function. The effect of inotropes on ventricular function is only one of many variables. As reviewed in detail in other chapters, heart rate, preload, and afterload are also major determinants of left ventricular function. The emphasis in this chapter will be on drugs whose primary effect is on cardiac muscle and not on the peripheral circulation, although many of the drugs, old and new, have combined effects. Documentation of ventricular function in humans is difficult, including separating the influence of preload and afterload from a direct positive inotropic effect. In most of the clinical studies, deduction of direct inotropic effect must be made from measurements of cardiac output, arterial pressure, and atrial and ventricu-

Ventricular Function, edited by David C. Warltier. Williams & Wilkins, Baltimore © 1995.

lar filling pressures. The few studies in which more sophisticated measurements have been made will be highlighted.

Any drug effective in treating a pathophysiological condition should ideally be able to reverse the biochemical mechanisms responsible for that condition. It has become apparent that a major factor in ventricular failure is altered intracellular calcium kinetics.[2] The central role of the calcium ion in cardiac muscle contraction has been adequately reviewed elsewhere (see Chapter 1). The classification of inotropic drugs used in this review is based on these mechanisms (Fig. 6–1). The process of regular rhythmic cardiac muscle contraction (which is the basis for ventricular function) is primarily controlled by the intracellular concentration of calcium. Although the extracellular calcium ion concentration is 10^{-3} M, the intracellular concentration al-

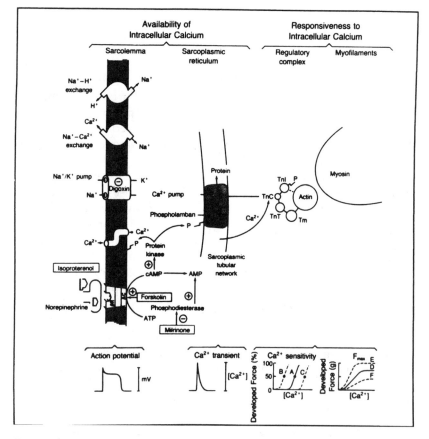

FIGURE 6-1. Schematic for regulation of cardiac contractile function. (*Reproduced with permission from Morgan JP. N Engl J Med 325:625–632, 1991*)

ternates between approximately 10^{-8} M(diastolic) and 10^{-6} M (systolic). The higher concentration is necessary to interact with troponin C, thereby allowing interaction of the actin and myosin filaments and to activate the actomyosin ATPase which is necessary for the energy utilization by the myocyte. Conversely, in order for the muscle to relax, this process must be reversed by an active decrease in the intracellular calcium ion concentration. These changes are governed by a complex series of interactions via the sarcolemma (cardiac cell membrane) and the sarcoplasmic reticular (SR) network (Fig. 6–1).

The first step in cardiac muscle contraction, excitation-contraction coupling, occurs when the cell membrane action potential depolarization opens the voltage-dependent calcium channels to allow the passive flux of calcium ions down the concentration gradient across the sarcolemma (Fig. 6–1). This calcium flux stimulates the release of additional calcium from the intracellular stores in the SR and results in the interaction with the contractile proteins referred to above. The decrease in intracellular calcium concentration is accomplished through active, energy-dependent uptake of calcium by the SR and extrusion of calcium through the sarcolemma by energy requiring ion pumps or exchangers. In addition to the calcium influx, a large influx of sodium into the cell occurs during depolarization. The intracellular concentration of sodium must also be decreased in order for the cell to repolarize. This is primarily accomplished by another energy-dependent pump, the sodium-potassium pump, and by sodium-calcium exchange which appears to be energy independent (Fig. 6–1)

Sympathetic nervous system activity is also an important physiological and pathophysiological regulator of cardiac muscle contractility. The major effects occur secondary to stimulation of the sarcolemmal β-adrenergic receptor which results in activation of membrane-bound adenylyl cyclase. The activated adenylyl cyclase then catalyzes the conversion of ATP to cyclic AMP (cAMP). cAMP further activates protein kinases which ultimately phosphorylate proteins in the sarcolemma, the SR, and the troponin-tropomyosin regulatory complex on the actin filament. These phosphorylations accentuate the effect of calcium on the contractile process and increase the influx of calcium through the calcium channels. cAMP also enhances diastolic relaxation by phosphorylating the regulatory subunit of the calcium pump in the SR, phospholamban, which stimulates the rate of reuptake of calcium into the SR during diastole. Phosphorylation of the troponin-tropomyosin complex also accelerates the dissociation of calcium from the contractile proteins which increases the rate of relaxation.

The recent availability of dye techniques to measure intracellular calcium ion concentrations and of human cardiac tissue from cardiac transplantation recipients and donors has allowed investigation into the biochemical mechanism of cardiac failure.[3,4] These studies strongly suggest that abnormal intracellular calcium kinetics are a major reason for ventricular failure from various etiologies and, in addition, that the etiology of the insufficiency is decreased activity or concentration of cAMP in these hearts. One of the mechanisms for the deficiency of cAMP in failing hearts is probably "downregulation" of β-adrenergic receptors. Bristow and colleagues first demonstrated that this occurs presumably as a result of continued high sympathetic nervous system activity in response to the decreased ventricular function.[5] Early studies suggested that cardiac β- and α- receptors were not downregulated, and consequently, the use of both β- and α-agonist drugs has received considerable investigation (see below).

A classification scheme for positive inotropic agents is as follows:

I. Drugs that increase intracellular calcium ion concentration:
   Calcium ion
   Calcium channel agonists (openers)
   Drugs that increase cardiac cyclic AMP:
      β-adrenergic agonists, (isoproterenol, epinephrine, norepinephrine, dopamine, dobutamine, ibopamine, dopexamine)
      Drugs that activate adenylyl cyclase (forskolin)
      Phosphodiesterase inhibitors (amrinone, milrinone, pimobendan, vesnarinone)
   Drugs that increase sodium influx:
      Inhibition of sodium/potassium pump (digitalis glycosides)
      Vesnarinone
   Drugs that prolong action potential duration (APD)
      Vesnarinone, α_1 adrenergic agonists
II. Drugs that increase the sensitivity of actomyosin to calcium ion:
      Pimobendan, vesnarinone, EMD 60263, α-adrenergic agonists, endothelin
III. Drugs that act through metabolic or endocrine pathways:
      Dichloroacetate, triiodothyronine

THE STUDIES

As indicated above, most of the studies to be reviewed will usually involve invasive measurement of cardiac output and derivatives, sometimes with more sophisticated estimates of left ventricular function using pressure volume loops and usually in patients with documented heart failure. The studies from Morgan's laboratory referred to above using isolated muscle from human heart transplant recipients and donors will also be reviewed for the insight they provide into mechanisms. A series of investigations from the Anesthesia Critical Care

Team at Bowman Gray Medical School studied patients after aorto-coronary bypass surgery, mostly without evidence of clinical heart failure, although some more recent studies investigated weaning from cardiopulmonary bypass. Finally, studies in chronically instrumented dogs from Warltier's laboratory at the Medical College of Wisconsin will be reviewed to demonstrate the effects of different inotropic drugs on healthy hearts with ventricular dysfunction produced by volatile anesthetics (Chapter 7). Most of the clinical studies have investigated patients with both ischemic and nonischemic heart failure. With some drugs and in some studies, this difference may be of significance. Another type of failing myocardium is the "stunned heart" most commonly observed after coronary revascularization procedures. This type of heart failure will also be briefly considered.

Calcium

Since there is considerable evidence that one of the mechanisms of heart failure is associated with decreased intracellular calcium concentration, it would seem logical to treat the syndrome with administration of calcium. In isolated muscle, calcium is very effective in both failing and nonfailing human hearts.[4] In chronically instrumented, healthy dogs, our laboratory reported minimal effects from the infusion of calcium chloride to awake animals.[6] Increasing blood calcium ion concentration to 1.77 mM partially reversed the cardiac depressant effects of several inhalation anesthetics. In a different experiment also conducted in chronically instrumented dogs, Pagel et al. first blocked the autonomic nervous system and then administered increasing doses of calcium chloride.[7] Under these circumstances there was a dose-related increase in heart rate, mean arterial pressure, system vascular resistance, and preload recruitable stroke work (PRSW), a relatively load-independent index of cardiac muscle function. On the other hand, there was no change in cardiac output or segment shortening. The high dose of calcium chloride (5 mg/kg) completely reversed the negative inotropic effect of both halothane and isoflurane in these autonomically blocked dogs.

Two studies in patients extubated and hemodynamically stable on the first postoperative day after coronary artery bypass graft surgery were reported from the Bowman Gray group.[8,9] Calcium chloride (10 mg/kg followed by 2 mg/kg/min or 1 mg/kg/min) only produced an increase in mean arterial pressure with no change in any other hemodynamic index. Another study from the same group conducted immediately after weaning from cardiopulmonary bypass without drug support except phenylephrine to maintain systolic arterial pressure above

90 mm Hg also reported the same response to 5 mg/kg of calcium.[10] It is of some interest that the cardiac index increased to the same extent as that observed with calcium therapy in a placebo group. There have been no studies of the effect of calcium in patients with documented heart failure or needing inotropic support during separation from cardiopulmonary bypass. The Bowman Gray patients all had normal ventricular function. These investigators concluded that calcium is never indicated in the treatment of ventricular failure unless ionized calcium is below 0.8 mM/liter.[11] However, another indication (which remains unstudied) may be to antagonize the effects of potassium cardioplegia.

Calcium Channel Agonists (Openers)

The Medical College of Wisconsin group has studied the effects of the calcium channel agonist Bay k 8644 on left ventricular function in chronically instrumented dogs with autonomic nervous system blockade.[12,13] The effects of opening the sarcolemmal calcium channel and thereby increasing the intracelluar calcium concentration appeared to be similar to their reported effects of infusing calcium chloride.[7] Dose-related increases in heart rate, mean arterial pressure, systemic vascular resistance, PRSW, and left ventricular dP/dt were reported without change in cardiac output or segment shortening, and the negative inotropic effects of isoflurane and halothane were completely reversed. There have been no reports of the use of calcium channel agonists in patients, predominately because the intravenous administration of these drugs produces not only an increase in intracellular calcium in cardiac muscle but also in vascular smooth muscle with a major vasoconstricting effect. In most patients with left ventricular dysfunction, such an effect is counterproductive to the desired increase in ventricular performance.

Drugs That Increase cAMP

β-adrenergic Agonists

Epinephrine

Isoproterenol is the only pure β-adrenergic agonist drug available, but it is rarely used for its inotropic effect because of concomitant potent chronotropic actions.[14] Although an increase in heart rate does increase contractility in cardiac muscle, in most circumstances of cardiac failure, such an increase in heart rate interferes with ventricular filling and increases myocardial oxygen consumption and, hence, is undesirable. All other β-adrenergic agonists have mixed effects. Norepinephrine is the physiological mediator of sympathetic nervous system β-stimulation of the heart, but because of its potent α-adrenergic activity and subsequent vasoconstriction, it is rarely used as a cardiac inotrope.[14] An endogenous catecholamine in frequent clinical use is epinephrine. Epinephrine's classical adrenergic profile is that of a predominate β_1- and β_2- agonist with lesser α_1 effects.[11] The initial concern about using epinephrine in patients with failing hearts was that tachycardia and increased systemic vascular resistance with increasing doses would interfere with the positive inotropic effect. However, with the use of calibrated infusion pumps and better monitoring techniques, epinephrine has become more popular when compared with the synthetic drugs which were introduced to replace it.

In their patients with normal ventricular function on the first postoperative day after coronary artery bypass graft surgery, the Bowman Gray group showed a dose-related increase in cardiac index and mean arterial pressure without changes in systemic vascular resistance or left ventricular filling pressures.[8] These investigators also noted that if epinephrine was administered during a calcium infusion, this positive inotropic effect was lost. Another study from the same group used a similar protocol in patients immediately after weaning from cardiopulmonary bypass but not requiring inotropic support other than phenylephrine to maintain arterial blood pressure.[10] Major concerns with this study were its short duration (6 min) and the fact that all patients were paced so that the effects on heart rate could not be ascertained. Epinephrine (30 ng/kg/min) produced significant increases in mean arterial pressure, cardiac index, and stroke volume without change in pulmonary artery pressures, central venous pressures, or systemic vascular resistance. Prior and coincident administration of calcium had no effect on the cardiovascular actions of epinephrine in contrast to the previous study. In a particularly interesting study, the same group of investigators compared the effects of epinephrine and dobutamine in patients on the first postoperative day.[15] Unfortunately this was neither random, simultaneous, nor blinded, and again, these were patients with normal ventricular function. Dobutamine (2.5 and 5.0 μg/kg/min) and epinephrine (10 and 30 ng/kg/min) were compared. Both drugs produced dose-related increases in cardiac index, stroke volume index, mean pulmonary artery pressure, and left ventricular stroke work, with dobutamine resulting in a higher cardiac index. In contrast to epinephrine, dobutamine caused a dose-related increase in heart rate and decrease in systemic vascular resistance. This study refuted the claim that a major advantage of dobutamine vs epinephrine was a positive inotropic effect without tachycardia.

Moran and colleagues studied the hemodynamic effects of epinephrine in a group of patients in septic shock after fluid resuscitation to a pulmonary artery occlusion pressure of >15 mm Hg.[16] If the patients could not maintain a systolic arterial pressure of 90 mm Hg, epinephrine was infused at a rate of 3 μg/min and titrated over the next 2 hours to obtain urine output >0.5 mL/kg/hour and restoration of systolic arterial pressure to >90 mm Hg. Secondarily, particular objective indices were also targeted: a cardiac index >4.5 liters/min/m²; oxygen delivery >600 liters/min/m²; and oxygen consumption >170 liters/min/m². All patients reached the clinical end points with epinephrine doses varying from 3 to 24 μg/minute. In addition, the objective indices were generally obtained although these responses were more variable. As the epinephrine dose increased so did heart rate, mean arterial pressure, cardiac index, stroke volume index, and oxygen delivery. There was no dose-response relationship for right atrial or pulmonary artery occlusion pressures nor for systemic vascular resistance. The authors concluded that epinephrine was an effective inotropic drug in patients with septic shock.[16]

Dopamine

Dopamine was the "magic" cardiovascular drug of the 1970s. Depending on the dose, it was touted to produce successively: renal artery vasodilation, β-adrenergic inotropic effects, and peripheral vasoconstriction via α-adrenergic mechanisms.[17] The ultimate actions of dopamine were highly dependent on the state of each patient's sympathetic nervous system. Early studies from the Mayo Clinic documented the efficacy of dopamine for inotropic support during emergence from cardiopulmonary bypass.[18,19] However, the population studied consisted primarily of patients with various types of valvular heart disease, and much of the effect appeared to be related to the vasodilating potential of dopamine rather than a positive inotropic action. One of the few human studies actually documenting the effect of inotropic drugs on cardiac muscle function was performed by Wechsler and colleagues.[20] Using implanted ultrasonic dimension crystals in patients with a normal cardiac output on ventilators 1 day after coronary artery bypass graft surgery, these investigators showed that equal doses of dopamine and dobutamine (2.5, 5, and 10 μg/kg/min) resulted in markedly different effects. Dobutamine produced dose-related increases in both the rate and extent of myocardial muscle shortening, whereas dopamine had no effect. Dopamine increased while dobutamine decreased peak left ventricular wall stress. In addition, dobutamine decreased while dopamine slightly increased systemic vascular resistance. Measurement of ventricular function by ultrasonic segment length or wall thickness guages is not entirely-load independent, and part of the effect of dobutamine may have been related to the decrease in afterload.

Dobutamine

The next magic inotrope to be developed dobutamine.[21] At low doses (less than 5 μg/kg/min) this drug was shown to be a selective β_1-agonist. β_2-activity appeared at higher doses and finally mild α-adrenergic agonism at very high doses. As with dopamine (and other drugs, see below) the relative influence of the peripheral vasodilating vs the direct inotropic effects on ventricular function was controversial. Initial reports suggested that significant inotropic effect could be obtained without increases in heart rate, but this is probably not true.[15] The discovery that β_1-adrenergic receptors were downregulated in patients with heart failure also cast some doubt on the specific usefulness of dobutamine.[5] Colucci and colleagues utilized an innovative approach to answer this question as well as investigate the direct cardiac effects of dobutamine by infusing this drug directly into the coronary circulation, thus eliminating (or markedly reducing) the systemic effect.[22] Since dobutamine has little or no effects on preload and afterload when administered by an intracoronary method, measurement of left ventricular dP/dt was a fairly accurate index of direct inotropic effect. Twenty-four patients with severe (NYHA III/IV) heart failure and eight patients with normal ventricular function were studied. Intracoronary dobutamine produced an increase in left ventricular dP/dt in patients with heart failure that was only 37% of that produced in patients with normal ventricular function (Fig. 6–2). Plasma norepinephrine levels were markedly elevated in the

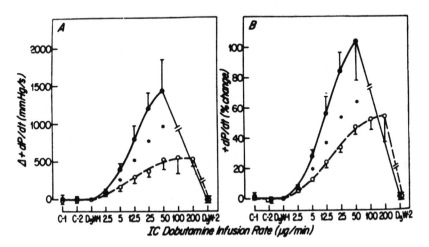

FIGURE 6-2. Effect of intracoronary dobutamine on left ventricular dP/dt in patients with (*open circle*) and without (*closed circle*) congestive heart failure. IC, intracoronary. (A) Absolute change. (B) Percentage change. (*Reproduced with permission from Colucci WS et al. J Clin Invest 81:1103–1110, 1988*)

patients with congestive heart failure, and the increase in dP/dt caused by intracoronary dobutamine was inversely related to resting plasma norepinephrine concentrations. Dobutamine caused a dose-related decrease in plasma norepinephrine. Dobutamine also affected ventricular function curves less in patients with heart failure.

In a particularly interesting study of the effect of dobutamine in healthy volunteers, Vanoverschelde and colleagues used two-dimensional echocardiography for assessing ventricular function and positron emission tomography to assess myocardial oxygen consumption.[23] Unfortunately these investigators studied only 1 dose of dobutamine which was infused at a range of 5 to 10 μg/kg/minute to double the rate-pressure product. Pressure-volume loops were constructed using ventricular volumes estimated from two dimensional echocardiography and ventricular pressure from carotid pulse recordings. Estimates of ventricular function were made by the ratio of end-systolic stress to end-systolic volume index (Ess/Esv) and the maximal slope of the pressure volume loop (E_{max}) (see Chapter 3). Other less load-independent estimates of ventricular function included ejection fraction and mean velocity of fiber shortening from analysis of the echocardiograms. Dobutamine caused a marked increase in heart rate and a significant increase in mean arterial pressure with decreased end-diastolic volume and end-systolic wall stress. Thus, the increases in ejection fraction and velocity of fiber shortening could have been related to the increase in heart rate and decrease in afterload (Fig. 6–3). However, the

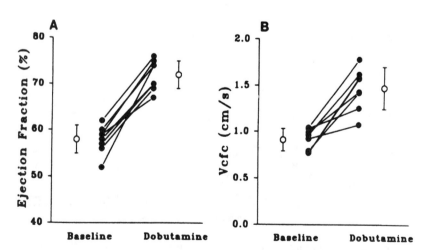

FIGURE 6-3. Effects of dobutamine on ejection fraction (A) and rate-adjusted mean velocity of fiber shortening (Vc cfc) (B) in healthy humans. (*Reproduced with permission from Vanoverschelde et al. Am J Physiol 265:H1884–H1892, 1993*)

relatively load-independent measures of ventricular function, E_{max}, and Ess/Esv suggested that there was, in fact, a true positive inotropic effect. In addition, there was a marked increase in myocardial oxygen consumption greater than that expected by changes in the normal physiological determinates of oxygen consumption, suggesting that dobutamine in healthy humans produces the same decrease in ventricular efficiency (oxygen wasting) as had been previously observed in animals and isolated hearts.

Ferrario et al. studied the effect of dobutamine (5 μg/kg/min) compared with volume loading in patients with right ventricular infarction within 48 hours of onset of symptoms. This patient group has been particularly difficult to treat and may have a higher incidence of mortality than patients with left ventricular infarction.[24] All patients had significant right ventricular dysfunction (cardiac index <1.6 liter/minute/m[2]; right atrial pressure >15 mm Hg with normal pulmonary capillary wedge pressure <15 mm Hg). Dobutamine produced a dose-related increase in heart rate, cardiac index, stroke volume, left and right ventricular stroke work, mean arterial pressure, and a decrease in systemic vascular resistance. In addition, after the study dobutamine therapy was continued, and all patients survived. Thus, dobutamine appears to be effective in treating right as well as left ventricular dysfunction. A major problem particularly in patients with ischemic heart disease is the increase in heart rate produced by most of the agents which increase cAMP. In an anesthetized dog preparation using implanted ultrasonic crystals for measurement of ventricular function, Warltier's laboratory showed that in the presence of a severe coronary artery stenosis, the deleterious effect of increasing doses of dobutamine on coronary blood flow and function of the ischemic area could be markedly improved by decreasing heart rate with a specific bradycardic agent, zatebradine.[25]

Ibopamine

The response of patients with heart failure to dopamine has been controversial (see above), but, nevertheless, other compounds with dopamine-like actions have been investigated. Ibopamine is a prodrug which is metabolized to epinine, a compound that produces dopamine receptor stimulation.[26] Neither of these drugs is likely to be very useful for the acute treatment of the failing heart. Rousseau et al. have studied the effects of intravenous epinine in patients with mild congestive heart failure and have constructed pressure volume-loops via conventional hemodynamic and angiographic techniques.[27] They showed rather convincingly that although epinine can produce increases in ejection fraction and cardiac and stroke volume index, this is predominately a result of decreased afterload. Two representative pressure-volume loops graphically demonstrate the lack of inotropic effect of epinine (Fig. 6–4).

Dopexamine

Dopexamine is a structural analog of dopamine which reportedly produces stimulation of both dopamine$_1$ and $_2$ receptors and relatively selective stimulation of the β-2 adrenergic receptor. In addition, there is some experimential evidence to suggest that this drug inhibits neuronal uptake of norepinephrine.[28] In a well conducted study, patients with severe (NYHA III/IV) congestive heart failure were given increasing doses of dopexamine (0.25 to 6 μg/kg/min).[29] The protocol was randomized, double-blinded, and performed on 3 separate days. Echocardiography was used to measure fractional circumferential fiber shortening. Dopexamine produced a dose-related increase in cardiac output, stroke volume index, heart rate (and ventricular ectopy), and a less pronounced increase in both circumferential fractional shortening and the rate of shortening. Marked decreases in systemic and pulmonary vascular resistances, pulmonary capillary wedge pressure, and right atrial pressure occurred simultaneously. Mean arterial pressure did not change, but there was a dose-related decrease in diastolic arterial pressure. Much of the increase in cardiac performance was undoubtedly due to afterload reduction, but in a study from the same laboratory, pure vasodilators used in a comparable patient population did not result in as much improvement in ventricular function. The investigators attribute this to β$_2$-agonist activity which theoretically should be more effective in patients with severe heart failure where β$_1$-receptors are downregulated.[5]

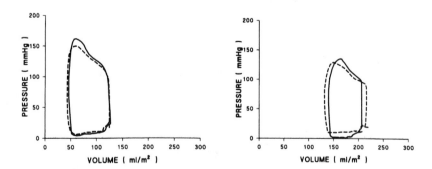

FIGURE 6-4. Effect of intravenous epinine infusion on pressure volume loops in patients with CHF. (*Left*) 0.5 μg/kg/minute. (*right*) 1 μg/kg/minute. (*Reproduced with permission from Rousseau et al. J Cardiovasc Pharmacol 19:155–162, 1992*)

Several studies have compared the effects of dopexamine with dopamine or dobutamine. Sonntag's group studied 20 males forelective coronary artery bypass graft surgery with no evidence of ventricular dysfunction.[30] They compared dopexamine (1 to 4 µg/kg/min) with dopamine (2.5 and 5 µg/kg/min) in separate groups of conscious patients before surgery. Both drugs produced a dose-related increase in cardiac index, but a much higher index was achieved with dopexmine. The latter was entirely related to increases in heart rate. Stroke volume index increased less with dopexamine than with dopamine. Other differences between the two drugs included a decrease in mean arterial pressure and systemic vascular resistance with dopexamine and an increase in mean arterial pressure, pulmonary artery pressure, and pulmonary capillary wedge pressure with dopamine. This study suggested that even in patients with normal ventricular function, β_2 stimulation from dopexamine results in marked chronotropic and perhaps less inotropic activity. Jaski and Peters studied 10 NYHA III digitalized patients comparing dobutamine (5 and 10 µg/kg/min) and dopexamine (2 and 4 µg/kg/min) in a randomized protocol.[31] A micromanometer was placed in the left ventricle for measurement of dP/dt. Both drugs produced dose-related increases in cardiac index, heart rate, and left ventricular dP/dt and decreases in preload (left and right ventricular filling pressures) and afterload (mean arterial pressure and systemic and pulmonary vascular resistances). There were no statistically significant differences between drug effects, but the improvement in stroke volume index tended to be associated with a greater decrease in systemic vascular resistance with dopexamine and a greater increase in left ventricular dP/dt with dobutamine, suggesting a greater inotropic effect with dobutamine (Fig 6–5 and 6–6). In addition, plasma norepinephrine levels were significantly increased by dopexamine but not affected by dobutamine, suggesting inhibition of norepinephrine reuptake by dopexamine. In a similar study, Baumann et al. observed similar effects of the two drugs.[32] Dobutamine produced a greater increase in heart rate and a higher mean arterial pressure while dopexamine resulted in a higher stroke volume index and greater decrease in systemic vascular resistance and pulmonary capillary wedge pressure. The hemodynamic effects of dopexamine were well maintained over a 48-hour infusion, while cardiac and stroke volume index progressively declined with dobutamine. The authors suggested that dopexamine predominantly caused vasodilation with no evidence of tachyphylaxis. Given the significant decreases in both preload and afterload in this study, it is doubtful that a primary inotropic effect caused by dopexamine was important in these patients. Thus, dopex-

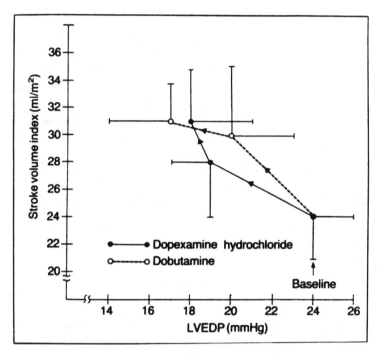

FIGURE 6-5. Comparative effects of dobutamine and dopexamine on left ventricular function at low and high doses. LVEDP, *left ventricular end-diastolic pressure.* (Reproduced with permission from Jaski BE, Peters C. Am J Cardiol 62:63C–67C, 1988)

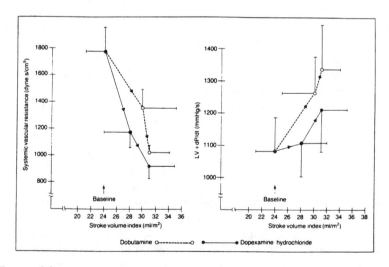

FIGURE 6-6. Improvement in left ventricular stroke volume associated with a trend to greater decreases in systemic vascular resistance with dopexamine and greater increases in left ventricular dP/dt with dobutamine. (*Reproduced with permission from Jaski BE, Paters C. Am J Cardiol 62:63C–67C, 1988*)

amine appears to be primarily a vasodilator in patients with heart failure.

Xamoterol

This drug is a β-adrenergic blocking agent with partial agonist activity. It was proposed to act as a β-agonist when intrinsic sympathetic activity was low and β-adrenergic blocking agent when sympathetic tone was high so that it should be an "ideal" drug, particularly in patients with ischemic heart disease. However, results with this drug have been controversial. A recent multicenter study showed increased mortality in patients with heart failure.[33] DeFeyter et al. studied patients with mild to moderate (NYHA II/III) left ventricular dysfunction secondary to previous myocardial infarction.[34] These investigators inserted a micromanometer in the left ventricle and used dP/dt and other indices to estimate ventricular function. The patients were studied at rest and during exercise; it was found that xamoterol increased systolic function and also enhanced indices of ventricular relaxation. Xamoterol had no effect on heart rate, mean arterial pressure, left ventricular end diastolic and peak systolic pressures, cardiac index, or pulmonary pressures. Time to anginal symptoms and the magnitude of ST segment depression was not different between placebo and drug treatments. Thus it is difficult to ascribe significant therapeutic advantages to this (and other) partial β-adrenergic agonists-antagonists, and their use remains undefined.

Drugs That Activate Adenylyl cyclase

Forskolin

This diterpene derivative is the prototype compound that activates adenylyl cyclase (Fig. 6–1). As such, forskolin produces an increase in cardiac (and other tissue) cAMP without an effect on the β-adrenergic receptor. In situations where there is β-receptor downregulation (such as congestive heart failure, see above) a drug acting through this mechanism might be useful. However, because of the ubiquitous effect of this compound on adenylyl cyclase in all tissues it has not been tested in humans. Bristow and coworkers studied the effects of forskolin in isolated heart muscle from cardiac transplant recipients and donors.[35] Forskolin was a potent activator of human cardiac adenylyl cyclase, producing maximal effects that were 4.8 and 6 times greater than isoproterenol in tissue from normal and failing hearts, respectively. The drug was also a potent positive inotrope in failing human myocardium. In contrast to the effect on adenylyl cyclase, the actions of isoproterenol and forskolin were similar except for the time course. Forskolin displayed a prolonged time to onset of action and a much prolonged time of action (45 min) in comparison to isoproterenol. The effects of forskolin and isoproterenol were also similar in anesthetized open chest dogs, but forskolin caused less increase in cardiac output than isoproterenol. In isolated muscle preparations, minimally effective doses of forskolin which produced elevated concentrations of intracellular cAMP markedly potentiated the effect of phosphodiesterase inhibitors in failing heart muscle.[4] No clinical usefulness for this compound has yet been demonstrated.

Phosphodiesterase Inhibitors

Amrinone and Milrinone

Although there are a number of specific phosphodiesterase inhibitors available throughout the world, only amrinone and milrinone are available for clinical use in the USA. Few studies have demonstrated significant differences between the effects of the different phosphodiesterase inhibitors except perhaps for dose and to a lesser extent pharmacokinetics.[36] This class of compounds belongs to the inotropes which act through increasing intracellular cAMP by interfering with cAMP breakdown (Fig. 6–1). Although they are called "selective phosphodiesterase II inhibitors," which supposedly restricts their action to cardiac muscle cells, without exception all of these compounds are also inhibitors of this enzyme in vascular smooth muscle and hence cause vasodilation.

The controversy continues over whether the vasodilating (and hence decreased afterload) effect of these drugs is more important than the positive inotropic effect to increase cardiac output, but there can be little question that these drugs do have significant positive inotropic actions. Two studies of patients with severe (NYHA III/IV) heart failure in the cardiac catheterization laboratory confirmed this. Konstam et al. compared the effect of nitroprusside and amrinone (3 mg/kg) on radio-nuclide-determined ventricular volumes and pressures.[37] In six of nine patients, the decrease in end-systolic volume produced by amrinone exceeded that predicted for a pure vasodilator based on the same patients' response to nitroprusside. In three of nine patients, the increase in cardiac index appeared to be predominately on the basis of vasodilation. Ludmer and colleagues used intracoronary injection of milrinone to study the direct inotropic effects of this agent.[38] Intracoronary infusion of milrinone produced a dose-related increase in left ventricular dP/dt, a good index of ventricular function in his type of experiment (Fig. 6–7). Other major determinates of ventricular function either did not change (systemic vascular resistance) or decreased (heart rate and left ventricular filling pressure) (Fig. 6–8). Since there was a significant increase in stroke volume and stroke work indices, the ventricular function curves plotting left ventricular filling pressure vs stroke work index also demonstrated a positive inotropic effect. On the other hand, amrinone increased *right* ventricular function (assessed by the end-systolic pressure-volume relationship) primarily by a decreased afterload similar to nitroprusside in the same patients (unfortunately with left but not right ventricular failure).[39]

It is generally accepted that the phosphodiestrase inhibitors produce both arterial and venous dilation. Levy and Bailey documented this in patients during cardiopulmonary bypass.[40] Amrinone (1.5 mg/kg) not only decreased systemic vascular resistance but also caused a progressive (over 10 min) decline in venous reservoir volume, thus documenting both arterial and venodilating effects of this drug. Several studies have also documented the positive inotropic effect of phospho-

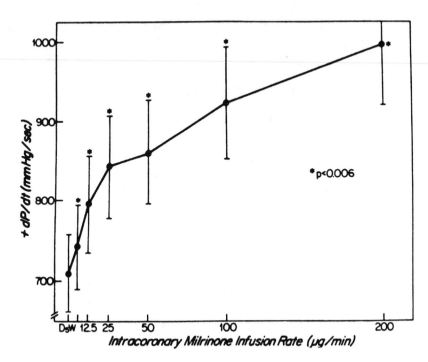

FIGURE 6-7. Effect of intracoronary infusion of milrinone on left ventricular dP/dt in patients with heart failure. (*Reproduced with permission from Ludmer et al. Circulation 73:130–137, 1986*)

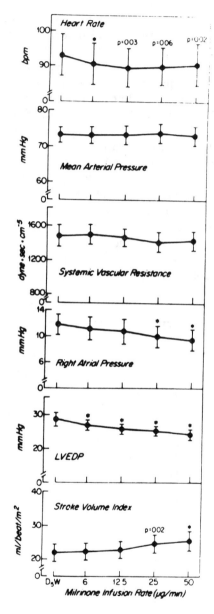

FIGURE 6-8. Hemodynamic effects of intracoronary infusion of milrinone in patients with congestive heart failure. (*Reproduced with permission from Ludmer et al. Circulation 73:130–137, 1986*)

diesterase inhibitors following cardiopulmonary bypass. The Bowman Gray group studied the effect of amrinone, initially in patients with normal left ventricular function on the first postoperative day after coronary artery bypass graft surgery.[41] Amrinone (0.75 and 2.25 mg/kg) produced increases in heart rate and cardiac index and decreases in mean arterial pressure, mean pulmonary artery pressure, pulmonary artery occlusion pressure, and systemic vascular resistance. The increase in cardiac index and decrease in cardiac filling pressure suggested a positive inotropic effect, although the effect of a decreased afterload could not be separated out in this study. In another group of patients with preoperative left ventricular dysfunction in a randomized double-blind study the effect of amrinone (1.5 mg/kg) was compared with placebo during weaning from cardiopulmonary bypass.[42] The end point was determined by the incidence of patients requiring administration of epinephrine for successful weaning. Epinephrine was required by 14 of 19 placebo patients, while only 1 of 20 amrinone patients needed other inotropic support. Most of the patients in both groups required a phenylephrine infusion to maintain systemic arterial pressure. Four of the 14 placebo patients needed amrinone in addition to epinephrine in order to achieve successful weaning.

Wright and Sherry studied the effect of milrinone (0.375, 0.5, and 0.75 µg/kg/min) for 12 hours in patients with a cardiac index <2.5 liters/min/m² and a pulmonary capillary wedge pressure of >8 mm Hg 2 hours following completion of cardiac surgery.[43] All patients were loaded with a bolus dose of 0.5 mg/kg. There was a significant increase in cardiac index, heart rate, left ventricular stroke work index, and stroke volume index during the first hour. This was accompanied by a marked decrease in systemic vascular resistance and a moderate decrease in mean arterial pressure and pulmonary capillary wedge pressure. All of these changes were sustained over the 12 hours of drug infusion and were maintained for 2 hours after discontinuing milrinone. At 4 hours after infusion, cardiac index had decreased but was still higher than baseline, whereas vascular resistance, heart rate, mean arterial pressure, and pulmonary capillary wedge pressure returned to baseline. Ventricular function curves suggested that ventricular function was increased with significant increases in stroke work and stroke volume index in the presence of a decrease in filling pressures. However, from these studies, the vasodilatory and inotropic factors cannot be separated. The Bowman Gray group compared the effects of amrinone (2.5 mg/kg) and epinephrine (30 ng/kg/min) in a group of patients immediately following cardiopulmonary bypass whose cardiac index and systemic arterial pressure were satisfactory and stable.[44]

Mean arterial pressure was maintained in all groups by infusion of phenylephrine. The design of the study was such that the drugs could be evaluated separately and together, and compared with a control group that received a placebo. Both epinephrine and amrinone produced equivalent increases in cardiac output, although the increase was more rapid with amrinone. Neither drug increased heart rate over the 10-minute observation period indicating the increase in cardiac output was secondary to a significant increase in stroke volume. The combination of amrinone and epinephrine produced a significantly greater increase in cardiac output and stroke volume as well as left ventricular stroke work. Systemic and pulmonary vascular resistances were maintained by epinephrine in the control group and decreased by both amrinone and amrinone plus epinephrine. Ejection fraction was also increased by amrinone and amrinone plus epinephrine but did not change with epinephrine alone. Epinephrine alone increased mean arterial pressure, but there was no change in arterial pressure in either of the amrinone groups. Only amrinone plus epinephrine decreased pulmonary capillary wedge pressure but right ventricular end diastolic volume was increased by both amrinone doses and epinephrine but not changed during control period. In fact, there was little to choose from between the 2 drugs in this patient population. A major observation was that the combination of the two drugs produced a greater positive inotropic effect than either drug alone.[42] It is worth noting, however, that left ventricular function (cardiac index) was normal and arterial pressure was supported with phenylephrine in these patients.

The last investigation relevant to surgical and anesthesia practice was conducted by the Medical College of Wisconsin group in autonomically blocked conscious dogs (this is one of the experimental preparations in which it is possible to actually analyze the effect of drugs on ventricular function by the use of implanted ultrasonic crystals).[45] Amrinone (1 mg/kg bolus followed by 10 to 80 μg/kg/min) was given to conscious animals and then on different days to the same animals anesthetized with 1.25 (MAC) isoflurane or halothane. In awake animals, amrinone produced the expected increase in cardiac output and decrease in left ventricular filling pressure. More importantly, amrinone caused a dose-related increase in left ventricular dP/dt, PRSW (a load-independent measure of contractile function), and velocity of segment shortening. There was a decrease in isovolumic relaxation time and an increase in rapid ventricular filling, suggesting a positive lusitropic effect as well. Amrinone produced similar effects in animals anesthetized with either isoflurane or halothane. However, in contrast to calcium chloride and the calcium channel openers,[7,13] amrinone did not completely reverse the effect of isoflurane on cardiac output and segment shortening velocity and the effect of halothane on dP/dt, segment shortening, cardiac output, PRSW, and segment shortening. It is of some interest that amrinone was able to more completely reverse the negative inotropic effects of isoflurane than halothane, consistent with the more potent effect of halothane on left ventricular function.[45]

A number of studies have compared the effects of amrinone or milrinone and dobutamine mostly in patients with refractory severe heart failure (NYHA III/IV). Monrad and colleagues also included nitroprusside in 10 patients.[46] The problem with this study was that it was not blinded and the drugs were given in the same order (nitroprusside, dobutamine, milrinone) to each patient. All three drugs produced the same 30 to 40% increase in cardiac index. Both nitroprusside and milrinone caused decreases in arterial pressure and systemic vascular resistance as well as both right and left heart filling pressures without a change in heart rate, coronary blood flow, or myocardial oxygen consumption. In contrast, dobutamine increased heart rate, coronary blood flow, and myocardial oxygen consumption without affecting mean arterial pressure, systemic vascular resistance, or filling pressures. The investigators concluded that milrinone produced a positive inotropic effect because there was less of a decrease in vascular resistance and mean arterial pressure with milrinone than with sodium nitroprusside. The combination of vasodilation and positive inotropy appeared to be more beneficial than the more pronounced inotropic effect of dobutamine in these patients. Gage et al. and Mager et al. studied both amrinone or milrinone and dobutamine in the same patients.[47,48] These investigations demonstrated similar effects characterized by increases in cardiac index and decreases in left ventricular filling pressure and systemic vascular resistance. In Gage's study, both drugs decreased mean arterial pressure, but amrinone produced a greater decrease in pressure than dobutamine. In contrast, Mager observed a greater reduction in blood pressure with dobutamine than with milrinone. There was also a greater increase in heart rate and less increase in stroke volume index as well as a slower response of filling pressures with dobutamine compared with milrinone. Milrinone produced a better maintenance of cardiac index over a prolonged period than did dobutamine in Mager's study.

Two other investigations randomized the administration of either milrinone or amrinone and dobutamine.[49,50] Biddle et al. in a multicenter study titrated either milrinone or dobutamine in an intensive care unit to achieve a cardiac index >2.15 liters/min/m^2 or pulmonary capillary wedge pressure <15 mm Hg by 48 hours.[50] These investigators observed similar effects of the two drugs at 24 and 48 hours. However, between 3 and 12 hours after drug administration, dobutamine caused more of an increase in heart rate and milrinone more of a decrease in capillary wedge pressure and mean arterial pressure. There was an equal incidence of troublesome ventricular arrhythmias. Marcus et al. observed a greater increase in heart rate and decrease in right atrial pressure with amrinone compared with dobutamine over a 48-hour period.[49] Stroke volume index was greater with dobutamine, but the pulmonary capillary wedge pressure was decreased in a higher percentage of amrinone-treated patients. All patients treated with amrinone diuresed over the 48-hour period, while only 78% of the dobutamine patients did so. They concluded that amrinone was a more effective drug in this patient population. Eichhorn et al. compared with the effect of dobutamine and milrinone on right ventricular function[51] using a protocol similar to that of their previous study of amrinone and nitroprusside.[39] There was no evidence of right ventricular dysfunction in these patients although all were in severe heart failure (NYHA III/IV). Both drugs produced significant increases in cardiac index and right ventricular ejection fraction, but milrinone accomplished this mostly by a decrease in right ventricular afterload with decreases in pulmonary artery pressure and pulmonary vascular resistance as well as systemic vascular resistance. Dobutamine did not change pulmonary artery pressure, pulmonary vascular resistance, or systemic vascular resistance.[51]

Whenever the combination of β-agonists (epinephrine, dobutamine) and phosphodiesterase inhibitors (amrinone, milrinone) has been studied an additive effect has been shown. Despite the fact that both drugs act through the same final common mechanism namely increase in cAMP, there appears to be a contractile reserve which is not mobilized individually by either drug. In particular, the intracoronary infusion of milrinone before dobutamine resulted in a marked potentiation of the effect of dobutamine in patients with severe heart failure.[22] Most investigations demonstrate that the phosphodiesterase inhibitors are more potent vasodilators than dobutamine.

Drugs That Increase Sodium Influx

The only useful positive inotropic drugs that inhibit the sodium-potassium sarcolemmal pump are the digitalis glycosides. These drugs are a mainstay for the chronic treatment of heart failure (see below), but there have been virtually no studies on the effect of digitalis in the acute treatment of heart failure. In a poorly designed study where either digoxin or dopamine was administered to patients in septic shock according to "doctors preference," 13 to 20 patients given a 10 μg/kg-bolus of digoxin showed a much greater increase in left ventricular stroke work with no change in ventricular filling pressure than 7 patients given a mean dose of 8 μg/kg/minute of dopamine.[52] The major indication for digoxin in the patient with acute heart failure is for control of heart rate during atrial fibrillation or atrial flutter.[11] It is the only effective antiarrhythmic drug under these circumstances that does not have a negative inotropic effect.

Another new compound that also produces an inotropic effect by increasing intracellular sodium concentration is vesnarinone.[53] This drug prolongs sodium channel opening which results in an increase in intracellular sodium. This effect still produces an increase in intracellular calcium concentration. It also has another mechanism and is not useful for acute treatment for heart failure but possibly for chronic therapy (see below).

Drugs That Prolong Action Potential Duration

There are a number of drugs that produce a positive inotropic effect (albeit small) by prolonging action potential duration of cardiac muscle. Prolongation of the action potential allows the voltage-dependent calcium channels to remain open for a longer period of time during the cardiac cycle, and this results in an increase in intracellular calcium concentration. Vesnarinone presumably has this effect. The positive inotropic effect of α_1-adrenergic agonists is partially mediated through prolongation of action potential duration as well.[54] Finally, the potassium channel blockers, a new class of antiarrhythmic drugs, also prolong action potential duration and hence hopefully may offer an effective antiarrhythmic drug without negative inotropic action and possibly with positive inotropic effects.[55] The reader will note that none of these compounds has been tested for acute treatment of heart failure and at this point are of academic interest only.

DRUGS THAT INCREASE THE SENSITIVITY OF THE CONTRACTILE PROTEINS TO CALCIUM

This is the newest area of pharmacological development of inotropic drugs. Many of these compounds also have other actions, especially phosphodiesterase-inhibiting properties. Most of the investigations to date have dealt with basic mechanisms and the treatment of chronic congestive heart failure, but there are two investigations that describe acute effects of these agents following intravenous administration. In one of the first studies of a reputedly pure myofibrillar calcium sensitizing drug known only as EMD60263, investigators at the cardiovascular research laboratory at the Thorax Center in Rotterdam described effects of this drug on function of segments of stunned myocardium.[56] They showed that increased calcium sensitization of myofibrils was particularly efficacious in reversing the effect of myocardial stunning (Fig. 6–9). "Stunned myocardium" represents a specific type of ven-

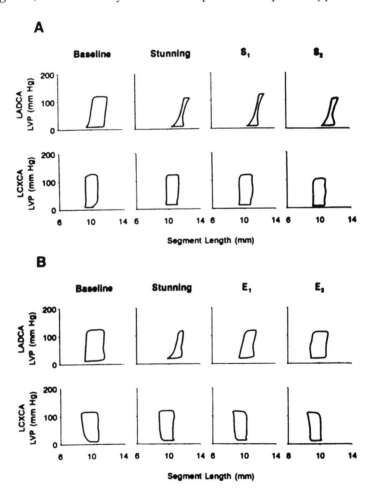

FIGURE 6-9. A representative left ventricular pressure/segment length loop in pigs with stunned and normal areas of myocardium. S_1 and S_2 are saline treated; E_1 and E_2 are treated with 0.75 mg/kg and 1.5 mg/kg of the myofibrillar calcium-sensitizing drug EMD60263. LADCA, left anterior descending coronary artery; LCXCA, left circumflex coronary artery; LVP, left ventricular pressure. (*Reproduced with permission from Soci et al. Circulation 90:959–969, 1994*)

tricular failure, but this class of drugs may be useful for other types as well. At the 1993 American Heart Association Meeting, a Japanese group presented several investigations of a new calcium sensitizing agent, MCI 154 in human heart failure patients using pressure-volume loops and the calculated E_{MAX} to estimate ventricular contractility. They showed that this new agent was as efficacious in increasing E_{MAX} as dobutamine but with considerably less oxygen cost.[57,58] Warltier's laboratory studied the effect of another experimental calcium sensitizer, levosimendan, on ventricular function in autonomically blocked animals in the conscious and anesthetized (isoflurane and halothane) states.[59] Similar to the most widely investigated of these compounds in clinical studies, pimobendan, levosimendan is also a phosphodiesterase inhibitor. Levosimendan produced dose-related increases in heart rate, cardiac output, segment shortening, velocity of segment shortening, PRSW and left ventricular dP/dt, and decreases in left ventricular filling pressure and systemic vascular resistance. Similar effects were observed in both isoflurane- and halothane-anesthetized dogs. In fact in this preparation, this drug was the only compound that was capable of increasing most indices of ventricular function above preanesthetized controls in halothane-anesthetized animals.

In addition to pimobendan, another calcium-sensitizing drug which is under active clinical investigation (see below), it is of some interest that both the endogenous cytokine endothelin[60] and the α_1-adrenergic agonist phenylephrine[54] also produce inotropic effects by increasing the sensitivity of contractile proteins to calcium. Both compounds appear to accomplish this effect by increasing intracellular pH (decreasing intracellular hydrogen ion concentration). In addition, the α_1-agonists also phosphorylate the contractile proteins. The clinical significance of these effects is still controversial. Landzberg et al. studied the effect of intracoronary phenylephrine in patients with normal and failing ventricles.[61] Intracoronary phenylephrine produced a dose-related increase in left ventricular dP/dt in both groups of patients but was less effective in those patients with heart failure. Phenylephrine was also considerably less effective than dobutamine especially in normal subjects. Phentolamine markedly decreased the positive inotropic effect of phenylephrine, more so in patients with heart failure than in the normal subjects. The observation that a positive inotropic effect remained albeit reduced after phentolamine suggested that phenylephrine may have some β-adrenergic agonist properties. On the other hand, there was no documentation of the degree of α-adrenergic blockade produced by a single dose of phentolamine. One might expect that the α-adrenergic-stimulating effect would predominate in patients with heart failure considering the downregulation of β-receptors.[5] The positive inotropic effect of phenylephrine complicates all studies in which a phenylephrine infusion has been used for control of systemic arterial pressure (see above).

AGENTS THAT ACT THROUGH METABOLIC OR ENDOCRINE PATHWAYS

Most of the investigations that have demonstrated beneficial effects of metabolic interventions in heart failure have related to improving myocardial energetics as a result of ischemia. However, a recent study demonstrated that manipulation of myocardial metabolism can produce positive inotropic effects.[62] Dichloroacetate (50 mg/kg) and dobutamine (5 to 12.5 μg/kg/min were administered to ten patients with severe (NYHA III/IV) heart failure. Hemodynamics and coronary blood flow and metabolism were studied over 30 minutes. Dichloroacetate increased stroke volume, stroke work, and minute work while at the same time oxygen consumption was decreased. Therefore, left ventricular efficiency was markedly improved. In contrast, although dobutamine caused similar increases in stroke volume and minute work, it was associated with an increase in myocardial oxygen consumption and a decrease in mechanical efficiency.Dichloroacetate stimulates pyruvate dehydrogenase, thereby increasing lactate and glucose metabolism and inhibiting fatty acid metabolism. The effect of dichloracetate appears to be primarily related to metabolism and oxygen kinetics rather than to a direct effect on left ventricular function.

There has been considerable recent interest in the effect of thyroid hormone on ventricular function, especially after cardiopulmonary bypass. Some investigators have shown a decrease in plasma-free triiodothyronine (T_3) in patients undergoing coronary artery bypass graft surgery. In studies limited by small numbers, Novitsky's group has shown that the administration of T_3 after coronary artery bypass graft surgery and through the first 24 hours was associated with a significantly reduced use of conventional inotropic drugs and diuretics and improved stroke volume and cardiac output in patients with normal left ventricular ejection fractions.[63] Morkin's group has been especially active in investigating the interaction of thyroid hormone and myocardial function, but most of their work has been in animals. One of their latest investigations in rats with ischemic heart failure demonstrated that adding a T_3 analogue (DITPA) with relatively low metabolic but preserved inotropic activity to therapy with captopril improved left ventricular performance above that observed with angiotensin-converting enzyme inhibition alone.[64] There continues to be considerable interest in the use of thyroid hormone in the immediate postoperative period after cardiac surgery, but thus far there is minimal published evidence for efficacy.

ADVANCES IN THE USE OF INOTROPIC DRUGS FOR THE CHRONIC THERAPY OF CONGESTIVE HEART FAILURE

There are several large outcome studies which indicate that the positive inotropic drugs digoxin and vesnarinone are effective for the chronic therapy of congestive heart failure,[65,66] but studies of other positive inotropic drugs including phosphodiesterase inhibitors and the partial β-adrenergic agonist-antagonist xamoterol have demonstrated adverse outcomes.[33,67] Even the positive studies with digitalis, vesnarinone, and pimobendan[68] have suggested that the doses of these drugs which are effective may, in fact, not produce a positive inotropic response. The beneficial effects are related not to an increase of contractile function of failing hearts but rather to modifying the body's reflex responses to heart failure.[69] Whether the introduction of the new class of positive inotropic agents which sensitize the contractile proteins to calcium will reverse this trend remains to be seen. Currently however, the major therapeutic use for positive inotropic drugs is for the short-term management of acute heart failure.

SUMMARY

At the present time, there are no clinically effective drugs for the treatment of left ventricular dysfunction that only improve the performance of the myocardial contractile proteins. The most useful drugs for the treatment of acute ventricular failure are the β-adrenergic agonists isoproterenol, epinephrine, dopamine, dobutamine, and possibly dopexamine. All of these drugs either through β_2-adrenergic receptor activation or other nonadrenergic-mediated vasodilation also produce their beneficial effect on cardiac performance by reducing ventricular afterload via systemic vasodilation. In many instances, it is difficult to separate which of these mechanisms is of greater importance for any particular group of patients. Previously published studies suggest that vasodilation is the predominate effect in right ventricular failure while a direct positive inotropic action is more important in left ventricular failure, but this is certainly not a general principle. Even in the same types of ventricular failure, the positive inotropic drugs have different effects in different studies. For instance, sometimes the phosphodiesterase inhibitors produce more vasodilation and less positive inotropic effect than dobutamine; in other studies, the reverse appears to be true. The major generalizations concerning the currently available drugs for the treatment of acute ventricular failure are: 1) If bradycardia is a major factor, isoproterenol or perhaps epinephrine may be the drug of choice; 2) In patients with ischemic heart failure, a profound vasodilation produced by phosphodiesterase inhibitors and dobutamine may be deleterious for coronary perfusion; 3) Adding β-adrenergic agonists to phosphodiesterase inhibitors produces at least an additive and occasionally a synergistic effect. This combination is probably optimal for the treatment of severe resistant heart failure, and 4) Perhaps the new drugs that sensitize the contractile proteins to calcium will prove to be more efficacious than previous drugs. However, this remains to be determined.

There is evidence that suggests that the most efficacious drugs for the chronic treatment of congestive heart failure do not rely on positive inotropic actions but rather may modify cardiovascular reflex responses to heart failure. The significance of the positive inotropic effect of predominately vasoconstricting compounds such as α_1-adrenergic receptor agonists, angiotensin II, and endothelin remains to be investigated.

REFERENCES

1. Dorlands Illustrated Medical Dictionary, 25th ed. Philadelphia, WB Saunders, p. 785. 1974
2. Morgan JP: Abnormal intracellular modulation of calcium as a major cause of cardiac contractile dysfunction. N Engl J Med 325:625–632, 1991
3. Morgan JP, Arny RE, Allen PD, et al: Abnormal intracellular calcium handling, a major cause of systolic and diastolic dysfunction in ventricular myocardium from patients with heart failure. Circulation 81(suppl III):21–32, 1990
4. Feldman MD, Copeles L, Gwathmey JK, et al: Deficient production of cyclic AMP: Pharmacologic evidence of an important cause of contractile dysfunction in patients with end-stage heart failure. Circulation 75:331–339, 1987
5. Bristow MR, Ginsburg R, Umans V, et al: Beta$_1$ and beta$_2$ adrenergic receptor subpopulations in non-failing and failing human ventricular myocardium: Coupling of both receptor subtypes to muscle contraction and selective beta$_1$ receptor down-regulation in heart failure. Circ Res 59:297–309, 1986
6. Hysing ES, Chelly JE, Jacobson L, et al: Cardiovascular effects of acute changes in extracellular ionized calcium concentration induced by citrate and $CaCl_2$ infusions in chronically instrumented dogs conscious and during enflurane, halothane and isoflurane anesthesia. Anesthesiology 72:100–104, 1990
7. Pagel PS, Kampine JP, Schmelling WT, Warltier DC: Reversal of volatile

anesthetic-induced depression of myocardial contractility by extracellular calcium also enhances left ventricular diastolic function. Anesthesiology 78:141–154, 1993

8. Zaloga GP, Strickland RA, Butterworth JF, et al: Calcium attenuates epinephrine's beta adrenergic effects in postoperative heart surgery patients. Circulation 81:196–200, 1990
9. Butterworth JF, Zaloga GP, Prielipp RC, et al: Calcium inhibits the cardiac stimulating properties of dobutamine but not of amrinone. Chest 101:174–180, 1992
10. Royster RL, Butterworth JF, Prielipp RC, et al: A randomized blinded placebo-controlled evaluation of calcium chloride and epinephrine for inotropic support after emergence from cardiopulmonary bypass. Anesth Analg 74:3–13, 1992
11. Zaloga GP, Prielipp RC, Butterworth JF, Royster RL: Pharmacologic cardiovascular support. Crit Care Clin N.A. 9:335–362, 1993
12. Wynsen JC, Gross GJ, Brooks HL, Warltier DC: Changes in adrenergic pressor responses by calcium channel modulation in conscious dogs. Am J Physiol 253:H531–H539, 1987
13. Pagel PS, Hetrick DA, Warltier DC: Left ventricular mechanical consequences of dihydroperidine calcium channel modulation in conscious anesthetized chronically instrumented dogs. Anesthesiology 81:190–208, 1994
14. Levy JH: Support of the perioperative failing heart with preexisting ventricular dysfunction: Currently available options. J Cardiothor Vas Anesth 7(suppl 2):46–51, 1993
15. Butterworth JF, Prielipp RC, Royster RL, et al: Dobutamine increases heart rate more than epinephrine in patients recovering from aortocoronary bypass surgery. J Cardiothorac Vasc Anesth 6:535–541, 1992
16. Moran JL, O'Fathartaigh MS, Peisach AR, et al: Epinephrine as an inotropic agent in septic shock: A dose-profile analysis. Crit Care Med 21:70–77, 1993
17. Goldberg LI: Dopamine-clinical uses of an endogenous catecholamine. N Engl J Med 291:707–710, 1976
18. Tinker JH, Tarhan S, White RD, et al: Dopamine for inotropic support during emergencies from cardiopulmonary bypass. Anesthesiology 44:281–286, 1976
19. Steen PA, Tinker JH, Pluth JR, et al: Efficacy of dopamine, dobutamine and epinephrine during emergence from cardiopulmonary bypass in man. Circulation 57:378–384, 1978
20. VanTrigt P, Spray TL, Pasque MK, et al: The comparative effects of dopamine and dobutamine on ventricular mechanics after coronary artery bypass grafting: A pressure-dimension analysis. Circulation 70(suppl 1):112–117, 1984
21. Leier CV, Unverferth DV: Drugs five years latter: Dobutamine. Ann Intern Med 99:490–496, 1983
22. Colucci WS, Dennis AR, Leatherman GF, et al: Intracoronary infusion of dobutamine to patients with and without severe congestive heart failure. J Clin Invest 81:1103–1110, 1988
23. Vanoverschelde JJ, Wijns W, Essamri B, et al: Hemodynamic and mechanical determinates of myocardial O_2 consumption in normal human heart: Effects of dobutamine. Am J Physiol 265:H1884–H1892, 1993
24. Ferrario M, Poli A, Previtali M, et al: Hemodynamics of volume loading compared with dobutamine in severe right ventricular infarction. Am J Cardiol 74:329–333, 1994

25. Wynsen JC, O'Brien PD, Warltier DC: Zatebradine, a specific bradycardiac agent enhances the positive inotropic actions of dobutamine in ischemic myocardium. J Am Coll Cardiol 23:233–241, 1994

26. Henwood J, Todd PA: Ibopamine: A preliminary review of its pharmacodynamic and pharmacokinetic properties and therapeutic efficacy. Drugs 36:11–31, 1988

27. Rousseau MF, Raigoso J, vanEyll C, et al: Effects of intravenous epinine administration on left ventricular systolic performance, coronary hemodynamics and circulating catecholamines in patients with heart failure. J Cardiovasc Pharmacol 19:155–162, 1992

28. Bass AS, Kohli JD, Lubbers N, Goldberg LI: Mechanisms mediating the positive inotropic and chronotropic changes induced by dopexamine in the anesthetized dog. J Pharmacol 242:940–944, 1987

29. Leier CV, Binkley PF, Carpenter J, et al: Cardiovascular pharmacology of dopexamine in low output congestive heart failure. Am J Cardiol 62:94–99, 1988

30. Stephan H, Sonntag H, Henning H, Yoshimine K: Cardiovascular and renal hemodynamic effects of dopexamine: Comparison with dopamine. Br J Anaesth 65:380–387, 1990

31. Jaski BE, Peters C: Inotropic vascular and neuroendocrine effects of dopexamine hydrochloride and comparison with dobutamine. Am J Cardiol 62:63C–67C, 1988

32. Baumann G, Felix SB, Flick SAL: Usefulness of dopexamine hydrochloride versus dobutamine in chronic congestive heart failure and effects on hemodynamics and urine output. Am J Cardiol 65:748–754, 1990

33. The Xamoterol in Severe Heart Failure Group: Xamoterol in severe heart failure. Lancet 336:1–6, 1993

34. DeFeyter PJ, Serruys PW, Suryapranata H, et al: Improvement of left ventricular contractility and relaxation with beta 1 adrenergic receptor partial agonist Xamoterol at rest and during exercise in patients with post-infarction left ventricular dysfunction. Circulation 81(suppl III):99–106, 1990

35. Bristow MR, Ginsburg R, Strosberg A, et al: Pharmacology and inotropic potential of forskolin in the human heart. J Clin Invest 74:212–213, 1984

36. Skoyles JR, Sherry KM: Pharmacology, mechanism of action and uses of selective phosphodiesterase inhibitors. Br J Anaesth 68:293–302, 1992

37. Konstam MA, Cowan SR, Weiland DS, et al: Relative contribution of inotropic and vasodilator effects to amrinone-induced hemodynamic improvement in congestive heart failure. Am J Cardiol 57:242–248, 1986

38. Ludmer PL, Wright RF, Arnold MO, et al: Separation of direct myocardial and vasodilator actions of milrinone administered by intracoronary infusion technique. Circulation 73:130–137, 1986

39. Konstam MA, Cowan SR, Salem DN: Effect of amrinone on right ventricular function: Predominance of afterload reduction. Circulation 74:359–366, 1986

40. Levy JH, Bailey JM: Amrinone: Its effect on vascular resistance and capacitance in human subjects. Chest 105:62–64, 1994

41. Prielipp RC, Butterworth JF, Zaloga GP, et al: Effects of amrinone on cardiac index venous, oxygen saturation and venous admixture in patients recovering from cardiac surgery. Chest 99:820–825, 1991

42. Butterworth JF, Royster RL, Prielipp RC, et al: Amrinone in cardiac surgical patients with left ventricular dysfunction. Chest 104:1660–1667, 1993

43. Wright EM, Sherry KM: Clinical and haemodynamic effects of milrinone in

the treatment of low cardiac output after cardiac surgery. Bri J Anaesth 67:585–590, 1991

44. Royster RL, Butterworth JF, Prielipp RC, et al: Combined inotropic effects of amrinone and epinephrine after cardiopulmonary bypass in humans. Anesth Analg 77:662–672, 1993

45. Pagel PS, Hetrick DA, Warltier DC: Amrinone enhances myocardial contractility and improves left ventricular diastolic function in conscious and anesthetized chronically instrumented dogs. Anesthesiology 79:753–765, 1993

46. Monrad ES, Bain DS, Smith HS, Lanoue AS: Milrinone, dobutamine and nitroprusside: Comparative effects on hemodynamics and myocardial energetics in patients with severe congestive heart failure. Circulation 73 (suppl III):168–174, 1986

47. Gage J, Rutman H, Lucido D, LeJemtel TH: Additive effects of dobutamine and amrinone on myocardial contractility in ventricular performance in patients with severe heart failure. Circulation 74:367–373, 1986

48. Mager G, Klocke RK, Kux A, et al: Phosphodiesterase 3 inhibition or adrenoreceptor stimulation: Milrinone as an alternative to dobutamine in the treatment of severe heart failure. Am Heart J 121:1974–1983, 1991

49. Marcus RH, Raw K, Patel J, et al: Comparison of intravenous amrinone and dobutamine in congestive heart failure due to idiopathic dilated cardiomyopathy. Am J Cardiol 66:1107–1112, 1990

50. Biddle TL, Benotti JR, Creager MA, et al: Comparison of intravenous milrinone and dobutamine for congestive heart failure secondary to either ischemic or dilated cardiomyopathy. Am J Cardiol 59:1345–1350, 1987

51. Eichhorn EJ, Konstam MA, Weiland DS, et al: Differential effects of milrinone and dobutamine on right ventricular preload, afterload and systolic performance in congestive heart failure secondary to ischemic or idiopathic dilated cardiomyopathy. Am J Cardiol 60:1329–1333, 1987

52. Nasraway SA, Rackow E, Astiz ME, et al: Inotropic response to digoxin and dopamine in patients with severe sepsis, cardiac failure and systemic hypoperfusion. Chest 95:612–615, 1989

53. Iijima T, Taira N: Membrane current changes responsible for the positive inotropic effect of OPC-8212 a new positive inotropic in single ventricular cells of guinea pig heart. J Pharmacol 240:657–62, 1987

54. Terzic A, Puceat M, Vassort G, Vogel SM: Cardiac alpha 1 adrenal receptors: An overview. Pharmacol Rev 45:147–176, 1993

55. Singh BN: Arrhythmia control of prolonging repolarization: The concept and its potential therapeutic impact. Eur Heart J 14(suppl H):14–23, 1993

56. Soei LK, Sassen LMA, Fan DS, et al: Myofibrillar Ca** sensitization predominantly enhnaces function and mechanical efficiency of stunned myocardium. Circulation 90:959–969, 1994

57. Mori M, Taeuchi T, Takoaka H, et al: Oxygen saving effect of Ca** sensitization with a new cardiotonic agent MCI 154 on human diseased hearts. Circulation 88 (Part 4, No. 2):I300, 1993

58. Mori M, Taeuchi T, Takoaka H, et al: Beneficial effect of new cardiotonic agent MC 154 on mechanoenergetics in human diseased heart. Circulation 88(Part 4, No. 2):I301, 1993

59. Pagel PS, Harkin CP, Hetrick DA, Warltier DC: Levosminedan (OR-1259) a myofilament calcium sensitizer enhances myocardial contractility but does not alter isovolumic relaxation in conscious and anesthetized dog. Anesthesiology 81:974–981, 1994

60. Kramer BK, Nishida M, Kelly RA, Smith TW: Endothelins: Myocardial actions of a new class of cytokines. Circulation 85:350–356, 1992

61. Landzberg JS, Parker JD, Gauthier DF, Colucci WS: Effects of myocardial alpha 1 adrenergic receptor stimulation and blockade on contractility in humans. Circulation 84:1608–1614, 1991

62. Bersin, Wolfe C, Kwasman M, et al: Improved hemodynamic function and mechanical efficiency in congestive heart failure with sodium dichloroacetate. J Am Coll Cardiol 23:1617–1624, 1994

63. Novitzky D, Cooper DKC, Barton CI, et al: Triiodothyronine as an inotropic agent after open heart surgery. J Thorac Cardiovasc Surg 98:972–978, 1989

64. Pennock GD, Raya TE, Bahl JJ, et al: Combination treatment with captopril and the thyroid hormone analog 3, 5-diiodothyropropionic acid. Circulation 88:1289–1298, 1993

65. Kelley RA, Smith TW: Digoxin in heart failure implications of recent trials. J Am Coll Cardiol 22(suppl A):107–112A, 1993

66. Feldman AM, Bristow MR, Parmley WW, et al: Effects of vesnarinone on morbidity and mortality in patients with heart failure. N Engl J Med 329:149–155, 1993

67. Packer M, Carver JR, Rodeheffer RJ, et al: Effect of oral milrinone on mortality in severe chronic heart failure: The PROMISES Study Research Group. N Engl J Med 325:1468–1475, 1991

68. Kubo SH, Gollub S, Burge R, et al: Beneficial effects of pimobendan on exercise tolerance and quality of life in patients with heart failure. Circulation 85:942–949, 1992

69. Packer M: The development of positive inotropic agents for chronic heart failure: How have we gone astray? J Am Coll Cardiol 22 (suppl A):119–126A, 1993

Paul S. Pagel
David C. Warltier

7 Anesthetics and Left Ventricular Function

VOLATILE ANESTHETICS AND SYSTOLIC FUNCTION IN NORMAL MYOCARDIUM

Modern volatile anesthetics, including halothane, enflurane, and isoflurane, depress myocardial contractility in a dose-dependent manner in the isolated and intact heart. Classic investigations conducted in the mid-1960s convincingly demonstrated that halothane produces dose-related depression of force-velocity relations and ventricular function curves in isolated cardiac muscle preparations[1,2] and intact, closed-chest dogs,[3] respectively. These findings supported the clinical observations of several investigators who reported halothane-induced circulatory depression in humans.[4–7] Enflurane[8] and isoflurane[9] also decreased maximal velocity of shortening (V_{max}), peak-developed force, and maximal rate of force development (+dF/dt) during isotonic contraction in isolated cat papillary muscles consistent with myocardial depression. These studies in vitro indicated that enflurane and isoflurane produced direct negative inotropic effects which probably contributed to the cardiovascular depression observed with these agents in vivo.[10,11]

Although the contention that volatile anesthetics depress intrinsic inotropic state in vitro was well established by these early studies,[1,8,9] controversy remained concerning the relative degree of myocardial de-

Ventricular Function, edited by David C. Warltier. Williams & Wilkins, Baltimore © 1995.

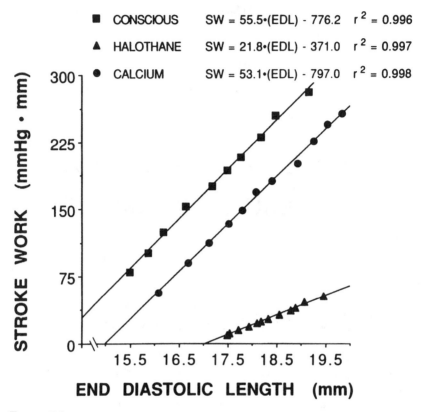

FIGURE 7-1. Regional stroke work (SW) vs end-diastolic segment length (EDL) relationship data in the conscious state, during 1.5 MACs of halothane, and following 5 mg·kg^{-1}·min^{-1} CaCl$_2$ during halothane anesthesia in a typical experiment. (*Reproduced with permission from Pagel PS et al. Anesthesiology 78:141–154,1993*)

pression produced by each of these agents. Iwatsuki and Shimosato[12] concluded that enflurane preserved contractility to a greater extent than halothane or methoxyflurane in vitro. Early studies of the cardiovascular effects of enflurane in humans suggested that enflurane produced minimal myocardial depression,[13–15] in direct contrast to halothane.[4–6] Other investigations used isovolumic and ejection phase measures of contractility and showed that enflurane and halothane caused very similar negative inotropic effects in dogs,[16–18] primates,[19] and humans.[11] These findings were later confirmed using the slope (E_{es}) of the end-systolic pressure-mid-axis diameter relation as a relatively loadindependent index of contractile state in chronically instru-

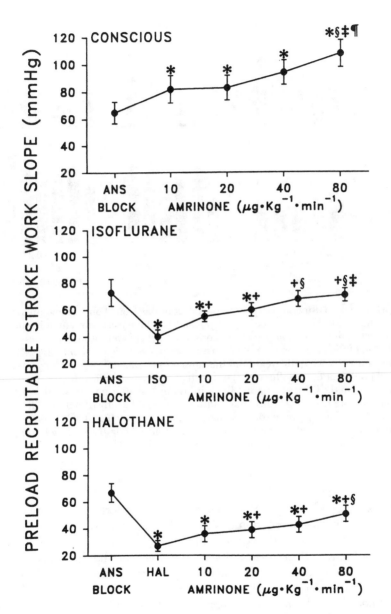

FIGURE 7-2. Preload recruitable stroke work slope (Mw) in conscious (*top panel*) and isoflurane- (ISO; *middle panel*) and halothane-anesthetized (HAL; *bottom panel*) dogs in the presence of pharmacological blockade of the autonomic nervous system (ANS *block*). *, significantly ($P < 0.05$) different from ANS block; †, significantly ($P < 0.05$) different from 1.25 MACs of isoflurane or halothane; §, significantly ($P < 0.05$) different from 10 $\mu g \cdot kg^{-1} \cdot min^{-1}$ amrinone; ‡, significantly ($P < 0.05$) different from 20 $\mu g \cdot kg^{-1} \cdot min^{-1}$ amrinone; ¶, significantly different from 40 $\mu g \cdot kg^{-1} \cdot min^{-1}$ amrinone. (*Reproduced with permission from Pagel PS et al. Anesthesiology 79:753–765, 1993*)

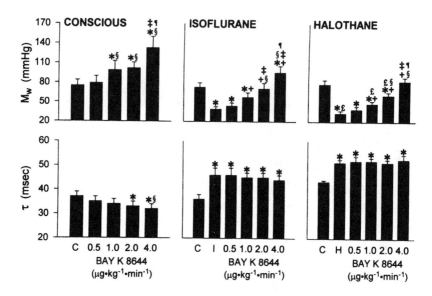

FIGURE 7-3. Histograms depicting the effect of Bay k 8644 on regional preload recruitable stroke work slope (*Mw; top panels*) and the time constant of isovolumic relaxation (τ; *bottom panels*) in conscious (*left column*), isoflurane-anesthetized (*middle column*), and halothane-anesthetized (*right column*) dogs. *, significantly (*P< 0.05*) different from the conscious (C) state; †, significantly (*P < 0.05*) different from isoflurane (*I*) or halothane (*H*); §, significantly (*P < 0.05*) different from the 0.5 μg·kg⁻¹·min⁻¹ Bay k infusion; ‡, significantly (*P < 0.05*) different from the 1.0 μg·kg⁻¹·min⁻¹ Bay k infusion; ¶, significantly (*P < 0.05*) different from the 2.0 μg·kg⁻¹·min⁻¹ Bay k infusion; £, significantly (*P < 0.05*) different from the corresponding value during isoflurane anesthesia. (*Reproduced with permission from Pagel PS et al. Anesthesiology 81:190–208, 1994*)

mented dogs.[20] Equi-MAC of halothane and enflurane were shown to depress contractile function to similar degrees in vivo.

In contrast to studies comparing the myocardial depressant effects of halothane with enflurane, several investigations have suggested differences in the degree of contractile depression produced by halothane and isoflurane in humans and experimental animals. Stevens et al.[10] examined the systemic hemodynamic effects of isoflurane in normocarbic, healthy volunteers and suggested that inasmuch as little change in cardiac output or the mean rate of ventricular ejection occurred with increasing doses of isoflurane, myocardial function must be relatively preserved. Nevertheless, dose-dependent declines in stroke volume were observed during isoflurane anesthesia which also occurred with halothane. Similar findings were reported in surgical patients.[21] Tarnow et al.[22] used left ventricular peak positive dP/dt to assess contrac-

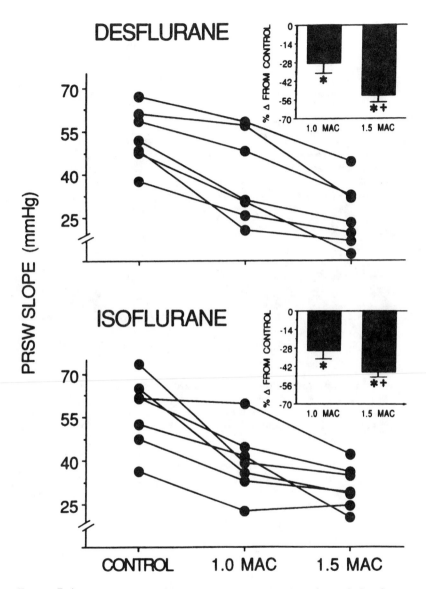

FIGURE 7–4.   Preload recruitable stroke work (PRSW) slope for each dog during control and at 1.0 and 1.5 end-tidal MACs of desflurane (*top*) and isoflurane (*bottom*). Insets depict percent changes from control. *, significantly (P < 0.05) different from control; †, significantly (P < 0.05) different from 1.0 MAC. (*Reproduced with permission from Pagel PS et al. Anesthesiology 74:900–907, 1991*)

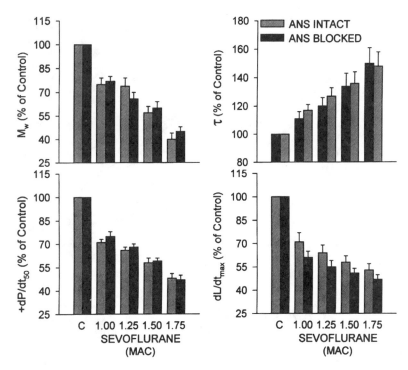

FIGURE 7-5. Comparison of the effects of sevoflurane on indices of left ventricular systolic and diastolic function in the absence and presence of autonomic nervous system (ANS) blockade (ANS-intact and ANS-blocked, respectively). Data are presented as percent of control before anesthesia (C). All data during sevoflurane in both ANS-intact and ANS-blocked groups are significantly ($P < 0.05$) different from C. At equivalent MAC, no differences between dogs with and without ANS function were observed. Mw, preload recruitable stroke work slope; τ, time constant of isovolumic relaxation; $dL/dtmax$, maximum segment lengthening velocity during rapid ventricular filling. (*Reproduced with permission from Harkin CP et al. Anesthesiology 81:156–167, 1994*)

tile state in geriatric patients and found less depression of contractility with isoflurane than with halothane. Interpretation of this study, however, was complicated by the presence of baseline intravenous anesthetics and neuromuscular blockade. M-mode transthoracic echocardiography has been used to noninvasively evaluate changes in fractional shortening and the mean velocity of circumferential fiber shortening during equi-MACs of halothane or isoflurane in healthy children.[23] Myocardial performance was decreased in a dose-dependent fashion when halothane was used but was not significantly altered when isoflurane was administered.[23] These studies strongly implied

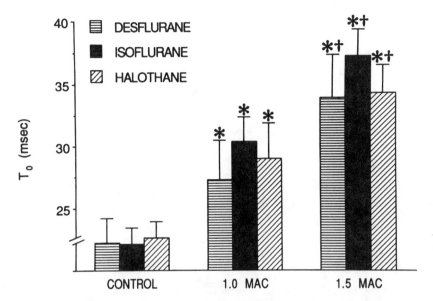

FIGURE 7-6. Effects of desflurane, isoflurane, and halothane on the time constant of isovolumic relaxation calculated using a zero decay assumption. *, significantly ($P < 0.05$) different from autonomically blocked, conscious control; †, significantly ($P < 0.05$) different from 1.0 MAC. (*Reproduced with permission from Pagel PS et al. Anesthesiology 74:1103–1114, 1991*)

that halothane depresses myocardial contractile function to a greater extent than equi-MAC isoflurane; however, lack of conscious control data, concomitant use of anesthetic adjuvants, differential direct and reflex effects of volatile anesthetics on the systemic circulation, and assessment of changes in contractile state using load-dependent or indirect indicators of left ventricular function represented important qualifications in these investigations.

Horan *et al*[24] Merin,[25] and Pagel et al.[18] used isovolumic indices of contractility to evaluate the effects of halothane and isoflurane on myocardial performance in chronically instrumented dogs. Horan et al.[24] showed significant differences in left ventricular dP/dt (40%) and maximum aortic acceleration (32%) when nearly equi-MAC halothane (1.0%) and isoflurane (1.2%) were directly compared in the same study. Similar differences in contractile function were inferred in separate investigations by Merin and coworkers[25,26] using nearly identical protocols, although the direct effects of the volatile anesthetics on the systemic circulation or reflex actions mediated through the autonomic nervous system could not be entirely excluded from the analysis. More recently, Pagel et al.[18] also demonstrated significant differences in con-

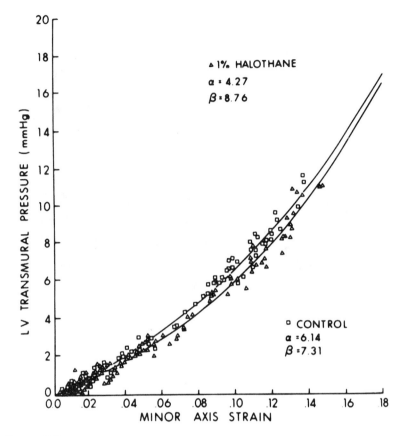

FIGURE 7-7. Left ventricular diastolic transmural pressure-Lagrangian strain relation in a conscious (*open squares*) and halothane-anesthetized (*open triangles*)
dog. The pressure-strain relation qualitatively shifted to the left during halothane
anesthesia, but this shift was not statistically significant, indicating that halothane
does not produce alterations in intrinsic myocardial stiffness. α, gain; β, modulus
of myocardial stiffness. (*Reproduced with permission from Van Trigt P et al. J
Thorac Cardiovasc Surg* 85:832–838, 1983)

tractility between isoflurane and halothane in dogs using left ventricular dP/dt_{max} and dP/dt_{50} in the presence and absence of autonomic
nervous system function, suggesting that differences in myocardial depression caused by these agents occurred independent of autonomic reflexes. These investigations strongly implied a difference between the
negative inotropic effects of halothane and isoflurane despite the use of
indices of contractile state which are influenced by heart rate and ventricular loading conditions.

This suspected difference in the negative inotropic effects of halo-

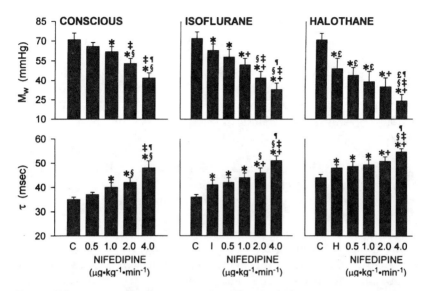

FIGURE 7-8. Histograms depicting the effect of nifedipine on regional preload recruitable stroke work slope (*Mw; top panels*) and the time constant of isovolumic relaxation (τ; *bottom panels*) in conscious (*left column*), isoflurane-anesthetized (*middle column*), and halothane-anesthetized (*right column*) dogs. *, significantly (P < 0.05) different from the conscious (C) state; †, significantly (P < 0.05) different from isoflurane (I) or halothane (H); §, significantly (P < 0.05) different from the 0.5 µg·kg⁻¹·min⁻¹ nifedipine infusion; ‡, significantly (P < 0.05) different from the 1.0 µg·kg⁻¹·min⁻¹ nifedipine infusion; ¶, significantly (P < 0.05) different from the 2.0 µg·kg⁻¹·min⁻¹ nifedipine infusion; £, significantly (P < 0.05) different from the corresponding value during isoflurane anesthesia. (*Reproduced with permission from Pagel PS et al. Anesthesiology 81:190–208,1994*)

thane and isoflurane was later quantified using the slope of the regional preload recruitable stroke work (PRSW) relation and a stroke work analog of the end-systolic pressure-segment length relationship (ES-PLR area) in chronically instrumented dogs with pharmacological blockade of the autonomic nervous system.[27] Isoflurane maintained a contractile state an average of 22% higher as compared to equi-MAC halothane using these models.[27] These findings were subsequently confirmed with a regional PRSW slope using end-tidal anesthetic concentrations in dogs with intact autonomic nervous system function,[28] indicating that differential depression of contractility by halothane and isoflurane was probably unrelated to differences in anesthetic-induced alterations in underlying autonomic tone. These results require qualification, however, because the incorporation of data from the entire cardiac cycle implicit in the PRSW relation does not exclude potential differential effects of halothane and isoflurane on diastolic mechanical properties from the analysis of systolic contractile behavior.[29] The negative inotropic actions of isoflurane and halothane are exacerbated by hypocalcemia,[30] Ca^{2+} channel-blocking agents,[31–33] or β_1-adrenoceptor antagonists[33] and can be reversed with administration of exogenous calcium,[30,34–36] cardiac phosphodiesterase inhibitors,[37,38] the Ca^{2+} channel agonist, Bay k 8644,[32] and a myofilament Ca^{2+} sensitizer, levosimendan.[39] The differential effects of halothane and isoflurane on myocardial contractility were maintained during depression or enhancement of the inotropic state produced by vasoactive drugs in the majority of these studies.

These findings in vivo are supported by a growing body of evidence in vitro that also implies a difference in the contractile depression caused by isoflurane and halothane based on differential modulation of intracellular calcium (Ca^{2+}) homeostasis at several subcellular targets within the cardiac myocyte (see Chapter 1).[40] Isoflurane and halothane have been shown to inhibit the transsarcolemmal Ca^{2+} transient resulting from membrane depolarization to differing degrees by affecting the function, reducing the number, or interfering with the dihydropyridine-binding sites of voltage-dependent Ca^{2+} channels.[41–46] This partial inhibition of Ca^{2+} influx via sarcolemmal Ca^{2+} channels responsible for the initiation of mechanical systole has several important consequences, including declines in the availability of Ca^{2+} for contractile activation, depression of Ca^{2+}-dependent Ca^{2+} release from the sarcoplasmic reticulum (SR), and reduction of the amount of Ca^{2+} that can be subsequently stored in the SR.[40] Volatile anesthetics also reduce the concentration of intracellular Ca^{2+} during systole by direct alteration of SR function. Isoflurane and halothane provoke enhanced leak of Ca^{2+} from the SR,[47,48] contributing to decreases in accumulation of intracellular Ca^{2+} during systole. Recent evidence suggests that halothane may cause a more pronounced SR Ca^{2+} leak than isoflurane[49] mediated in part by a differential activation at the SR Ca^{2+} release channel.[50] This represents another important mechanism by which halothane depresses myocardial contractility to a greater extent than isoflurane. Volatile anesthetics may also differentially modify the responsiveness of contractile proteins to activator Ca^{2+}, although recent studies fail to support this hypothesis.[39,51–53]

The cardiovascular effects of desflurane have been the subject of intense research in recent years. Desflurane produces a systemic and coronary hemodynamic profile which is remarkably similar to that of isoflurane during steady-state conditions[54]; however, desflurane may also produce transient tachycardia and hypertension concomitant with rapid changes in the inspired anesthetic concentration.[55,56] Using isovolumic and ejection phase measures of contractility, several investi-

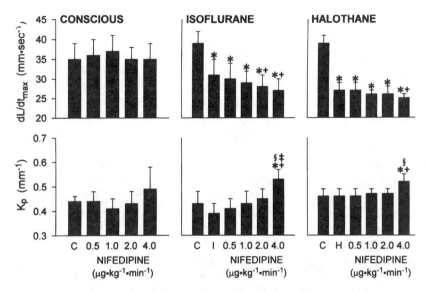

FIGURE 7-9. Histograms depicting the effects of nifedipine on maximum segment lengthening velocity (*dL/dtmax; top panels*) and the regional chamber stiffness constant (K_p; *bottom panels*) in conscious (*left column*), isoflurane-anesthetized (*middle column*), and halothane-anesthetized (*right column*) dogs. *, significantly ($P < 0.05$) different from the conscious (C) state; †, significantly ($P < 0.05$) different from isoflurane (I) or halothane (H); §, significantly ($P < 0.05$) different from the 0.5 µg·kg⁻¹·min⁻¹ nifedipine infusion; ‡, significantly ($P < 0.05$) different from the 1.0 µg·kg⁻¹·min⁻¹ nifedipine infusion. (*Reproduced with permission from Pagel PS et al. Anesthesiology 81:190–208, 1994*)

gators[18,57–59] concluded that desflurane and isoflurane depress myocardial function to nearly equivalent degrees. This contention was supported by investigations from our laboratory using the slope of the PRSW relation as an assay of intrinsic inotropic state in chronically instrumented dogs. In these studies, desflurane and isoflurane decreased myocardial contractility equally in the presence[60] and absence[61] of autonomic nervous system reflexes. These observations were further supported by Boban et al.[62] in the isolated guinea pig heart. The cardiovascular stimulation associated with rapid changes in inspired desflurane concentrations may lead to transient increases in myocardial contractility resulting from augmentation of sympathetic nervous system tone in humans; however, this hypothesis has yet to be systematically examined.

The cardiovascular effects of another new volatile anesthetic, sevoflurane, have been incompletely studied. Bernard et al.[63] compared the systemic and coronary hemodynamic actions of sevoflurane to those produced by isoflurane in dogs. Using dP/dt_{max} as an index of inotropic state, the investigators demonstrated that the effect of sevoflurane on myocardial contractile function was virtually indistinguishable from that produced by isoflurane.[63] Other reports in humans[64] and experimental animals[65,66] have supported these findings and have suggested that sevoflurane may produce less cardiac depression than halothane. A recent study using transthoracic and transesophageal echocardiography also demonstrated that sevoflurane causes less myocardial depression than equi-MAC enflurane in volunteers using the heart rate-corrected velocity of circumferential fiber shortening vs left ventricular end-systolic wall stress relation as a noninvasively derived index of contractile state.[67] An investigation from our laboratory examined the effects of sevoflurane on myocardial contractility in the presence and absence of autonomic nervous system tone using the slope of the regional PRSW relation as an index of contractile state.[68] Sevoflurane decreased contractile function to approximately 40 to 45% of control values at 1.75 MAC. This magnitude of myocardial depression has been previously reported by our laboratory for isoflurane and desflurane using an identical experimental preparation.[60,61] Thus, modern volatile anesthetics appear to depress contractile state in normal ventricular myocardium in the following order: halothane = enflurane > isoflurane = desflurane = sevoflurane.

VOLATILE ANESTHETICS AND DIASTOLIC FUNCTION

The actions of potent inhalational anesthetics on diastolic function in the normal heart have been incompletely studied. Cardiac function during diastole has become the focus of intense experimental and clinical research in recent years because of increasing awareness that left ventricular performance during this phase of the cardiac cycle significantly influences the mechanical activity of the heart. Although abnormalities in diastolic function can usually be directly linked to systolic dysfunction, cardiac failure may result from primary diastolic dysfunction in the absence of or before the appearance of alterations in left ventricular systolic function in a variety of disease processes, including ischemic heart disease, hypertrophic or infiltrative cardiomyopathy, and hypertensive heart disease.[69] Halothane, isoflurane, enflurane, and the new volatile anesthetics, desflurane and sevoflurane, produce dose-related prolongation of isovolumic relaxation in vivo.[68,70-72] This delay of isovolumic relaxation is associated with declines in early ventricular filling[32,36,37,39,68] but probably is not of sufficient magnitude to interfere with overall chamber stiffness. The significance of delayed

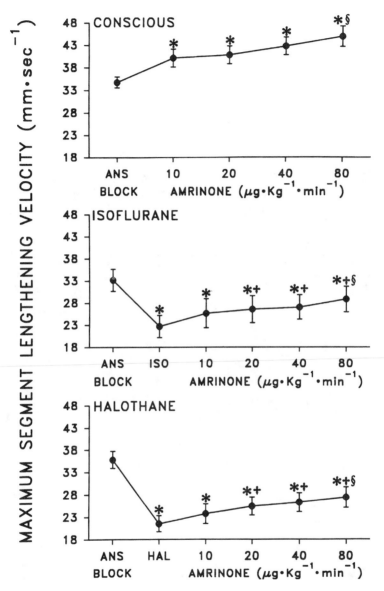

FIGURE 7-10. The time constant of isovolumic relaxation (τ) in conscious (*top panel*) and isoflurane- (*ISO; middle panel*) or halothane- (*HAL; bottom panel*) anesthetized dogs in the presence of pharmacological blockade of the autonomic nervous system (*ANS block*). *, significantly ($P < 0.05$) different from ANS block; †, significantly ($P < 0.05$) different from 1.25 MACs of isoflurane or halothane; §, significantly ($P < 0.05$) different from 10 μg·kg^{-1}·min^{-1} amrinone; ‡, significantly ($P < 0.05$) different from 20 μg·kg^{-1}·min^{-1} amrinone. (*Reproduced with permission from Pagel PS et al. Anesthesiology 79:753–765, 1993*)

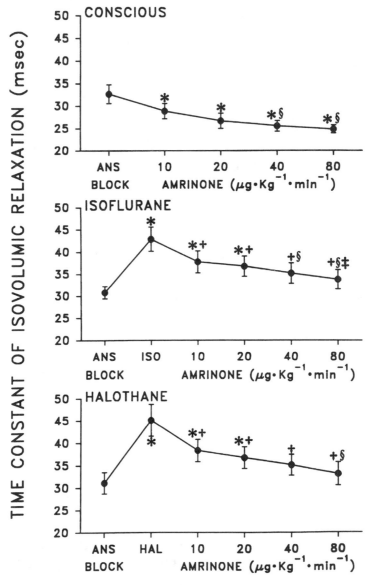

FIGURE 7-11. Maximum segment lengthening velocity during rapid ventricular filling (*dL/dtmax*) in conscious (*top panel*) and isoflurane (ISO; *middle panel*) or halothane (HAL; *bottom panel*) anesthetized dogs in the presence of pharmacological blockade of the autonomic nervous system (ANS *block*). *, significantly (P < 0.05) different from ANS block; †, significantly (P < 0.05) different from 1.25 MACs of isoflurane or halothane; §, significantly (P < 0.05) different from 10 μg·kg⁻¹·min⁻¹ amrinone. (*Reproduced with permission from Pagel PS et al. Anesthesiology 79:753–765, 1993*)

relaxation to early coronary blood flow has also not been thoroughly investigated with volatile anesthetics. Coronary flow is highest during this period of diastole, and an experimental study in dogs has suggested that delays in isovolumic relaxation lead to impairment of flow during halothane anesthesia.[71]

Isoflurane, desflurane, and sevoflurane do not alter invasively derived regional myocardial or chamber stiffness,[68,72] indicating that intrinsic ventricular distensibility may be unchanged by these agents. Although some indirect evidence suggests that halothane affects diastolic compliance, this conclusion has been disputed by more recent investigations using invasively derived measures of passive ventricular filling. Halothane decreases myocardial compliance in isolated rat left ventricular muscle subjected to paired electrical stimulation in vitro.[73] Increases in left ventricular end-diastolic volume as assessed with high-speed, biplane cineradiography are also observed following administration of halothane to dogs.[74] Halothane, but not morphine sulfate nor regional major conduction blockade, results in depression of stroke volume at equivalent left ventricular end-diastolic pressures following cardiopulmonary bypass in acutely instrumented swine. The latter finding indirectly suggests a halothane-induced decrease in ventricular compliance.[75] In contrast, dynamic stiffness of the series elastic element of myocardium was unaltered by halothane in isolated cat papillary muscle.[1] No differences in passive compliance (characterized by a monoexponential pressure-volume relationship) were observed during administration of 1 vs 2 MACs of halothane to acutely instrumented, open-chest dogs.[76] Halothane (1 to 2%) did not change the end-diastolic-minor axis strain relationship, indicating that halothane does not alter end-diastolic myocardial stiffness.[77] Halothane but not isoflurane nor desflurane was shown to produce a significant increase in passive regional chamber stiffness calculated using a monoexponential ventricular pressure-segment length relationship.[72] This effect was not dose-dependent and may have resulted secondary to increases in left ventricular end-diastolic pressure and decreases in systolic contractile performance and heart rate.[78] The actions of enflurane on diastolic compliance have yet to be thoroughly characterized. Thus, although volatile anesthetics have been shown to prolong isovolumic relaxation and impede early ventricular filling in a dose-related fashion, it seems unlikely that these agents, with the possible exception of halothane, affect overall ventricular compliance in vivo.

Relaxation of cardiac muscle requires the removal of Ca^{2+} from the troponin C binding sites, allowing dissociation of actin-myosin cross-bridges and restoration of the inhibitory action of the troponin-tropomyosin regulatory complex (see Chapter 1). Removal of Ca^{2+} from the intracellular environment of the contractile proteins is accomplished by adenosine triphosphate (ATP)-dependent Ca^{2+} pumps in the SR and the sarcolemmal membrane and by sarcolemmal exchange of sodium (Na+) for Ca^{2+}.[79] Because Ca^{2+} extrusion mechanisms are enzyme and energy-dependent, the process of Ca^{2+} uptake by the SR and extrusion from the myoplasm is relatively slow compared with the delivery of activator Ca^{2+} during systole. Relaxation proceeds very rapidly under normal circumstances because of the high concentration of Ca^{2+} pumps in the SR. However, the potential for the myoplasm to accumulate Ca^{2+} clearly exists when energy supplies are diminished or when functional abnormalities of the sarcolemmal membrane, the SR, the troponin-tropomyosin regulatory proteins, or the contractile filaments are present. Such a Ca^{2+} release-sequestration mismatch may impair relaxation.[80,81] Altered binding of Ca^{2+} to troponin C may also represent a factor in the kinetics of Ca^{2+} removal from the myoplasm.[82] The mechanical consequences of impaired relaxation may be partially manifested by attenuation of early ventricular filling and decreased chamber compliance.[83]

Abnormalities in intracellular Ca^{2+} homeostasis resulting from downregulation or dysfunction of Ca^{2+} channels in the sarcolemma and the SR and altered structural integrity of and response to activator Ca^{2+} by contractile proteins are characteristic findings in failing myocardium associated with diastolic dysfunction.[84] The mechanisms responsible for the negative lusitropic effects of volatile anesthetics have yet to be fully described but probably involve acute alteration of similar subcellular targets.[40] Volatile anesthetics partially inhibit voltage-dependent transsarcolemmal Ca^{2+} influx,[41–45,85] precipitating declines in Ca^{2+}-dependent Ca^{2+} release from and subsequent storage of Ca^{2+} in the SR.[40] These actions cause net decreases in the amount of Ca^{2+} available for contractile activation[86] and depress the activity of Ca^{2+}-dependent calmodulin kinase II, an enzyme which stimulates phosphorylation of the troponin I subunit of the troponin-tropomyosin regulatory complex and the regulatory proteins of the SR (phospholamban) and sarcolemmal Ca^{2+} ATPases.[87] Phosphorylation of these key intracellular moieties leads to declines in Ca^{2+} affinity for troponin C, increased Ca^{2+} uptake by the SR, and enhanced Ca^{2+} extrusion from the myoplasm through the sarcolemmal membrane, respectively, thereby accelerating relaxation of the cardiac myocyte. Thus, volatile anesthetic-induced declines in Ca^{2+} availability not only lead to depression of myocardial contractility but also may contribute to delays in relaxation concomitant with decreased activity of Ca^{2+}-dependent calmodulin kinase II. Potent inhalational anesthetics also disrupt intracellular Ca^{2+} regulation by direct functional alteration of the SR. Volatile anesthetics have been shown to enhance Ca^{2+} leakage from this organelle,[47–49] mediated in part by activation of the SR Ca^{2+} release channel.[50] These ef-

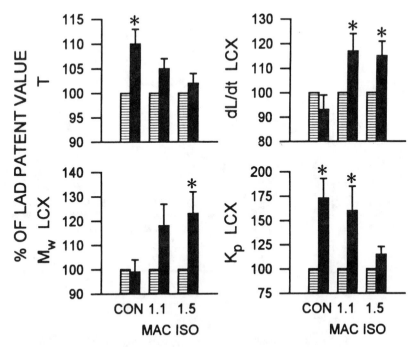

FIGURE 7-12.   Histograms depicting the influence of left anterior descending coronary artery (LAD) occlusion on the time constant of isovolumic relaxation (T), preload recruitable stroke work slope (Mw) in the perfusion territory of the left circumflex coronary artery (LCX), LCX regional maximum segment lengthening velocity during rapid ventricular filling (dL/dt), and LCX regional chamber stiffness (Kp) before (LAD patent) and during (LAD occluded) 2-minute occlusion of the LAD in the conscious state (CON) and during 1.1 and 1.5 MACs of isoflurane (ISO) anesthesia. *, significantly ($P < 0.05$) different from corresponding LAD patent value. (*Reproduced with permission from Pagel PS et al. Anesth Analg, in press, 1995*)

fects may effectively prolong diastolic Ca^{2+} clearance and delay relaxation. Volatile anesthetics have recently been demonstrated to inhibit the activity of plasma membrane Ca^{2+} ATPases in red blood cells.[88] In cardiac muscle, this inhibition of energy-dependent Ca^{2+} transport may also lead to prolonged relaxation. Thus, volatile anesthetics acutely produce abnormal handling of intracellular Ca^{2+} during systole and diastole, mechanisms which are probably responsible for depression of myocardial contractility, prolongation of isovolumic relaxation, and delayed early ventricular filling observed in vivo.

A recent series of experiments examined the interaction of pharmacological modulators of myocardial Ca^{2+} regulation and volatile

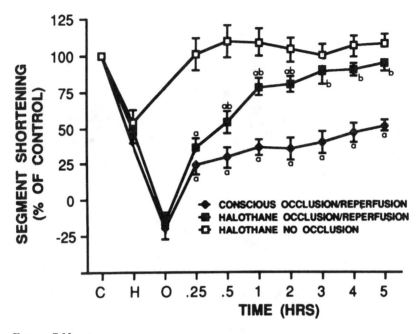

FIGURE 7-13. Segment shortening data (expressed as a percent of control) during coronary artery occlusion (O) and at various times following reperfusion in the conscious (C) and halothane-anesthetized (H) states. Comparisons are made at various time points to those animals anesthetized with halothane for 2.25 hours and allowed to emerge from anesthesia over a 5-hour period but not undergoing coronary artery occlusion and reperfusion. (*Reproduced with permission from Warltier et al. Anesthesiology 69:552–565, 1988*)

anesthetics on left ventricular systolic and diastolic function. The negative lusitropic properties of volatile anesthetics were reversed by exogenous calcium chloride.[36] In contrast, the slow Ca^{2+} channel antagonist, nifedipine, exacerbated volatile anesthetic-induced diastolic dysfunction, causing prolongation of isovolumic relaxation and attenuation of early ventricular filling.[32] These investigations emphasized the importance of the intracellular Ca^{2+} concentration in the determination of both systolic and diastolic performance. Amrinone, a cardiac phosphodiesterase III (PDE) inhibitor, enhanced isovolumic relaxation and rapid ventricular filling in the presence of volatile anesthetics,[37] consistent with the cyclic adenosine monophosphate (cAMP)-induced, protein kinase A-mediated phosphorylation of the SR regulatory protein, phospholamban, and the troponin I subunit of the troponin-tropomyosin complex.[89–91] In contrast, levosimendan, a myofilament Ca^{2+} sensitizer with PDE III-inhibiting activity, did not alter volatile anesthetic-induced increases in the time constant of isovolumic relaxation (τ).[39] These findings indicated that stabilization of Ca^{2+}-induced changes in troponin C produced by levosimendan[92] blunted anticipated declines in τ associated with the direct positive inotropic effect of the drug. Similar findings were observed with administration of Bay k 8644, a Ca^{2+} channel agonist. Bay k 8644 caused dose-dependent increases in myocardial contractility in anesthetized dogs but did not reverse abnormalities in isovolumic relaxation and early ventricular filling.[32] Under these conditions, the combination of increased SR permeability to Ca^{2+} produced by volatile anesthetics[47,48] and Bay k 8644[93] may have caused inefficient SR sequestration of Ca^{2+} and precipitated relative delays in relaxation which could not be overcome by the positive inotropic effects of the Ca^{2+} channel agonist. The diastolic functional effects of levosimendan and Bay k could not be completely explained by alterations in systemic hemodynamics[94] produced by these vasoactive drugs in the presence of isoflurane and halothane. Thus, the experiments with levosimendan and Bay k 8644 demonstrated that reversal of volatile anesthetic-induced depression of myocardial contractility is not always accompanied by improvement of indices of diastolic performance and provided indirect evidence to support the hypothesis that abnormalities in diastolic function caused by potent inhalational anesthetics are not solely related to depression of systolic function in normal myocardium.

MECHANICAL EFFECTS OF VOLATILE ANESTHETICS IN CARDIAC DISEASE

The effects of isoflurane[9] and enflurane[95] on the mechanics of isolated cat papillary muscle from normal hearts and those with congestive heart failure precipitated by chronic exposure to pressure overload have been compared. Decreases in V_{max} and $+dF/dt$ were observed in both groups in response to isoflurane and enflurane; however, papillary muscles from failing hearts demonstrated significantly greater depression than those from normal hearts. The findings demonstrated that the combined negative inotropic effects of volatile anesthetics and failing myocardium were more pronounced than the actions of isoflurane or enflurane alone.[9,95] The investigations also provided important experimental evidence to support the hypothesis that patients with underlying global contractile dysfunction may be more sensitive to the myocardial depressant properties of volatile anesthetics. In experimental models of regional myocardial ischemia[96] or infarction,[97] however, declines in contractile function caused by volatile anesthetics were well tolerated and did not precipitate frank systolic dysfunction.

These studies implied that the extent of regional ischemia or infarction may be an important factor in determining the overall functional consequences imposed by volatile anesthetics.

Volatile anesthetics may have beneficial effects during myocardial ischemia and reperfusion injury. Halothane attenuated ST segment changes caused by brief coronary artery occlusion[98,99] and decreased ST segment elevation to a greater extent than propranolol and sodium nitroprusside despite producing similar hemodynamic effects.[99] Halothane reduced myocardial infarct size after ligation of the left anterior descending (LAD) coronary artery in dogs.[100] Enflurane decreased lactate production by canine hearts with an 80% LAD stenosis when perfusion pressure was artificially controlled.[101] A recent investigation from our laboratory[102] examined the effects of isoflurane and desflurane on regional contractile function in ischemic (perfusion territory of the LAD) and nonischemic (myocardium perfused by the left circumflex (LCX) coronary artery) zones during brief (2-min) LAD occlusion using the PRSW relation in chronically instrumented dogs. The preliminary findings of this study suggested that mechanical compensation in the normal LCX zone during acute LAD ischemia is not depressed and may actually be enhanced in the presence of isoflurane and desflurane. In addition, regional indices of rapid ventricular filling and chamber stiffness in the normal zone were not adversely affected by these anesthetics during brief LAD occlusion, indicating that diastolic properties are also preserved during isoflurane and desflurane anesthesia.

Halothane,[103–105] enflurane,[106] and isoflurane[105] decreased myocardial reperfusion injury and improved functional recovery after global ischemia in isolated hearts. Volatile anesthetics have also been shown to enhance systolic functional recovery of stunned myocardium when these agents are administered prior to and during,[107] but not after,[108,109] brief periods of myocardial ischemia in vivo. Isoflurane-induced improvement of regional myocardial contractility in ischemia-reperfusion injury is accompanied by preservation of high-energy phosphate levels.[110] Halothane, isoflurane, and enflurane have been shown to attenuate the effect of oxygen-derived free radicals on the development of left ventricular isovolumic pressure in isolated rabbit hearts, suggesting that volatile anesthetics may protect myocardium against free radical-induced damage by limiting intracellular Ca^{2+} accumulation.[111] In addition, halothane preserved contractile function and ultrastructural integrity in isolated rat hearts during reperfusion after normothermic cardioplegic arrest, protective effects which were attributed to a reduction in excessive intracellular Ca^{2+} accumulation.[112]

The mechanisms responsible for volatile anesthetic-induced cardioprotection during myocardial ischemia and reperfusion are incompletely understood. Because potent inhalational agents cause direct negative inotropic and chronotropic effects and decrease left ventricular afterload, the beneficial effects of volatile anesthetics may be attributed to a favorable reduction in myocardial oxygen demand required for active contraction with concomitant relative preservation of energy-dependent vital cellular processes. However, halothane also exerts protective effects during complete functional arrest induced by cardioplegia, indicating that preferential alterations in myocardial oxygen supply-demand relations are not solely responsible for the antiischemic actions of this anesthetic.[112] Halothane may significantly lower excessive intracellular Ca^{2+} during reperfusion via a direct decline in the net transsarcolemmal Ca^{2+} transient resulting from partially inhibited voltage-dependent Ca^{2+} channel activity[41–46] or an indirect reduction of oxygen-derived free radical formation.[111] Although some evidence exists supporting the hypothesis that the slow Ca^{2+} channel plays a role in ischemia and reperfusion-induced Ca^{2+} accumulation,[113,114] other studies using Ca^{2+} channel antagonists indicate that the Ca^{2+} channel is not involved in this process.[115,116] It also appears unlikely that volatile anesthetics reduce the concentration of intracellular Ca^{2+} during reperfusion by effects on the SR because these agents contribute to increases in SR calcium leak[47,48] and enhance Ca^{2+} flux through the Ca^{2+} release channel of this organelle in normal myocardium.[50] The cardioprotective effects of volatile anesthetics may be mediated through sodium $(Na+)$-Ca^{2+} exchange mechanisms during reperfusion[112] or activation of ATP-dependent potassium channels $(K+_{ATP})$,[117,118] but experimental evidence for these hypotheses has yet to be established.

NITROUS OXIDE AND LEFT VENTRICULAR FUNCTION

Determination of the effects of nitrous oxide on myocardial contractility in vivo has been a technically difficult task, and the obtained results are controversial. Experiments in isolated heart preparations have demonstrated that nitrous oxide causes a direct negative inotropic effect.[119] Previous investigations conducted in healthy experimental animals have supported[120–125] the contention that nitrous oxide is a direct negative inotrope; however, other studies have failed to verify this conclusion.[77,126,127] Conflicting results have also been observed in healthy volunteers.[128–136] Evidence that nitrous oxide possesses direct myocardial depressant actions appears to be more uniform in humans with heart disease[137–141] and in experimental models of coronary artery disease in dogs,[142,143] but this issue remains unsettled as well.[137,144,145]

Several persistent difficulties with previous investigations conducted in vivo have contributed to these contradictory results. Observed changes in contractile function may be influenced by the direct actions of nitrous oxide on the systemic circulation or by reflex effects mediated by the autonomic nervous system[120,132] because nitrous oxide may increase sympathetic nervous system tone.[146-148] Studies using nitrous oxide alone are difficult to perform and interpret because this gas does not produce total anesthesia at partial pressures less than one atmosphere.[128,129,136,137,149,150] Protocols examining the effects of nitrous oxide in combination with other volatile anesthetics, opioids, or benzodiazepines are diverse, often difficult to directly compare, and have implied that nitrous oxide may have differential effects on myocardial function, depending on the baseline anesthetic.[20,126,127,131-135,139-141] The underlying health of the patient or animal population studied appears to influence the obtained results when the effects of nitrous oxide on contractile function are evaluated.[151] Lastly, lack of a reliable, load-insensitive measure of myocardial contractility has allowed only qualitative assessment of the effects of nitrous oxide on intrinsic inotropic state in the majority of investigations.

The regional PRSW relationship has been used in a recent reexamination of the effects of nitrous oxide on myocardial contractility in autonomically blocked, chronically instrumented dogs anesthetized with isoflurane or sufentanil. The results of this investigation[125] indicated that nitrous oxide produces dose-related depression of myocardial contractile state in the presence of either volatile or opioid-based anesthesia when underlying autonomic nervous system activity is eliminated. (Fig. 7–14) The degree of depression of PRSW slope with 70% nitrous oxide was 28 and 41% with sufentanil and isoflurane anesthesia (Fig. 7–14), respectively, indicating that 70% nitrous oxide decreased myocardial contractility to approximately the same extent as 1 MAC of isoflurane.[27,61] These nitrous oxide-induced myocardial depressant effects may be negated in vivo by concomitant increases in sympathetic tone.

The actions of nitrous oxide on ventricular diastolic function have been incompletely studied in vitro and remain completely uncharacterized in vivo. Carton et al.[152] examined the effects of nitrous oxide on contractility and relaxation in ferret papillary muscle. No changes in the rates of isometric or isotonic relaxation in twitches of equal amplitude were observed in response to nitrous oxide administration. In addition, although modest nitrous oxide-induced increases in maximal lengthening velocity ($-V_{max}$) and maximal rate of decline of force ($-dF/dt$) were observed, these changes in lusitropic state occurred concomitant with direct decreases in contractile state. Thus, the investigators[152] demonstrated that while nitrous oxide produces direct negative

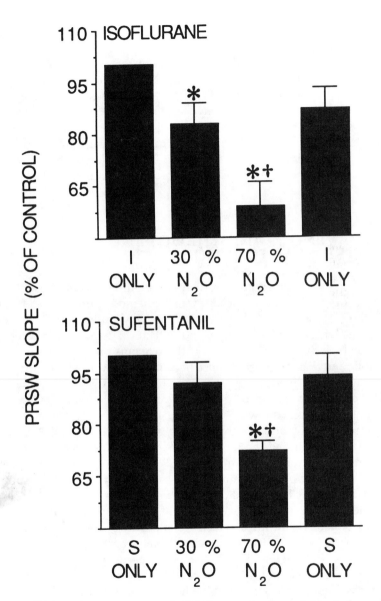

FIGURE 7-14. Effects of nitrous oxide (N2O) on preload recruitable stroke work (PRSW) slope in the presence of isoflurane (*top panel*) and sufentanil (*bottom panel*) as presented as a percent of control (I or S only, respectively). *, significantly ($P < 0.05$) different from I or S only; †, significantly ($P < 0.05$) different from I or S plus 30% N_2O. (*Adapted with permission from Pagel PS et al. Anesthesiology* 73:1148–1157, 1990)

inotropic effects, this anesthetic gas did not modify myocardial relaxation in vitro.

Recent evidence in barbiturate-anesthetized, open-chest dogs suggests that nitrous oxide impairs functional recovery of stunned myocardium.[153] Nitrous oxide-induced sympathetic nervous system activation[147,154] and imbalances of myocardial oxygen supply and demand represent potential mechanisms by which nitrous oxide delays contractile recovery of postischemic, reperfused myocardium. Further research will be required in order to describe the actions of nitrous oxide on left ventricular systolic and diastolic function in other forms of heart disease.

INTRAVENOUS ANESTHETICS AND LEFT VENTRICULAR FUNCTION

The effects of intravenous anesthetics, including barbiturates, etomidate, propofol, and ketamine, on systemic hemodynamics and left ventricular systolic function have been extensively studied. Ironically, despite the widespread and long-standing clinical use of barbiturates for anesthetic induction, the actions of these agents on specific indices of systolic and diastolic performance have not been well established. Barbiturates, including thiopental and methohexital, decrease indirect indices of myocardial contractility in vivo.[155–159] Thiopental and methohexital have been shown to decrease the slope of a noninvasively derived approximation of the end-systolic pressure-volume relationship (ESPVR) in anesthetized patients.[160–162] Several simplifying assumptions were used to estimate the ESPVR which cloud interpretation of the results and make quantitative assessment of changes in contractility difficult.[163] Thiopental decreases ventricular dP/dt_{max} in a dose-related manner in the isolated heart[164] and depresses the tension development and the force-velocity relationship of atrial[165] and ventricular muscle[166,167] in vitro. These actions have been attributed to inhibition of transsarcolemmal Ca^{2+} flux and subsequent declines in availability of intracellular Ca^{2+} for contractile activation.[165–170] These direct negative inotropic actions combine with barbiturate-induced increases in venous capacitance[171] and transient decreases in central sympathetic nervous system tone to produce the characteristic decreases in mean arterial pressure and cardiac output observed clinically during the administration of these agents.[171,172] Further study using relatively load-independent indices of myocardial contractility such as the ESPVR or PRSW derived invasively in experimental animals or humans would provide quantitative insight into the relative effects of barbiturates on systolic ventricular performance. The actions of barbiturates on ventricular diastolic function in vivo have yet to be described; however, barbiturate-induced alterations in intracellular Ca^{2+} homeostasis may have an impact on diastolic performance as well as systolic function.

The hallmark of induction of anesthesia with etomidate is remarkable stability of systemic and pulmonary hemodynamics. Investigations in normal patients[173-175] and those with cardiovascular disease[175-177] have repeatedly demonstrated that etomidate produces little change in hemodynamics. Modest decreases in mean arterial pressure, presumably resulting from declines in central sympathetic nervous system tone, venous return, and peripheral metabolism,[178] have been reported with higher doses of etomidate in patients with cardiac disease without apparent negative inotropic effects.[175,176] Etomidate has been shown to have little effect on myocardial contractility of isolated normal[179] and cardiomyopathic[180] rat papillary muscle, presumably by maintaining the availability of intracellular Ca^{2+} for contractile activation in vitro.[181] Etomidate also causes little or no myocardial depression in isolated hearts[164] and dogs[182-184] as evaluated with isovolumic and ejection phase indices of contractility. However, the effects of etomidate on more load-independent measures of contractile state have yet to be established. The actions of etomidate on diastolic function have not been specifically described in vivo.

Induction or maintenance of anesthesia with propofol is associated with significant decreases in systemic arterial pressure.[185] Propofol-induced hypotension results from a combination of venous and arterial vasodilation[186,187] and mild direct negative inotropic effects[188,189] (Fig. 7–15). A growing body of evidence obtained in vitro in isolated papillary muscle preparations[159,190] and in vivo in dogs[183] and humans[160-162] suggests that propofol causes less myocardial depression than equipotent doses of thiopental and methohexital. In chronically instrumented dogs, propofol was found to cause no change in isovolumic relaxation or regional chamber stiffness even at doses which far exceed the usual clinical range required for anesthesia, indicating that this intravenous anesthetic does not alter diastolic function (Fig. 7–16).[191] These findings are indirectly supported by two recent investigations in isolated guinea pig ventricular muscle[190] and rat papillary muscle.[192] Propofol produces moderate changes in intrinsic myocardial contractility by depressing voltage-dependent transsarcolemmal Ca^{2+} entry and late Ca^{2+} release from sarcoplasmic reticulum.[190] In addition, although propofol impairs uptake of Ca^{2+} by the sarcoplasmic reticulum to a small extent, no change in the rate constant of exponential decay of isometric force has been observed in vitro.[192] These results are consistent with the hypothesis that propofol does not alter the functional integrity of the sarcoplasmic reticulum with the exception of modest decreases in Ca^{2+} uptake. Thus, although propofol produces some effects on intracellular

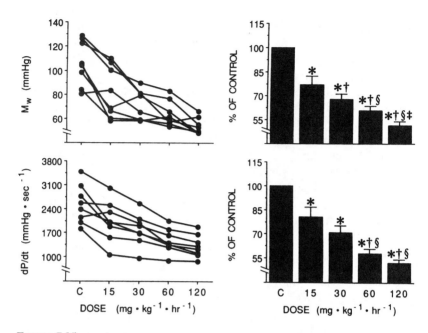

FIGURE 7-15. Preload recruitable stroke work slope (*Mw, top left panel*) and left ventricular dP/dt (*bottom left panel*) for each dog and cumulative data represented as a percent of control (*right panels*) during control (C) and at 15, 30, 60, and 120 mg·kg^{-1}·hr^{-1} infusions of propofol. *, significantly ($P < 0.05$) different from control; †, significantly ($P < 0.05$) different from 15 mg·kg^{-1}·hr^{-1} propofol infusion; §, significantly ($P < 0.05$) different from 30 mg·kg^{-1}·hr^{-1} propofol infusion; ‡, significantly ($P < 0.05$) different from 60 mg·kg^{-1}·hr^{-1} propofol infusion. (*Reproduced with permission from Pagel PS and Warltier DC. Anesthesiology 78:100–108, 1993*)

Ca^{2+} homeostasis during systole and diastole, these perturbations appear to cause only modest derangements in myocardial contractility[189] and no change in lusitropic state.

Ketamine has been used with widespread success in the induction of anesthesia in certain patients with hemodynamic compromise.[193] The observation that ketamine can lead to acute hemodynamic decompensation in a subset of critically ill patients with impaired function of the sympathetic nervous system[194] has stimulated exploration of the direct effects of this intravenous anesthetic on cardiovascular function. Ketamine produces dramatic increases in heart rate and arterial pressure in most patients which can be attributed to the central and peripheral sympathomimetic actions of this drug.[193] Ketamine blocks the reuptake of monoamines including norepinephrine into adrenergic nerves, a mechanism of action similar to that of cocaine[195,196] Depletion

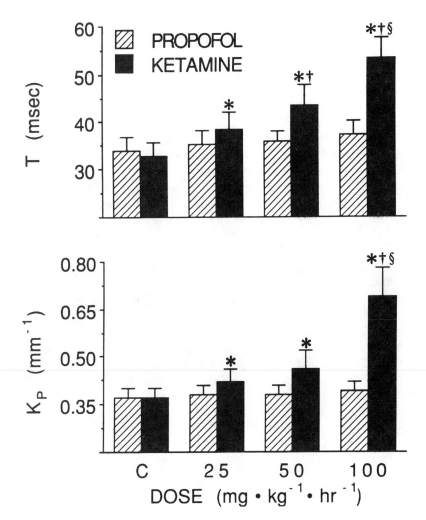

FIGURE 7-16. Effects of propofol and ketamine on the time constant (*T*) of isovolumic relaxation (*top panel*) and regional chamber stiffness (*Kp; bottom panel*). *, significantly ($P < 0.05$) different from the autonomically blocked conscious (C) control; †, significantly ($P < 0.05$) different from 25 mg·kg⁻¹·hr⁻¹ dose; §, significantly ($P < 0.05$) different from 50 mg·kg⁻¹·hr⁻¹ dose. (*Adapted with permission from Pagel PS et al. Anesthesiology 76:419–425, 1992*)

of catecholamines may unmask the direct vasodilator and myocardial depressant actions of ketamine independent of sympathomimetic effects. This has been postulated as the potential mechanism of hemodynamic collapse after administration of ketamine in some patients.[194,197] The direct effects of ketamine on myocardial contractility in vivo have been difficult to interpret because changes in contractile state are often masked by ketamine-induced increases in sympathetic tone.[193,197–199] However, ketamine has been shown to produce direct myocardial depressant actions as assessed with the regional PRSW slope in dogs with pharmacological blockade of the autonomic nervous system.[200] This observation is supported by investigations in vitro[201–205] demonstrating ketamine-induced negative inotropic effects when normal adrenergic nerve transmission is impaired. The direct myocardial depression caused by ketamine probably occurs as a result of inhibition of transsarcolemmal Ca^{2+} influx and subsequent decreases in intracellular Ca^{2+} availability without changes in myofibrillar Ca^{2+} sensitivity.[203,204] Ketamine also produces abnormalities in indices of diastolic function in a dose-related manner, prolonging isovolumic relaxation and increasing regional chamber stiffness.[191] Thus, cardiovascular collapse observed in the catecholamine-depleted patient during induction of anesthesia with ketamine[194] may be related not only to depression of systolic performance but also to direct alterations of ventricular diastolic function.

The effects of anesthetic-induced abnormalities in systolic and diastolic function in the heart with impaired mechanical performance have yet to be explored in other experimental models or patients with preexisting left ventricular dysfunction and represents an important goal of future research. It is highly likely that anesthetic agents even in low doses will exacerbate preexisting left ventricular dysfunction and attenuate cardiac performance by negative inotropic and lusitropic actions. Further study in both experimental and clinical settings of myocardial ischemia and infarction and cardiomyopathy are required to provide a more comprehensive understanding of the left ventricular systolic and diastolic mechanical interactions between anesthetics and these pathological states.

Acknowledgements

The authors thank Doug Hettrick, John Tessmer, and Dave Schwabe for superb technical assistance. This work was supported by US PHS grant HL 36144 and Anesthesiology Research Training Grant GM 08377.

References

1. Sugai N, Shimosato S, Etsten BE: Effect of halothane on force-velocity relations and dynamic stiffness of isolated heart muscle. Anesthesiology 29:267–274, 1968
2. Goldberg AH, Ullrick WC: Effects of halothane on isometric contractions of isolated heart muscle. Anesthesiology 28:838–845, 1967

3. Shimosato S, Li TH, Etsten B: Ventricular function during halothane anesthesia in closed chest dog. Circ Res 12:63–75, 1963
4. Severinghaus JW, Cullen SC: Depression of myocardium and body oxygen consumption with fluothane. Anesthesiology 19:165–177, 1958
5. Deutsch S, Linde HW, Dripps RD, Price HL: Circulatory and respiratory actions of halothane in normal man. Anesthesiology 23:631–638, 1962
6. Eger EI II, Smith NT, Stoelting RK, Cullen DJ, Kadis LB, Whitcher CE: Cardiovascular effects of halothane in man. Anesthesiology 32:396–409, 1970
7. Sonntag H, Donath U, Hillebrand W, Merin RG, Radke J: Left ventricular function in conscious man and during halothane anesthesia. Anesthesiology 48:320–324, 1978
8. Shimosato S, Sugai N, Iwatsuki N, Etsten BE: The effect of Ethrane on cardiac muscle mechanics. Anesthesiology 30:513–518, 1969
9. Kemmotsu O, Hashimoto Y, Shimosato S: Inotropic effects of isoflurane on mechanics of contraction in isolated cap papillary muscles from normal and failing hearts. Anesthesiology 39:470–477, 1973
10. Stevens WC, Cromwell TH, Halsey MJ, Eger EI II, Shakespeare TF, Bahlman SH: The cardiovascular effects of a new inhalation anesthetic, Forane, in human volunteers at constant arterial carbon dioxide tension. Anesthesiology 35:8–16, 1971
11. Calverley RK, Smith NT, Prys-Roberts C, Eger EI II, Jones CW: Cardiovascular effects of enflurane anesthesia during controlled ventilation in man. Anesth Analg 57:619–628, 1978
12. Iwatsuki N, Shimosato S: Diethyl ether and contractility of isolated cat heart muscle. Comparison of inotropic effects of five anesthetics at equipotent levels. Br J Anaesth 43:420–426, 1971
13. Marshall BE, Cohen PJ, Klingenmaier CH, Neigh JL, Pender JW: Some pulmonary and cardiovascular effects of enflurane (Ethrane) anesthesia with varying $PaCO_2$ in man. Br J Anaesth 43:996–1002, 1971
14. Graves CL, Downs NH: Cardiovascular and renal effects of enflurane in surgical patients. Anesth Analg 53:898–903, 1974
15. Levesque PR, Nanagas V, Shanks C, Shimosato S: Circulatory effects of enflurane in normocarbic human volunteers. Can Anaesth Soc J 21:580–585, 1974
16. Merin RG, Kumazawa T, Luka NL: Enflurane depresses myocardial function, perfusion, and metabolism in the dog. Anesthesiology 45:501–507, 1976
17. Horan BF, Prys-Roberts C, Hamilton WK, Roberts JG: Haemodynamic responses to enflurane anesthesia and hypovolaemia in the dog, and their modification by propranolol. Br J Anaesth 49:1189–1197, 1977
18. Pagel PS, Kampine JP, Schmeling WT, Warltier DC: Comparison of the systemic and coronary hemodynamic actions of desflurane, isoflurane, halothane, and enflurane in the chronically instrumented dog. Anesthesiology 74:539–551, 1991
19. Ritzman JR, Erickson HH, Miller ED Jr: Cardiovascular effects of enflurane and halothane on the rhesus monkey. Anesth Analg 55:85–91, 1976
20. Van Trigt P, Christian CC, Fagraeus L, Spray TL, Peyton RB, Pellom GL, Wechsler AS: Myocardial depression by anesthetic agents (halothane, enflurane and nitrous oxide): Quantitation based on end-systolic pressure-dimension relations. Am J Cardiol 53:243–247, 1984
21. Graves CL, McDermott RW, Bidwai A: Cardiovascular effects of isoflurane in surgical patients. Anesthesiology 41:486–489, 1974
22. Tarnow J, Bruckner JB, Eberlein HJ, Hess W, Patschke D: Haemodynamics

and myocardial oxygen consumption during isoflurane (Forane) anaesthesia in geriatric patients. Br J Anaesth 48:669–675, 1976

23. Wolf WJ, Neal MB, Peterson MD: The hemodynamic and cardiovascular effects of isoflurane and halothane anesthesia in children. Anesthesiology 64:328–333, 1986

24. Horan BF, Prys-Roberts C, Roberts JG, Bennett MJ, Foex P: Haemodynamic responses to isoflurane anaesthesia and hypovolaemia in the dog, and their modification by propranolol. Br J Anaesth 49:1179–1187, 1977

25. Merin RG: Are the myocardial function and metabolic effects of isoflurane really different from those of halothane and enflurane? Anesthesiology 55:398–408, 1981

26. Merin RG, Kumazawa T, Luka NL: Myocardial function and metabolism in the conscious dog and during halothane anesthesia. Anesthesiology 44: 402–415, 1976

27. Pagel PS, Kampine JP, Schmeling WT, Warltier DC: Comparison of end-systolic pressure-length relations and preload recruitable stroke work as indices of myocardial contractility in the conscious and anesthetized, chronically instrumented dog. Anesthesiology 73:278–290, 1990

28. Pagel PS, Nijhawan N, Warltier DC: Quantitation of volatile anesthetic-induced depression of myocardial contractility using a single beat index derived from maximal ventricular power. J Cardiothorac Vasc Anesth 7:688–695, 1993

29. Kass DA, Maughan WL; From "Emax" to pressure-volume relations: A broader view. Circulation 77:1203–1212, 1988

30. Hysing ES, Chelly JE, Jacobson L, Doursout MF, Merin RG: Cardiovascular effects of acute changes in extracellular ionized calcium concentration induced by citrate and $CaCl_2$ infusions in chronically instrumented dogs, conscious and during enflurane, halothane, and isoflurane anesthesia. Anesthesiology 72:100–104, 1990

31. Merin RG, Chelly JE, Hysing ES, Rogers K, Dlewati A, Hartley CJ, Abernethy DR, Doursout MF: Cardiovascular effects of and interaction between calcium blocking drugs and anesthetics in chronically instrumented dogs. IV. Chronically administered oral verapamil and halothane, enflurane, and isoflurane. Anesthesiology 66:140–146, 1987

32. Pagel PS, Hettrick DA, Warltier DC: Left ventricular mechanical consequences of dihydropyridine calcium channel modulation inconscious and anesthetized chronically instrumented dogs. Anesthesiology 81:190–208, 1994

33. Makela VHM, Kapur PA: Amrinone and verapamil-propranolol induced cardiac depression during isoflurane anesthesia in dogs. Anesthesiology 66:792–797, 1987

34. Price HL: Calcium reverses myocardial depression caused by halothane: Site of action. Anesthesiology 41:576–579, 1974

35. Denlinger JK, Kaplan JA, Lecky JH, Wollman H: Cardiovascular responses to calcium administered intravenously to man during halothane anesthesia. Anesthesiology 42:390–397, 1975

36. Pagel PS, Kampine JP, Schmeling WT, Warltier DC: Reversal of volatile anesthetic-induced depression of myocardial contractility by extracellular calcium also enhances left ventricular diastolic function. Anesthesiology 78:141–154, 1993

37. Pagel PS, Hettrick DA, Warltier DC: Amrinone enhances myocardial contractility and improves left ventricular diastolic function in conscious and anesthetized chronically instrumented dogs. Anesthesiology 79:753–765, 1993

38. Makela VHM, Kapur PA: Amrinone blunts cardiac depression caused by enflurane or isoflurane anesthesia in the dog. Anesth Analg 66:215–221, 1987
39. Pagel PS, Harkin CP, Hettrick DA, Warltier DC: Levosimendan (OR-1259), a myofilament calcium sensitizer, enhances myocardial contractility but does not alter isovolumic relaxation in conscious and anesthetized dogs. Anesthesiology 81:974–987, 1994
40. Rusy BF, Komai H: Anesthetic depression of myocardial contractility: A review of possible mechanisms. Anesthesiology 67:745–766, 1987
41. Bosnjak ZJ, Kampine JP: Effects of halothane on transmembrane potentials, Ca^{2+} transients, and papillary muscle tension in the cat. Am J Physiol 251:H374–H381, 1986
42. Bosnjak ZJ, Aggarwal A, Turner LA, Kampine JM, Kampine JP: Differential effects of halothane, enflurane, and isoflurane on Ca^{2+} transients and papillary muscle tension in guinea pigs. Anesthesiology 76:123–131, 1992
43. Lynch C III, Vogel S, Sperelakis N: Halothane depression of myocardial slow action potentials. Anesthesiology 55:360–368, 1981
44. Lynch C III: Differential depression of myocardial contractility by halothane and isoflurane in vitro. Anesthesiology 64:620–631, 1986
45. Eskinder H, Rusch NJ, Supan FD, Kampine JP, Bosnjak ZJ: The effects of volatile anesthetics on L- and T-type calcium channel currents in canine cardiac Purkinje cells. Anesthesiology 74:919–926, 1991
46. Drenger B, Heitmiller ES, Quigg M, Blanck TJJ: Depression of calcium channel blocker binding to rat brain membranes by halothane. Anesth Analg 74:758–761, 1992
47. Blanck TJJ, Peterson CV, Baroody B, Tegazzin V, Lou J: Halothane, enflurane, and isoflurane stimulate calcium leakage from rabbit sarcoplasmic reticulum. Anesthesiology 76:813–821, 1992
48. Frazier MJ, Lynch C III: Halothane and isoflurane effects on Ca^{2+} fluxes of isolated myocardial sarcoplasmic reticulum. Anesthesiology 77:316–323, 1992
49. Wheeler DM, Katz A, Rice RT, Hansford RG: Volatile anesthetic effects on sarcoplasmic reticulum Ca content and sarcolemmal Ca flux in isolated rat cardiac cell suspensions. Anesthesiology 80:372–382, 1994
50. Connelly TJ, Coronado R: Activation of the Ca^{2+} release channel of cardiac sarcoplasmic reticulum by volatile anesthetics. Anesthesiology 81:459–469, 1994
51. Housmans PR, Murat I: Comparative effects of halothane, enflurane, and isoflurane at equipotent anesthetic concentrations on isolated ventricular myocardium of the ferret. I. Contractility. Anesthesiology 69:451–463, 1988
52. Housmans PR, Murat I: Comparative effects of halothane, enflurane, and isoflurane at equipotent anesthetic concentrations on isolated ventricular myocardium of the ferret. II. Relaxation. Anesthesiology 69:464–471, 1988
53. Blanck TJJ, Chiancone E, Salviati G, Heitmiller ES, Verzili D, Luciani G, Colotti G: Halothane does not alter Ca^{2+} affinity of troponin C. Anesthesiology 76:100–105, 1992
54. Warltier DC, Pagel PS: Cardiovascular and respiratory actions of desflurane: Is desflurane different from isoflurane? Anesth Analg 75:S17–S31, 1992
55. Weiskopf RB, Moore MA, Eger EI II, Noorani M, McKay L, Chortkoff B, Hart PS, Damask M: Rapid increase in desflurane concentration is associated with greater transient cardiovascular stimulation than with rapid in-

crease in isoflurane concentration in humans. Anesthesiology 80:1035–1045, 1994

56. Ebert TJ, Muzi M: Sympathetic hyperactivity during desflurane anesthesia in healthy volunteers. A comparison with isoflurane. Anesthesiology 79:444–453, 1993

57. Merin RG, Bernard JM, Doursout MF, Cohen M, Chelly JE: Comparison of the effects of isoflurane and desflurane on cardiovascular dynamics and regional blood flow in the chronically instrumented dog. Anesthesiology 74:568–574, 1991

58. Weiskopf RB, Holmes MA, Eger EI II, Johnson BH, Rampil IJ, Brown JG: Cardiovascular effects of I653 in swine. Anesthesiology 69:303–309, 1988

59. Weiskopf RB, Cahalan MK, Eger EI II, Yasuda N, Rampil IJ, Ionescu P, Lockhart SH, Johnson BH, Freire B, Kelley S: Cardiovascular actions of desflurane in normocarbic volunteers. Anesth Analg 73:143–156, 1991

60. Pagel PS, Kampine JP, Schmeling WT, Warltier DC: Evaluaton of myocardial contractility in the chronically instrumented dog with intact autonomic nervous system function: Effects of desflurane and insoflurane. Acta Anaesthesiol Scand 37:203–210, 1993

61. Pagel PS, Kampine JP, Schmeling WT, Warltier DC: Influence of volatile anesthetics on myocardial contractility in vivo: Desflurane versus isoflurane. Anesthesiology 74:900–907, 1991

62. Boban M, Stowe DF, Buljubasic N, Kampine JP, Bosnjak ZJ: Direct comparative effects of isoflurane and desflurane in isolated guinea pig hearts. Anesthesiology 76:775–780, 1992

63. Bernard JM, Wouters PF, Doursout MF, Florence B, Chelly JE, Merin RG: Effects of sevoflurane and isoflurane on cardiac and coronary dynamics in chronically instrumented dogs. Anesthesiology 72:659–662, 1990

64. Frink EJ Jr, Malan TP, Atlas M, DiNardo JA, Brown BR Jr: Hemodynamic changes during sevoflurane or isoflurane anesthesia in ASA I and ASA II surgical patients (abstr). Anesthesiology 75:A156, 1991

65. Lerman J, Oyston JP, Gallagher TM, Miyasaka K, Volgyesi GA, Burrows FA: The minimum alveolar concentration (MAC) and hemodynamic effects of halothane, isoflurane, and sevoflurane in newborn swine. Anesthesiology 73:717–721, 1990

66. Azari DM, Cork RC, Conzen P, Vollmar B, Kramer TH: Inotropic effects of sevoflurane compared to isoflurane and halothane (abstr). Anesthesiology 77:A628, 1992

67. Kikura M, Ikeda K: Comparison of effects of sevoflurane-nitrous oxide and enflurane-nitrous oxide on myocardial contractility in humans. Load-independent and noninvasive assessment with transesophageal echocardiography. Anesthesiology 79:235–243, 1993

68. Harkin CP, Pagel PS, Kersten JR, Hettrick DA, Warltier DC: Direct negative inotropic and lusitropic effects of sevoflurane. Anesthesiology 81:156–167, 1994

69. Grossman W: Diastolic dysfunction and congestive heart failure. Circulation 81(2suppl):III1–7, 1990

70. Humphrey LS, Stinson DC, Humphrey MJ, Finney RS, Zeller PA, Judd MR, Blanck TJJ: Volatile anesthetic effects on left ventricular relaxation in swine. Anesthesiology 73:731–738, 1990

71. Doyle RL, Foex P, Ryder WA, Jones LA: Effects of halothane on left ventricular relaxation and early diastolic coronary blood flow in the dog. Anesthesiology 70:660–666, 1989

72. Pagel PS, Kampine JP, Schmeling WT, Warltier DC: Alteration of left ven-

tricular diastolic function by desflurane, isoflurane, and halothane in the chronically instrumented dog with autonomic nervous system blockade. Anesthesiology 74:1103–1114, 1991

73. Goldberg AH, Phear WPC: Halothane and paired stimulation: Effects on myocardial compliance and contractility. J Appl Physiol 28:391–396, 1970

74. Rusy BF, Moran JE, Vongvises P, Lattanand S, MacNab M, Much DR, Lynch PR: The effects of halothane and cyclopropane on left ventricular volume determined by high-speed biplane cineradiography in dogs. Anesthesiology 36:369–373, 1972

75. Moores WY, Weiskopf RB, Baysinger M, Utley JR: Effects of halothane and morphine sulfate on myocardial compliance following total cardiopulmonary bypass. J Thorac Cardiovasc Surg 81:163–170, 1981

76. Greene ES, Gerson JI: One versus two MAC halothane anesthesia does not alter the left ventricular diastolic pressure-volume relationship. Anesthesiology 64:230–237, 1986

77. Van Trigt P, Christian CC, Fagraeus L, Peyton RB, Jones RN, Spray TL, Pasque MK, Pellom GL, Wechsler AS: The mechanism of halothane-induced myocardial depression: Altered diastolic mechanics versus impaired contractility. J Thorac Cardiovasc Surg 85:832–838, 1983

78. Brower RW, Merin RG: Left ventricular function and compliance in swine during halothane anesthesia. Anesthesiology 50:409–415, 1979

79. Morgan JP, MacKinnon R, Briggs M, Gwathmey JK: Calcium and cardiac relaxation. In Grossman W, Lorell BH (eds): Diastolic Relaxation of the Heart: Basic Research and Current Applications for Clinical Cardiology, pp. 17–26. Boston, Martinus Nijhoff, 1988

80. Nakamura Y, Tonomura Y: The binding of ATP to the catalytic and the regulatory site of Ca^{2+}, Mg^{2+}-dependent ATPase of the sarcoplasmic reticulum. J Bioenerg Biomembr 14:307–318, 1982

81. Smith VE, Katz AM: Inotropic and lusitropic abnormalities in the genesis of heart failure. Eur Heart J 4(suppl A):7–17, 1983

82. Smith VE, Zile MR: Relaxation and diastolic properties of the heart. In The Heart and Cardiovascular System: Scientific Foundations pp. 1353–1367. Fozzard HA, Haber E, Jennings RB, Katz AM, Morgan HE New York, Raven Press, 1991

83. Pagel PS, Grossman W, Haering JM, Warltier DC: Left ventricular diastolic function in the normal and diseased heart: Perspectives for the anesthesiologist (First of two parts). Anesthesiology 79:836–854, 1993

84. Morgan JP: Abnormal intracellular modulation of calcium as a major cause of cardiac contractile dysfunction. N Engl J Med 325:625–632, 1991

85. Bosnjak ZJ, Supan FD, Rusch NJ: The effects of halothane, enflurane, and isoflurane on calcium current in isolated canine ventricular cells. Anesthesiology 74:340–345, 1991

86. Housmans PR: Negative inotropy of halogenated anesthetics in ferret ventricular myocardium. Am J Physiol 259:H827–H834, 1990

87. Vittone L, Cingolani HE, Mattiazzi RA: The link between myocardial contraction and relaxation: The effects of calcium antagonists. J Mol Cell Cardiol 17:255–263, 1985

88. Kosk-Kosicka D, Roszczynska G: Inhibition of plasma membrane Ca^{2+}-ATPase activity by volatile anesthetics. Anesthesiology 79:774–780, 1993

89. Hicks MJ, Shigekawa M, Katz AM: Mechanism by which cyclic adenosine 3':5'-monophosphate-dependent protein kinase stimulates calcium transport in cardiac sarcoplasmic reticulum. Circ Res 44:384–391, 1979

90. Gaide MS, Fitterman WS, Wiggins JR, Myerburg RJ, Cameron JS, Bassett AL: Amrinone relaxes potassium-induced contracture of failing right ventricular muscle of cats. J Cardiovasc Pharmacol 5:335–340, 1983
91. Katz AM: Cyclic adenosine monophosphate effects on the myocardium: A man who blows hot and cold with one breath. J Am Coll Cardiol 2:143–149, 1983
92. Ovaska M, Haikala H, Lundstrom K, Korkolainen T, Taskinen J, Linden IB: Studies on calcium-dependent binding of simendan to troponin complex and troponin C (abstr). J Mol Cell Cardiol 24(suppl I):S260, 1992
93. Hryshko LV, Kobayashi T, Bose D: Possible inhibition of canine ventricular sarcoplasmic reticulum by BAY K 8644. Am J Physiol 257:H407–H414, 1989
94. Gilbert JC, Glantz SA: Determinants of left ventricular filing and of the diastolic pressure-volume relation. Circ Res 64:827–852, 1989
95. Kemmotsu O, Hashimoto Y, Shimosato S: The effects of fluroxene and enflurane on contractile performance of isolated papillary muscles from failing hearts. Anesthesiology 40:252–260, 1974
96. Lowenstein E, Foex P, Francis CM, Davies WL, Yusuf S, Ryder WA: Regional ischemic ventricular dysfunction in myocardium supplied by a narrowed coronary artery with increasing halothane concentration in the dog. Anesthesiology 55:349–359, 1981
97. Prys-Roberts C, Roberts JG, Foex P, Clarke TN, Bennett MJ, Ryder WA: Interaction of anesthesia, beta-receptor blockade, and blood loss in dogs with induced myocardial infarction. Anesthesiology 45:326–329, 1976
98. Bland JHL, Lowenstein E: Halothane-induced decrease in experimental myocardial ischemia in the non-failing canine heart. Anesthesiology 45:287–293, 1976
99. Gerson JI, Hickey RF, Bainton CR: Treatment of myocardial ischemia with halothane or nitroprusside-propranolol. Anesth Analg 61:10–14, 1982
100. Davis RF, DeBoer LW, Rude RE, Lowenstein E, Maroko PR: The effect of halothane anesthesia on myocardial necrosis, hemodynamic performance, and regional myocardial blood flow in dogs following coronary artery occlusion. Anesthesiology 59:402–411, 1983
101. Van Ackern K, Vetter HO, Bruckner UB, Madler C, Mittman U, Peter K: Effects of enflurane on myocardial ischaemia in the dog. Br J Anaesth 57:497–504, 1985
102. Pagel PS, Hettrick DA, Warltier DC: Isoflurane alters the left ventricular mechanical effects of acute regional myocardial ischemia in dogs. Anesth Analg, 80:S363, 1995
103. Buljubasic N, Stowe DF, Marijic J, Roerig DL, Kampine JP, Bosnjak ZJ: Halothane reduces release of adenosine, inosine, and lactate with ischemia and reperfusion in isolated hearts. Anesth Analg 76:54–62, 1993
104. Coetzee A, Brits W, Genade S, Lochner A: Halothane does have protective properties in the isolated ischemic rat heart. Anesth Analg 73:711–719, 1991
105. Marijic J, Stowe DF, Turner LA, Kampine JP, Bosnjak ZJ: Differential protective effects of halothane and isoflurane against hypoxic and reoxygenation injury in the isolated guinea pig heart. Anesthesiology 73:976–983, 1990
106. Freedman BM, Hamm DP, Everson CT, Wechsler AS, Christian CM II: Enflurane enhances postischemic functional recovery in the isolated rat heart. Anesthesiology 62:29–33, 1985
107. Warltier DC, Gross GJ, Brooks HL, Preuss KC: Improvement of postis-

chemic, contractile function by the calcium channel blocking agent nitrendipine in conscious dogs. J Cardiovasc Pharmacol 12(suppl 4):S120–S124, 1988

108. Mattheussen M, Rusy BF, Van Aken H, Flameng W: Recovery of function and adenosine triphosphate metabolism following myocardi ischemia induced in the presence of volatile anesthetics. Anesth Analg 76:69–75, 1993

109. Belo SE, Mazer CD: Effect of halothane and isoflurane on postischemic "stunned" myocardium in the dog. Anesthesiology 73:1243–1251, 1990

110. Kanaya N, Fujita S: The effects of isoflurane on regional myocardial contractility and metabolism in "stunned" myocardium in acutely instrumented dogs. Anesth Analg 79:447–454, 1994

111. Tanguay M, Blaise G, Dumont L, Beique G, Hollmann C: Beneficial effects of volatile anesthetics on decrease in coronary flow and myocardial contractility induced by oxygen-derived free radicals in isolated rabbit hearts. J Cardiovasc Pharmacol 18:863–870, 1991

112. Lochner A, Harper IS, Salie R, Genade S, Coetzee AR: Halothane protects the isolated rat myocardium against excessive total intracellular calcium and structural damage during ischemia and reperfusion. Anesth Analg 79:226–233, 1994

113. Allshire A, Cobbald PH: Ca^{2+} flux into metabolically deprived cardiomyocytes. Biochem Soc Trans 15:960, 1987

114. Nayler WG, Panagiotopoulos S, Elz JS, Daly MJ: Calcium-mediated damage during post-ischaemic reperfusion. J Mol Cell Cardiol 20(suppl 2):41–54, 1988

115. Watts JA, Koch DC, LaNoue KF: Effects of Ca^{2+} antagonism on energy metabolism: Ca^{2+} and heart function after ischemia. Am J Physiol 238:H909–H916, 1980

116. Murphy JG, Smith TW, Marsh JD: Mechanisms of reoxygenation induced calcium overload in cultured chick embryo heart cells. Am J Physiol 254:H1133–1141, 1988

117. Larach DR, Schuler HG: Potassium channel blockade and halothane vasodilation in conducting and resistance coronary arteries. J Pharmacol Exp Ther 267:72–81, 1993

118. Cason B, Hickey R, Shubayev I: Isoflurane-induced coronary vasodilation is mediated by glibenclamide-sensitive potassium channels. Anesthesiology, 81:1245–1255, 1994

119. Stowe DF, Monroe SM, Marijic J, Bosnjak ZJ, Kampine JP: Comparison of halothane, enflurane, and isoflurane with nitrous oxide on contractility and oxygen supply and demand in isolated hearts. Anesthesiology 75:1062–1074, 1991

120. Craythorne NW, Darby TD: The cardiovascular effects of nitrous oxide in the dog. Br J Anaesth 37:560–565, 1965

121. Eisele JH, Trenchard D, Stubbs J, Guz A: The immediate cardiac depression by anaesthetics in conscious dogs. Br J Anaesth 41:86–93, 1969

122. Lundborg RO, Milde JH, Theye RA: Effect of nitrous oxide on myocardial contractility of dogs. Can Anaesth Soc J 13:361–367, 1966

123. Thorburn J, Smith G, Vance JP, Brown DM: Effect of nitrous oxide on the cardiovascular system and coronary circulation of the dog. Br J Anaesth 51:937–942, 1979

124. Diedericks J, Leone BJ, Foex P: Regional differences in left ventricular wall motion in the anesthetized dog. Anesthesiology 70:82–90, 1989

125. Pagel PS, Kampine JP, Schmeling WT, Warltier DC: Effects of nitrous oxide on myocardial contractility as evaluated by the preload recruitable

stroke work relationship in chronically instrumented dogs. Anesthesiology 73:1148–1157, 1990

126. Smith NT, Corbascio AN: The cardiovascular effects of nitrous oxide during halothane anesthesia in the dog. Anesthesiology 27:560–566, 1966

127. Coetzee A, Fourie P, Bolliger C, Badenhorst E, Rebel A, Lombard C: Effect of N_2O on segmental left ventricular function and effective arterial elastance in pigs when added to a halothane-fentanyl-pancuronium anesthetic technique. Anesth Analg 69:313–322, 1989

128. Eisele JH, Smith NT: Cardiovascular effects of 40 percent nitrous oxide in man. Anesth Analg 51:956–963, 1972

129. Eriksen S, Johannsen G, Frost N: Effects of nitrous oxide on systolic time intervals. Acta Anaesthesiol Scand 24:74–78, 1980

130. Hill GE, English JE, Lunn J, Stanley TH, Sentker CR, Loeser E, Liu WS, Kawamura R, Bidwai AV, Hodges M: Cardiovascular responses to nitrous oxide during light, moderate, and deep halothane anesthesia in man. Anesth Analg 57:84–94, 1978

131. Wong KC, Martin WE, Hornbein TF, Freund FG, Everett J: The cardiovascular effects of morphine sulfate with oxygen and with nitrous oxide in man. Anesthesiology 38:542–549, 1973

132. Smith NT, Eger EI II, Stoelting RK, Whayne TF, Cullen D, Kadis LB: The cardiovascular and sympathomimetic responses to the addition of nitrous oxide to halothane in man. Anesthesiology 32:410–421, 1970

133. Smith NT, Calverley RK, Prys-Roberts C, Eger EI II, Jones CW: Impact of nitrous oxide on the circulation during enflurane anesthesia in man. Anesthesiology 48:345–349, 1978

134. Bahlman SH, Eger EI II, Smith NT, Stevens WC, Shakespeare TF, Sawyer DC, Halsey MJ, Cromwell TH: The cardiovascular effects of nitrous oxide-halothane anesthesia in man. Anesthesiology 35:274–285, 1971

135. Dolan WM, Stevens WC, Eger EI II, Cromwell TH, Halsey MJ, Shakespeare TF, Miller RD: The cardiovascular and respiratory effects of isoflurane-nitrous oxide anaesthesia. Can Anaesth Soc J 21:557–568, 1974

136. Lichtenthal P, Philip J, Sloss LJ, Gabel R, Lesch M: Administration of nitrous oxide in normal subjects. Evaluation of systems of gas delivery for their clinical use and hemodynamic effects. Chest 72:316–322, 1977

137. Stoelting RK, Gibbs PS: Hemodynamic effects of morphine and morphine-nitrous oxide in valvular heart disease and coronary-artery disease. Anesthesiology 38:45–52, 1973

138. Eisele JH, Reitan JA, Massumi RA, Zelis RF, Miller RR: Myocardial performance and N_2O analgesia in coronary-artery disease. Anesthesiology 44:16–20, 1976

139. Lappas DG, Buckley MJ, Laver MB, Daggett WM, Lowenstein E: Left ventricular performance and pulmonary circulation following addition of nitrous oxide to morphine during coronary-artery surgery. Anesthesiology 43:61–69, 1975

140. Lunn JK, Stanley TH, Eisele J, Webster L, Woodward A: High dose fentanyl anesthesia for coronary artery surgery: Plasma fentanyl concentrations and influence of nitrous oxide on cardiovascular responses. Anesth Analg 58:390–395, 1979

141. Wynne J, Mann T, Alpert JS, Green LH, Grossman W: Hemodynamic effects of nitrous oxide administered during cardiac catheterization. JAMA 243:1440–1442, 1980

142. Leone BJ, Philbin DM, Lehot JJ, Foex P, Ryder WA: Gradual or abrupt nitrous oxide administration in a canine model of critical coronary stenosis

induces regional myocardial dysfunction that is worsened by halothane. Anesth Analg 67:814–822, 1988

143. Ramsay JG, Arvieux CC, Foex P, Philbin DM, Jeavons P, Ryder WA, Jones LA: Regional and global myocardial function in the dog when nitrous oxide is added to halothane in the presence of critical coronary artery constriction. Anesth Analg 65:431–436, 1986

144. Cahalan MK, Prakash O, Rulf ENR, Cahalan MT, Mayala APG, Lurz FC, Rosseel P, Lachitjaran E, Siphanto K, Gussenhoven EJ, Roelandt JRTC: Addition of nitrous oxide to fentanyl anesthesia does not induce myocardial ischemia in patients with ischemic heart disease. Anesthesiology 67:925–929, 1987

145. Slavik JR, LaMantia KR, Kopriva CJ, Prokop E, Ezekowitz MD, Barash PG: Does nitrous oxide cause regional wall motion abnormalities in patients with coronary artery disease? An evaluation by two-dimensional transesophageal echocardiography. Anesth Analg 67:695–700, 1988

146. Sellgren J, Ponten J, Wallin BG: Percutaneous recording of muscle nerve sympathetic activity during propofol, nitrous oxide, and isoflurane anesthesia in humans. Anesthesiology 73:20–27, 1990

147. Ebert TJ, Kampine JP: Nitrous oxide augments sympathetic outflow: Direct evidence from human peroneal nerve recordings. Anesth Analg 69:444–449, 1989

148. Ebert TJ: Differential effects of nitrous oxide on baroreflex control of heart rate and peripheral sympathetic nerve activity in humans. Anesthesiology 72:16–22, 1990

149. Thornton JA, Fleming JS, Goldberg AD, Baird D: Cardiovascular effects of 50 percent nitrous oxide and 50 percent oxygen mixture. Anaesthesia 28:484–489, 1973

150. Falk RB Jr, Denlinger JK, Nahrwold ML, Todd RA: Acute vasodilation following induction of anesthesia with intravenous diazepam and nitrous oxide. Anesthesiology 49:149–150, 1978

151. Eisele JH Jr: Cardiovascular effects of nitrous oxide. In Eger EI II (ed): Nitrous Oxide/N2O, pp. 125–156. New York, Elsevier, 1985

152. Carton EG, Wanek LA, Housmans PR: Effects of nitrous oxide on contractility, relaxation and the intracellular calcium transient of isolated mammalian ventricular myocardium. J Pharmacol Exp Ther 257:843–849, 1991

153. Siker D, Pagel PS, Pelc LR, Kampine JP, Schmeling WT, Warltier DC: Nitrous oxide impairs functional recovery of stunned myocardium in barbiturate-anesthetized, acutely instrumented dogs. Anesth Analg 75:539–548, 1992

154. Rorie DK, Tyce GM, Sill JC: Increased norepinephrine release from dog pulmonary artery caused by nitrous oxide. Anesth Analg 65:560–564, 1986

155. Seltzer JL, Gerson JI, Allen FB: Comparison of the cardiovascular effects of bolus v. incremental administration of thiopentone. Br J Anaesth 52:527–30, 1980

156. Sonntag H, Hellberg K, Schenk HD, Donath U, Regensburger D, Kettler D, Duchanova H, Larsen R: Effects of thiopental (Trapanal) on coronary blood flow and myocardial metabolism in man. Acta Anaesthesiol Scand 19:69–78, 1975

157. Reiz S, Balfors E, Friedman A, Haggmark S, Peter T: Effects of thiopentone on cardiac performance, coronary hemodynamics and myocardial oxygen consumption in chronic ischemic heart disease. Acta Anaesthesiol Scand 25:103–110, 1981

158. Fischler M, Dubois C, Brodaty D, Schlumberger S, Melchior JC, Guilmet D, Vourc'h G: Circulatory responses to thiopentone and tracheal intubation in patients with coronary artery disease. Effects of pretreatment with labetalol. Br J Anaesth 57:493–496, 1985

159. Conway CM, Ellis DB: The haemodynamic effects of short acting barbiturates. Br J Anaesth 41:534–542, 1969

160. Mulier JP, Wouters PF, Van Aken H, Vermaut G, Vandermeersch E: Cardiodynamic effects of propofol in comparison with thiopental: Assessment with a transesophageal echocardiographic approach. Anesth Analg 72:28–35, 1991

161. Lepage J-YM, Pinaud ML, Helias JH, Cozian AY, Le Normand Y, Souron RJ: Left ventricular performance during propofol and methohexital anesthesia: Isotopic and invasive cardiac monitoring. Anesth Analg 73:3–9, 1991

162. Gauss A, Heinrich H, Wilder-Smth OHG: Echocardiographic assessment of the haemodynamic effects of propofol: A comparison with etomidate and thiopentone. Anaesthesia 46:99–105, 1991

163. Coddens J, DeLoof T: End-systolic pressure-volume relationship and arterial elastance: The optimal method to evaluate myocardial contractile effects of anesthetic agents? [Letter]. Anesth Analg 74:165, 1992

164. Stowe DF, Bosnjak ZJ, Kampine JP: Comparison of etomidate, ketamine, midazolam, propofol, and thiopental on function and metabolism of isolated hearts. Anesth Analg 74:547–558, 1992

165. Azari DM, Cork RC: Comparative myocardial depressive effects of propofol and thiopental. Anesth Analg 77:324–329, 1993

166. Davies AE, McCans JL: Effects of barbiturate anesthetics and ketamine on the force-frequency relation of cardiac muscle. Eur J Pharmacol 59:65–73, 1979

167. Frankl WS, Poole-Wilson PA: Effects of thiopental on tension development, action potential, and exchange of calcium and potassium in rabbit ventricular myocardium. J Cardiovasc Pharmacol 3:554–565, 1981

168. Ikemoto Y: Reduction by thiopental of the slow-channel-mediated action potential of canine papillary muscle. Pfulgers Arch 372:285–286, 1977

169. Komai H, Rusy BF: Differences in the myocardial depressant action of thiopental and halothane. Anesth Analg 63:313–318, 1984

170. Blanck TJJ, Stevenson RL: Thiopental does not alter Ca^{2+} uptake by cardiac sarcoplasmic reticulum. Anesth Analg 67:346–348, 1988

171. Eckstein JW, Hamilton WK, McCammond JM: The effect of thiopental induction on peripheral venous tone. Anesthesiology 22:525–528, 1961

172. Flickinger H, Fraimow W, Cathcart RT, Nealon TF Jr: Effect of thiopental induction on cardiac output in man. Anesth Analg 40:693–700, 1961

173. Patschke D, Bruckner JB, Eberlein HJ, Hess W, Tarnow J, Weymar A: Effects of althesin, etomidate and fentanyl on haemodynamics and myocardial oxygen consumption in man. Can Anaesth Soc J 24:57–69, 1977

174. Criado A, Maseda J, Navarro E, Escarpa A, Avello F: Induction of anaesthesia with etomidate. Haemodynamic study of 36 patients. Br J Anaesth 52:803–806, 1980

175. Gooding JM, Corssen G: Effect of etomidate on the cardiovascular system. Anesth Analg 56:717–719, 1977

176. Gooding JM, Weng JT, Smith RA, Berninger GT, Kirby RR: Cardiovascular and pulmonary responses following etomidate induction of anesthesia in patients with demonstrated cardiac disease. Anesth Analg 58:40–41, 1979

177. Colvin MP, Savege TM, Newland PE, Weaver EJ, Waters AF, Brookes JM, Inniss R: Cardiorespiratory changes following induction of anaesthesia with etomidate in patients with cardiac disease. Br J Anaesth 51:551–556, 1979

178. Prakash O, Dhasmana KM, Verdouw PD, Saxena PR: Cardiovascular effects of etomidate with emphasis on regional myocardial blood flow and performance. Br J Anaesth 53:591–599, 1981

179. Riou B, Lecarpentier Y, Chemla D, Viars P: *In Vitro* effects of etomidate on intrinsic myocardial contractility in the rat. Anesthesiology 72:330–340, 1990

180. Riou B, Lecarpentier Y, Viars P: Effects of etomidate on the cardiac papillary muscle of normal hamsters and those with cardiomyopathy. Anesthesiology 78:83–90, 1993

181. Komai H, DeWitt DE, Rusy BF: Negative inotropic effects of etomidate in rabbit papillary muscle. Anesth Analg 64:400–404, 1985

182. Brussel T, Theissen JL, Vigfusson G, Lunkenheimer PP, Van Aken H, Lawin P: Hemodynamic and cardiodynamic effects of propofol and etomidate: Negative inotropic properties of propofol. Anesth Analg 69:35–40, 1989

183. De Hert SG, Vermeyen KM, Adriaensen HF: Influence of thiopental, etomidate, and propofol on regional myocardial function in the normal and acute ischemic heart segment in dogs. Anesth Analg 70:600–607, 1990

184. Kissin I, Motomura S, Aultman DF, Reves JG: Inotropic and anesthetic potencies of etomidate and thiopental in dogs. Anesth Analg 62:961–965, 1983

185. Sebel PS, Lowdon JD: Propofol: A new intravenous anesthetic. Anesthesiology 71:260–277, 1989

186. Muzi M, Berens RA, Kampine JP, Ebert TJ: Venodilation contributes to propofol-mediated hypotension in humans. Anesth Analg 74:877–883, 1992

187. Rouby JJ, Andreev A, Leger P, Arthaud M, Landault C, Vicaut E, Maistre G, Eurin J, Gandjbakch I, Viars P: Peripheral vascular effects of thiopental and propofol in humans with artificial hearts. Anesthesiology 75:32–42, 1991

188. Coetzee A, Fourie P, Coetzee J, Badenhorst E, Rebel A, Bolliger C, Uebel R, Wium C, Lombard C: Effect of various propofol plasma concentrations on regional myocardial contractility and left ventricular afterload. Anesth Analg 69:473–483, 1989

189. Pagel PS, Warltier DC: Negative inotropic effects of propofol as evaluated by the regional preload recruitable stroke work relationship in chronically instrumented dogs. Anesthesiology 78:100–108, 1993

190. Park WK, Lynch C III: Propofol and thiopental depression of myocardial contractility: A comparative study of mechanical and electrophysiologic effects in isolated guinea pig ventricular muscle. Anesth Analg 74:395–405, 1992

191. Pagel PS, Schmeling WT, Kampine JP, Warltier DC: Alteration of canine left ventricular diastolic function by intravenous anesthetics in vivo: Ketamine and propofol. Anesthesiology 76:419–425, 1992

192. Riou B, Besse S, Lecarpentier Y, Viars P: In vitro effects of propofol on rat myocardium. Anesthesiology 76:609–616, 1992

193. White PF, Way WL, Trevor AJ: Ketamine—its pharmacology and therapeutic uses. Anesthesiology 56:119–136, 1982

194. Waxman K, Shoemaker WC, Lippmann M: Cardiovascular effects of anesthetic induction with ketamine. Anesth Analg 59:355–358, 1980

195. Lundy PM, Gverzdys S, Frew R: Ketamine: Evidence of tissue specific inhibition of neuronal and extraneuronal catecholamine uptake processes. Can J Physiol Pharmacol 63:298–303, 1985

196. Salt PJ, Barnes PK, Beswick FJ: Inhibition of neuronal and extraneuronal uptake of noradrenaline by ketamine in the isolated perfused rat heart. Br J Anaesth 51:835–838, 1979

197. Schwartz DA, Horwitz LD: Effects of ketamine on left ventricular performance. J Pharmacol Exp Ther 194:410–414, 1975

198. Tweed WA, Minuck M, Mymin D: Circulatory response to ketamine anesthesia. Anesthesiology 37:613–619, 1972

199. Ivankovich AD, Miletich DJ, Reimann C, Albrecht RF, Zahed B: Cardiovascular effects of centrally administered ketamine in goats. Anesth Analg 53:924–933, 1974

200. Pagel PS, Kampine JP, Schmeling WT, Warltier DC: Ketamine depresses myocardial contractility as evaluated by the preload recruitable stroke work relationship in chronically instrumented dogs with autonomic nervous system blockade. Anesthesiology 76:564–572, 1992

201. Cook DJ, Carton EG, Housmans PR: Mechanism of the positive inotropic effect of ketamine in isolated ferret ventricular papillary muscle. Anesthesiology 74:880–888, 1991

202. Cook DJ, Housmans PR, Rorie DK: Effect of ketamine HCl on norepinephrine disposition in isolated ferret ventricular myocardium. J Pharmacol Exp Ther 261:101–107, 1992

203. Kongsayreepong S, Cook DJ, Housmans PR: Mechanism of the direct, negative inotropic effect of ketamine in isolated ferret and frog ventricular myocardium. Anesthesiology 79:313–322, 1993

204. Rusy BF, Amuzu JK, Bosscher HA, Redon D, Komai H: Negative inotropic effect of ketamine in rabbit ventricular muscle. Anesth Analg 71:275–278, 1990

205. Urthaler F, Walker AA, James TN: Comparison of the inotropic action of morphine and ketamine studied in canine cardiac muscle. J Thorac Cardiovasc Surg 72:142–149, 1976

Matthew J. A. Benson
Michael K. Cahalan
Manfred D. Seeberger
Damon C. Sutton
Kathryn Rouine-Rapp

8 | The Echocardiographic Assessment of Left Ventricular Function

Left ventricular function is vital for and predictive of survival. Despite advances in patient assessment and care, cardiac morbidity continues to be the leading cause of perioperative death.[1,2] Moreover, as the surgical patient population continues to age and the incidence of coronary artery disease and other diseases associated with aging increases, a greater number of patients with left ventricular dysfunction will require anesthesia. Therefore, anesthesiologists must be able to assess left ventricular function in order to employ appropriate treatment modalities.

Intraoperative transesophageal echocardiography (TEE) was first used to assess left ventricular function,[3] and currently, high-resolution TEE technology allows anesthesiologists to view cardiac filling and ejection in real time throughout surgery. This chapter reviews TEE assessment of left ventricular function: first, global left ventricular function, cardiac output, ejection fraction, and assessment of acute hypotension; and second, assessment of regional function and myocardial ischemia.

GLOBAL LV FUNCTION

TEE can assess global left ventricular function indirectly by measurement of cardiac output, stroke volume, or ejection fraction. In addition,

Ventricular Function, edited by David C. Warltier. Williams & Wilkins, Baltimore © 1995.

TEE can measure those factors that directly affect ventricular function: preload, contractility, and afterload. At the moment, most intraoperative assessment is qualitative: digital storage of the images allows rapid side-by-side comparison of images obtained at different times (Fig. 8–1). Recently, automated systems for quantitative analysis of left ventricular function have been introduced which allow for potential continuous comparisons with enhanced precision.

Automated Analysis of LV Filling and Ejection

Automated edge or border detection (ABD) is a hardware-based algorithm that processes acoustic data before compression into video format. Previous efforts to characterize blood and myocardial tissue, on the basis of their different ultrasound-scattering properties, have been hampered by noise (coherent speckle) in the returning signal.[4–8] This coher-

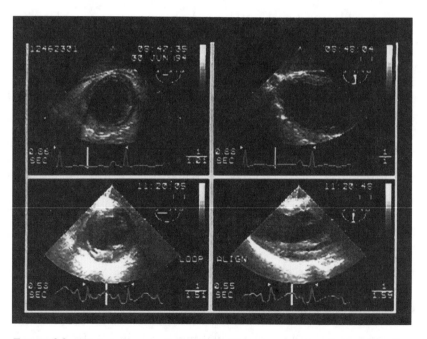

FIGURE 8-1. Digital storage and playback of four separate views for rapid qualitative analysis. The *top* two images (midpapillary short- and long-axis views) are taken from the prebypass period. The *bottom* two images are the same views taken after coronary grafting has occurred. The loops are of one RR interval and played back so that the RR interval occurs over the same time period to eliminate the effect of change in heart rate.

ent speckle is reduced in the ABD system by integrating the backscatter in the returning signal, facilitating the accurate description of the boundary between high (myocardium) and low (blood) signal power.

Optimal image quality is first obtained by appropriate adjustment of the controls of the ultrasonograph. Then the ABD system is activated, which highlights the derived endocardial borders automatically. Automatic border detection is optimized by adjusting time-gain compensations and lateral gain controls. Within a user-defined region of interest (containing the left ventricle but excluding other cardiac chambers), the ABD system sums the cross-sectional area of blood in each video frame (30 per sec) and displays this information as continuously updated plots of area and derived variables, such as fractional area change and rate of change of area vs time (Fig. 8–2).

The performance of the ABD system depends critically on image quality and operator intervention for selection of appropriate time-gain compensation settings. Even when border detection is deemed excellent, some areas of myocardium in the septum and posterior wall may be identified as blood and not tissue, leading to an overestimate of end-

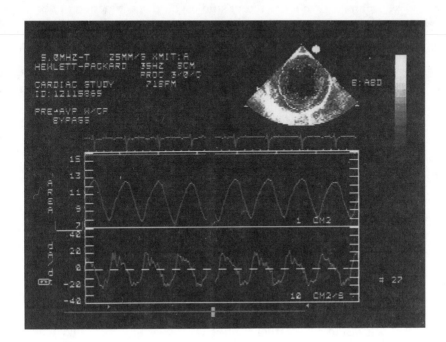

FIGURE 8-2. Automatic border detection (*ABD*) with the endocardial border highlighted within an area of interest. The *top curve* depicts the area with time. The *bottom curve* depicts the first derivative (*dA/dt*).

systolic area. This problem of myocardial dropout, or anisotropy, may be decreased by use of a lower frequency transducer and by drawing a "tight" region of interest around the endocardial border at end diastole. Also, the endocardial border tracking may be disrupted by marked changes in cardiac size or position because the region of interest and gain control settings are fixed at specified depths of the scan.

We have recently found that in 72 to 86% of adult patients monitored with intraoperative TEE, ABD estimates of end-diastolic (EDA) and end-systolic areas (ESAs) fall within the limits expected of an expert, but in a fraction of the time.[9] However, because ABD slightly underestimated EDA and overestimated ESA, its estimates of fractional area change were unacceptably higher than measurements by an expert. In the other 14 to 28% of patients, problems with cavity area estimation were confirmed by comparison to independent off-line expert measurements and could be predicted by recognition of inadequate border detection in the real-time images.

ABD estimates of left ventricular EDAs and ESAs exclude the papillary muscles because the ABD system correctly recognizes the papillary muscles as tissue and not blood. This is in contrast to standard measurement techniques that include the papillary muscles in the cavity area estimation. In more recent studies, on-line estimation of beat-to-beat changes in stroke volume have been shown to be determined by ABD.[10]

Cardiac Output Determination

Although viewing TEE images of left ventricular filling and ejection gives one an immediate method to detect marked changes in cardiac output, our recent studies suggest this practice may be unreliable.[11] Fortunately, substantial research using Doppler has established that TEE can measure cardiac output. Investigators have studied flows in the main pulmonary artery and across the mitral valve. Initial results were somewhat disappointing,[12] but subsequent studies excluding patients with tricuspid regurgitation (known to confound thermodilution) were more promising.[13] These investigations suggest that TEE should have a bias of near zero and limits of agreement of less than 1 liter/minute when compared with thermodilution, for detecting absolute cardiac output. The one drawback of Doppler estimation is that not all patients have suitable anatomy for these measurements; failure rates range from 8 to 24%.[13–15]

In contrast to these earlier studies, Darmon et al.[16] were able to determine the cardiac output in all patients using a transgastric long-axis view of the left ventricular outflow tract. Not only were these investigators able to acquire adequate Doppler signals in all patients, but they achieved excellent concordance with the thermodilution cardiac output (limits of agreement of 0.91 1/min). These investigators used continuous wave Doppler and a triangular model of the aortic valve (Fig. 8–3). Compared to the usual circular model, the correlation coefficient improved from $r = 0.88$ to $r = 0.93$.

Ejection Fraction Determination

Using TEE to obtain quantitative ejection fraction (EF) by nonautomated techniques is time-consuming and consequently mainly a research tool. The accuracy of TEE estimation of EF varies. When compared to radionuclide EF, TEE has a correlation coefficient of $r= 0.80$.[17] When compared to measures of EF by transthoracic echocardiography, TEE estimation initially reached good correlation ($r = 0.98$).[18] In a sub-

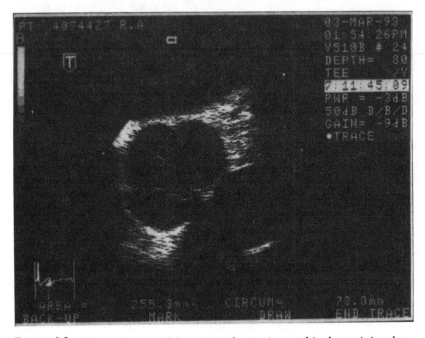

FIGURE 8-3. Triangular area of the aortic valve tracing used in determining the cardiac output. The area (A) is given by the following formula: $A = 0.5 \cos 30°.S^2$, where S = the average length of the three sides of the valve. (*Reproduced with permission from Darmon PL et al. Anesthesiology 80:796–805,1994*)

sequent sample, this correlation was not as good ($r = 0.83$), presumably because of the problem with imaging the apex when using TEE. Another technique, the left ventricular fractional area change ([EDA − ESA]/EDA) measured at the midpapillary short-axis view is a reasonable approximation of EF. Ejection fraction is clearly preload and afterload-dependent and as such should be viewed cautiously as an index of overall ventricular performance. However, it is still an excellent predictor of survival in patients with coronary artery disease and is widely used in the preoperative assessment of high-risk patients.

There are other echocardiographic techniques that have been shown to correlate reasonably well with the EF,[19,20] but these tend to be used off-line because of their labor intensity. One technique that is relatively easy to use and has been shown to have high sensitivity and specificity has been described by Ohte et al.[21] The shortest distance between the mitral leaflets coaptation and the interventricular septum at end-systole (MVC-IVS distance) is measured. An MVC-IVS distance of greater than or equal to 30 mm suggests left ventricular dysfunction (EF less than 50%) with high sensitivity (94.4%) and specificity (90.6%), while a value less than 30 mm suggests that left ventricular performance is likely to be within normal limits.

3D-TEE Assessment of LV Filling and Ejection

The technique of 3D-TEE is a promising one (Fig. 8–4). The accuracy of volume and EF measurement is comparable to that of other currently used clinical approaches such as radionuclide scintigraphy and angiography.[17,22-26] 3D imaging also promises substantial advantages in the evaluation of regional function as well, avoiding the criticism of 2D-TEE, that only one plane is viewed.[27] However, ongoing problems with 3D imaging include the need for an external frame of reference, the requirement to scan the apex more consistently, and the time-consuming effort to collate images (minutes to hours).

Assessment of Preload

TEE can provide accurate estimates of left ventricular preload. For instance, Harpole et al. studied 12 patients during resection of abdominal aortic aneurysm[28] and showed excellent correlation between echocardiographic and radionuclide estimates of left ventricular volume as a measure of filling. Interestingly, in contrast, virtually no correlation was observed between estimates from either of these techniques and pulmonary artery pressure. However, if severe segmental wall motion

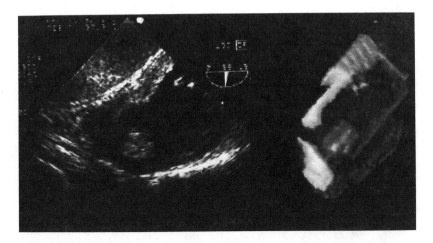

FIGURE 8-4. Conventional 2D (left) image and 3D (*right*) image of the left ventricle showing a left ventricular myxoma. Note the apparent ventricular septal defect in the 3D image due to dropout caused by the very echo-dense myxoma. (*Courtesy of Drs. Foster and Stainback*)

abnormalities are present, information from a single cross-section may not be adequate.

Using TEE to assess preload avoids the assumption that left ventricular end-diastolic volume (true preload) and left ventricular end-diastolic pressure as reflected by the pulmonary capillary wedge pressure are consistently related during surgery. For instance, Kalman et al. studied 23 patients during elective abdominal vascular surgery.[29] These investigators compared pulmonary capillary wedge pressure and radionuclide estimates of left ventricular end-diastolic volume preoperatively, during aortic cross-clamping, and immediately after unclamping the aorta. Following unclamping, wedge pressure was unchanged, but left ventricular end-diastolic volume decreased significantly, suggesting a marked decrease in ventricular diastolic compliance. Concomitantly, blood pressure and cardiac output decreased. In this clinical setting, the authors point out that use of pulmonary capillary wedge pressure data might result in inappropriate therapy (e.g., inotropic support instead of volume administration).

Surprisingly, TEE also provides practical ways to estimate left ventricular filling pressure. By placing the Doppler cursor at the junction of the left atrium and left superior pulmonary vein, Kuecherer et al. demonstrated that the systolic fraction of pulmonary venous flow into the left atrium was inversely correlated with left atrial pressure.[30] The proximity of the TEE transducer to the pulmonary veins permits excellent Doppler recordings of their flow which is biphasic (systolic and diastolic) in nature. A systolic fraction of flow of less than 55% was a specific and sensitive marker of left atrial pressure greater than 15 mm Hg. This can be easily recognized in real time as predominance of flow during diastole (Fig. 8–5). Unfortunately, this specificity and sensitivity decrease in patients who have significant mitral regurgitation, nonsinus rhythms, and marked changes in left ventricular contractility.

In a separate study, Kusumoto et al. noted that at low or normal left atrial pressures the interatrial septum transiently reverses its normal rightward curvature during the exhalation phase of positive pressure ventilation (because for just this moment the right atrial pressure exceeds the left atrial pressure).[31] Absence of this reversal of septal movement has a positive predictive value of 0.97 for a left atrial pressure of greater than 15 mm Hg. TEE cannot quantitatively measure left atrial pressure, but this technique appears able to reliably identify clinically significant elevations of left ventricular preload.

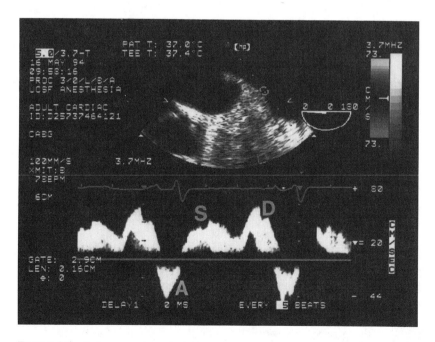

FIGURE 8-5. Pulse wave Doppler of the left upper pulmonary vein. This displays an abnormal pattern of diastolic dominance suggesting an elevated left atrial pressure. S, systolic flow; D, diastolic flow; A, flow reversal with atrial contraction.

Assessment of the Hypotensive Surgical Patient

Qualitative estimates of left ventricular filling and ejection serve as a practical guide for administration of fluids and inotropes during a sudden, severe decrease in arterial pressure. In some ultrasonographs, computer technology converts the echocardiographic images from one cardiac cycle into digital code and then plays the cycle repeatedly for side-by-side comparison with other cardiac cycles captured at previous times during surgery. This juxtapositioning of images greatly facilitates the qualitative evaluation of changes in ventricular performance and the prompt diagnosis of the etiology of hypotension (Table 8–1). When arterial vasodilatation is considered the apparent cause of hypotension and vasoconstrictor therapy is planned, severe aortic regurgitation, mitral regurgitation, and ventricular septal defect can be ruled out first by TEE. These abnormalities can produce exactly the same left ventricular filling and ejection pattern as severe arterial vasodilation but require different therapy.

Assessment of Contractility

A practical and reliable real-time measure of myocardial contractility would be useful for evaluating the effects of coronary revascularization, myocardial preservation techniques, and drugs on ventricular performance. Unfortunately, most echocardiographic indices of contractility, such as the end-systolic wall stress dimension and end-systolic wall stress rate-corrected velocity of fiber shortening are dependent on loading conditions.

In contrast, the ventricular pressure to volume ratio at end-systole is relatively insensitive to cardiac loading and varies directly with changes in ventricular contractility.[32-34] The introduction of ABD (see above) has made it possible to obtain a pressure/volume analysis in real time from TEE and peripheral arterial pressure. The values of end-

TABLE 8–1.   TEE AND THE ETIOLOGY OF HYPOTENSION

	LV Filling	LV Ejection
Hypovolemia	↓↓	↑↑
Cardiac depression	↑↑	↓↓
Arterial vasodilatation	Adequate	↑↑
Severe mitral regurgitation	Adequate	↑↑
Severe aortic incompetence	Adequate or ↑↑	↑ or ↔
Large ventricular septal defect	Adequate or ↑	↑↑

systolic pressure estimated by peripheral pressure[35,36] and ESA from the area-vs-time ABD plot can be collected during a rapid change in preload, afterload or contractility produced by administration of glyceryl trinitrate, phenylephrine or dobutamine and plotted (Fig. 8–6). Alternatively, these parameters can be monitored in real time in cardiac surgery patients in whom load and contractility may be expected to vary rapidly.[37] A key advantage of this method over other load-independent indices of contractility (such as the preload recruitable stroke work index[38]; see Chapters 3 and 4) is that the area beneath the end-systolic pressure-dimension relationship does not require left ventricular pressure measurement and can be obtained relatively noninvasively from TEE and peripheral arterial pressure.[39]

Assessment of Diastolic Function

Although it is well recognized that diastolic dysfunction often precedes the impairment of systolic function,[40,41] there are no direct methods to monitor either ventricular relaxation or compliance intraoperatively. However, TEE allows indirect measures of diastolic function by analysis of the velocity of flow of blood through the mitral valve. Normally, early diastolic filling (the "E"-wave) predominates (Fig. 8–7). When the rate of ventricular relaxation is impaired, the E-wave is reduced, and

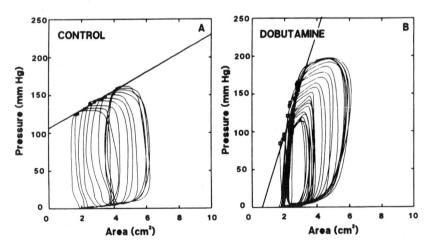

FIGURE 8-6. Pressure-area curves showing the relationship between change in the ABD-derived area and the systemic arterial pressure. The introduction of an inotrope (dobutamine) shifts the slope of the end-systolic pressure area curve up and to the left, representing an increase in contractility. (*Reproduced with permission from Gorcsan J III et al. J Am Coll Cardiol 23:242–252,1994*)

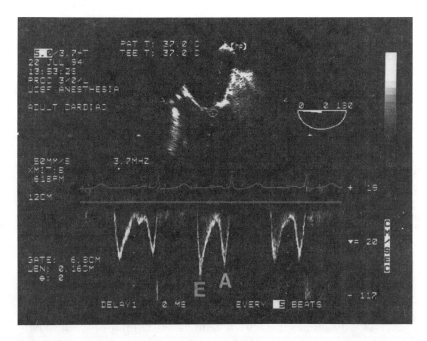

FIGURE 8-7. Pulsed wave Doppler through a normal mitral valve. *E*, E-wave, early diastolic flow; *A*, A-wave, atrial systole flow.

most ventricular filling occurs during atrial systole, causing A-wave dominance. In contrast, when the compliance of the ventricle is reduced but the rate of relaxation is normal, the E-wave is increased and the A-wave reduced. With age, the ventricle has a normal decrease in rate of relaxation, resulting in a normal pattern of A-wave dominance in the aged. However, if the ventricle has a pathological process causing decreased compliance (leading to an increase in the E-wave) the waveforms begin to appear more like the normal pattern of the young. Thus, in the elderly a "normal" pattern (pseudonormalization) is actually abnormal. Other derived indices, such as peak and integrated velocities of early diastolic filling and atrial contraction and their ratios and acceleration and deceleration times of early filling have been studied. Unfortunately, no simple relationship exists between these indices and diastolic function, because all relationships are confounded by ventricular loading,[42–44] heart rate,[45,46] and contractility.[43,44,47] Other influences include autonomic blockade,[48] cardiopulmonary bypass,[49] and various other determinants of ventricular compliance[50] and relaxation,[43,44,51] as well as atrial compliance.[52–54]

Color flow imaging shows that the transmitral flow is initially directed to the left ventricular apex and then turns 180° to the left ventricular outflow tract. Pulse wave Doppler in the outflow tract confirms this biphasic flow pattern. Pai and Shah[55] have compared this flow pattern to that across the mitral valve and showed a linear relationship between the rate of the diastolic flow wave propagation inside the left ventricle and its stiffness. They also postulated this relationship to be independent of heart rate and preload. In a similar analysis of flow Brun et al.[56] also demonstrated that flow propagation within the left ventricle is related to stiffness and state of relaxation. These preliminary studies will require further verification before their clinical implications are clear.

Assessment of Afterload

TEE derived end-systolic wall stress is a better measure of left ventricular afterload than is systemic vascular resistance, because the former incorporates ventricular dimension, pressure, and wall thickness.[36,57,58] The problem with systemic vascular resistance as a measure of afterload is that it assumes that the left ventricle is a nonpulsatile pump with steady-state hemodynamic characteristics. A better estimate of afterload is end-systolic meridional wall stress. Smith and colleagues showed this measure of afterload to have a strong association with intraoperative myocardial ischemia in a study of patients undergoing carotid endarterectomy.[59] Systolic blood pressure was maintained at the preoperative level in patients randomized to two experimental groups: one using phenylephrine and the other a "light" anesthesia. A 40% higher wall stress (despite comparable blood pressures) and a 2 1/2-fold higher incidence of ischemia were found in the group receiving phenylephrine, indicating the importance of wall stress as a deter-

TABLE 8–2.   TEE AND THE DIAGNOSIS OF ISCHEMIA

	Wall Thickening	Δ in Radius[a]
0. No view		
1. Normal or hyperkinetic	Marked	>30% ↓
2. Mild hypokinesis	Moderate	10–30% ↓
3. Severe hypokinesis	Minimal	<10, >0% ↓
4. Akinesis	None	No Δ
5. Dyskinesis	Thinning	↑

[a] Percent change in the radius (midpapillary short-axis view) from the imaginary center of the left ventricle to the endocardium during systole. Ischemia is diagnosed by a two-class worsening of segmental function.

minant of oxygen demand and myocardial ischemia. Unfortunately, calculation of systolic wall stress is tedious and not yet available in any automated system. Qualitatively the wall stress can often be inferred by knowledge of the preload (ventricular size) and ejection status and presence of valvular regurgitation during a critical event such as hypotension (Table 8–1).

REGIONAL LV FUNCTION

Assessment of Regional Perfusion

No reliable, quantifiable index of tissue perfusion is currently available, either to assess baseline disease or the efficacy of coronary artery bypass graft surgery. Sonicated Renografin-76 microbubbles have been used with TEE[60] with good results. However, this agent must be injected into the aortic root or coronary arteries. Various other agents that can be injected peripherally are currently being tested.

Assessment of Regional Systolic Contraction

In 1935, segmental wall motion abnormalities were shown to occur during cessation of myocardial blood flow in an animal model.[61] Since then they have been shown to occur within seconds of the onset of regional ischemia,[61–63] simultaneously with regional lactate production,[64] and before (and even in the absence of) changes on the surface electrocardiogram.[65] Not only are segmental wall motion abnormalities indicative of ischemia (Table 8–2) but in some clinical settings, prognostic of survival after myocardial infarction.[66] The location of wall motion abnormalities via TEE also provides an indication of the coronary arteries involved and the ultimate site of infarction (Fig. 8–8).

Other than ischemia, no pathophysiological process produces such acute changes in segmental myocardial contraction. Until the advent of TEE, anesthesiologists could not detect these changes because they had no way of directly monitoring myocardial contraction. Beaupre et al.[67] first reported the use of this technique for intraoperative detection of myocardial infarction when they noted a new anteroseptal wall motion abnormality after cardiopulmonary bypass that persisted until the conclusion of surgery. Within 18 hours, an anteroseptal myocardial infarction was confirmed by changes in the echocardiogram.

Subsequently, Smith et al.[68] used TEE in 50 patients undergoing coronary artery or major vascular surgery. At predetermined intervals, echocardiograms and multilead echocardiograms (limb leads, aug-

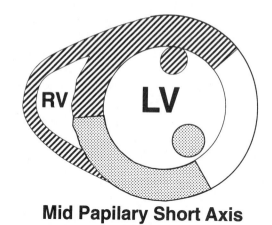

Mid Papilary Short Axis

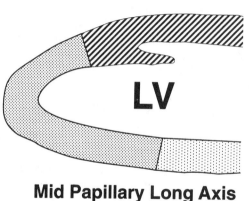

Mid Papillary Long Axis

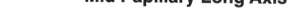

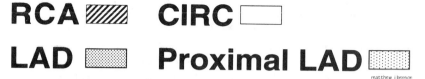

FIGURE 8-8. A drawing of the midpapillary short and long axes showing the territory supplied by the coronary arteries. *RV*, right ventricle; *LV*, left ventricle; *LAD*, Left anterior descending artery; *CIRC*, circumflex coronary artery; *RCA*, right coronary artery.

mented leads, and V5) were recorded, both of which were evaluated by "blinded" observers. Intraoperatively, six patients had ST segment changes diagnostic of myocardial ischemia ($\geq$0.1 mV deviation), while 24 had new segmental wall motion abnormalities indicative of myocardial ischemia. No patient experienced an ST segment change before or in the absence of a new wall motion abnormality. In three of the six patients who experienced ST segment alterations, the segmental wall motion abnormality occurred minutes before the electrocardiographic change. Three of the 50 patients suffered intraoperative myocardial infarctions, and all had a wall motion abnormality develop and persist until the end of surgery in the corresponding area of myocardium. Only one of these patients had intraoperative ST segment change diagnostic of ischemia. Ten patients without coronary disease were also studied, and none of these patients developed segmental wall motion abnormalities. In the 50 patients with coronary disease, 97% of the echocardiograms were analyzed, but inadequate resolution or an inappropriate cross-section prevented analysis in the other 3%. In contrast, only 86% of the electrocardiograms could be analyzed because of the onset of bundle branch block or paced rhythm.

Leung et al.[69] found comparable results in a similar study in which continuous TEE and 2-lead Holter recordings were used in patients undergoing coronary artery surgery. In both studies, however, hemodynamics were not shown to be predictive of ischemia or postoperative cardiac complications. Thus, in patients with coronary artery disease, myocardial ischemia can be detected more frequently with TEE than with electrocardiography, and when new abnormalities of wall motion persist through the conclusion of surgery they should be viewed as prognostic signs for cardiovascular complications.

The insensitivity of hemodynamics for the detection of myocardial ischemia, in particular pulmonary capillary wedge pressure, has been previously demonstrated.[70] In 98 patients anesthetized with high doses of opioids, 12-lead electrocardiography and TEE identified 14 patients experiencing ischemia before the start of coronary artery surgery (all 14 had TEE-detected segmental wall motion abnormalities) and 10 also had ST segment changes). Concomitant with the onset of ischemia, pulmonary capillary wedge pressure increased 3.5 $\pm$ 4.8 mm Hg. However, many patients without ischemia experienced similar increases in wedge pressure. In fact, an increase of 3 mm Hg in pulmonary capillary wedge pressure had a sensitivity of 33% and a positive predictive value of 16% for detection of myocardial ischemia in this patient population.

In contrast to these studies, Eisenberg et al.[71] found very poor concordance between continuous intraoperative 2-lead or 12-lead electrocardiography and TEE monitoring in the diagnosis of myocardial ischemia. Only 17 of 174 (10%) of the total episodes of ischemia were detected by all three monitors. The concordance between TEE and the 2-lead or 12-lead electrocardiograms was 16%, and between 2-lead and 12-lead only 37%, with the 2-lead system actually detecting almost twice as many episodes of ischemia as either the 12-lead system or TEE (122 vs 74 vs 72 episodes, respectively). These results are in marked contrast to other studies which have compared echocardiography and electrocardiography for the detection of myocardial ischemia during intraoperative monitoring,[59,68–70] myocardial infarction,[66] stress testing,[72] and coronary angioplasty.[73,74]

The authors offer no explanation for this striking lack of concordance. However, because they found no independent value for TEE or the 12-lead electrocardiogram in predicting postoperative cardiac complications, they concluded that TEE and 12-lead electrocardiography are of unproven worth in monitoring for myocardial ischemia in noncardiac surgical patients. We would offer a number of cautions regarding this conclusion. First, the electrocardiograms were evaluated continuously while the TEE images only intermittently. Second, only about half of the patients had definite evidence of coronary artery disease, and only 11 patients had significant outcomes thought to be directly attributable to coronary artery disease. Third, the anesthesiologists were not permitted to view any of the monitors being studied (they used their standard electrocardiography system with which they detected a total of eight patients having myocardial ischemia). Thus, other monitoring advantages of TEE could not be utilized. Finally, the TEE data were interpreted by consensus evaluation and not by multiple independent observers. We have noted that the concordance between electrocardiographic and TEE evidence of ischemia is better when two independent readers are used to review the echocardiograms[59,68,70] than when only one reader or a consensus of two simultaneous readers is used.[71,75]

There are a number of general limitations of TEE in the diagnosis of ischemia (Table 8–3). Even when an area of myocardium is clearly in view, its segmental contraction can be difficult to evaluate if the entire heart rotates or translates markedly during systole, or if discoordinated contraction occurs due to bundle branch block or ventricular pacing. Consequently, a valid system for assessing segmental wall motion abnormalities must first compensate for global motion of the heart (usually done by a "floating" frame of reference) and then evaluate both regional endocardial motion and myocardial thickening. Unfortunately, no currently available automated wall motion analysis system has proven adequate for TEE images. However, Sklenar et al.[76] have described a computer-aided approach for measuring left ventricular wall thickening and endocardial motion and curvature during an entire systolic contraction sequence. It delineates the endocardial and epicardial

TABLE 8–3. LIMITATIONS OF TEE DIAGNOSIS OF ISCHEMIA

SWMAa Artifacts	SWMAs Not Caused by Acute Ischemia
1. Changed cross-section	1. Preload[85]
2. Translation	2. Afterload[b]
3. Discoordination	3. Tethering
4. Anisotropy	4. Stunning

aSWMA, segmental wall motion abnormality.
bSubtle SWMA even with large increases in afterload.[84]

borders without manual tracing and may enable on-line quantitative analysis of wall movement.

Interpretation of septal motion is most often confounded by discoordinated contraction. When the septum is viable and nonischemic, it will appreciably thicken during systole, although its inward motion may begin slightly before or after inward motion of the other walls of the ventricle. Thus, new wall motion abnormalities can be detected during bundle branch block, ventricular pacing, and marked global movements of the heart, but not by assessment of endocardial motion alone.

All segmental wall motion abnormalities are not indicative of myocardial ischemia (Table 8–3). Because of biological differences in normal patients, not all hearts contract normally, and not all parts of the same heart contract to the same degree.[77] Myocardial infarction, previous cardiac surgery,[78] and myocarditis can cause wall motion abnormalities, but a new acute, decrease or cessation of segmental contraction, for example, as occurs during surgery, is almost certainly due to myocardial ischemia. One exception to this rule is myocardial stunning or prolonged, postischemic ventricular dysfunction. When ischemia has been prolonged, full restoration of blood flow may occur minutes to hours before return of normal segmental contraction.[79] Does a new regional contractile deficit detected immediately after coronary artery bypass graft surgery represent inadequate revascularization and ongoing ischemia or stunned myocardium from inadequate cooling during bypass? Inadequate revascularization may require placement of additional grafts, while stunned myocardium requires only supportive measures until function ultimately returns. Echocardiographic contrast agents capable of readily delineating myocardial blood flow are not yet clinically available but do appear quite promising.[80–83] At present when faced with this clinical dilemma, graft status is reevaluated and the new wall motion abnormality watched for signs of improvement. If deterioration of function occurs, graft status is questionable, or systemic hemodynamics are unstable, then additional revascularization is provided if possible.

Another possible cause of acute segmental wall motion abnormalities is unmasking of areas of previous scarring by changes in afterload. For instance, a marked increase in arterial pressure might retard contraction in an already damaged segment of myocardium more than in a normal segment. Three observations make this an unlikely explanation for the wall motion alterations reported in the studies above. First, only marked changes in segmental contraction were taken as indicative of ischemia. Indeed, Buffington and Coyle,[84] in a canine model, demonstrated that a large increase in afterload only produces a subtle change in wall movement of stunned myocardium. Second, previous studies have not found any consistent correlation between hemodynamic aberrations and new wall motion abnormalities. In contrast to these observations, Seeberger et al.[85] demonstrated an appearance of regional dysfunction with severe reduction in preload. In general, anesthesiologists prevent marked changes in loading conditions. Third, the vast majority of new segmental wall motion abnormalities occurred in segments of myocardium with normal contraction at baseline (after induction of anesthesia). Thus, acute changes in left ventricular loading probably require an intervention by the anesthesiologist, and can cause myocardial ischemia, but alone are not an explanation for new wall motion abnormalities.

Tethering or systolic dysfunction of nonischemic myocardium adjacent to ischemic or infarcted myocardium is also commonly mentioned as another cause of "artifactual" changes in wall motion. Tethering probably accounts for the consistent overestimation of infarct size by echocardiography when compared to postmortem studies. However, Force et al.,[86] using an improved analysis system, found that segmental contraction is normal to within 1 cm of the ischemic area. Thus, tethering may actually help in the intraoperative detection of myocardial ischemia by making a new wall motion abnormality involve an area of myocardium slightly larger than the true area of ischemia. Tethering alone is not responsible for new wall motion abnormalities in the absence of acute myocardial ischemia.

Monitoring segmental wall motion from a single short-axis monitoring position will miss ischemia confined to the right ventricle, apex, or base of the left ventricle. Shah et al.[87] recently studied 94 patients intraoperatively or in the intensive care unit with biplane TEE and found abnormalities of wall motion in either the longitudinal long-axis or transverse short-axis images of the left ventricle in 20 patients. Segmental wall motion abnormalities in seven patients were visible only in the longitudinal plane. However, multiple transverse cuts through the left ventricle at different heights may provide similar information.[88]

One limitation of using TEE as a monitor of ischemia is the need for constant vigilance. Obviously, it would be easier if the occurrence of ischemia could be predicted. Preoperative stress echocardiography, either by atrial pacing or administration of positive chronotropic drug, may be able to define the high-risk patient and thus enable a higher level of vigilance. However, preoperative stress testing is not always possible. Up to one-third of operations are urgent or emergent.[89] For these patients, intraoperative stress echocardiography may define those at high risk of ischemia.[90] Another benefit of stress echocardiography may be to assess the adequacy of revascularization.[91]

Other echocardiographic signs suggestive of ischemia include the onset of mitral regurgitation[92] (particularly involving the posterior papillary muscle) or decreasing EF and other load-dependent indicators of contractility. Unfortunately, abnormal mitral valve inflow indices, such as mitral regurgitation, are not specific to ischemia and have been shown to be dependent on sample volume position, preload and afterload, contractility, heart rate, rhythm, P-Q interval, left atrial to left ventricular pressure gradient, mitral valve size and geometry, and other factors.[40,41]

SUMMARY

TEE is used to assess the left ventricle in both qualitative and quantitative manners. Qualitative assessment can guide administration of fluids and inotropic drugs and monitor left ventricular function intraoperatively. For instance, left ventricular hypovolmia or depression are easily recognized by directly noting a small end-diastolic area or low EF, respectively. Appropriate therapy can be instituted and continuously monitored. New applications and technical improvements in TEE continue at a remarkable rate. Future versions of automatic border detection technology are likely to address the problem of anisotropy, require less user intervention, and incorporate three-dimensional information from multiplane probes to produce real-time estimates of left ventricular volumes. The raw information in the returning signal is likely to be further analyzed to allow characterization of ischemic, but still viable, tissue. Coupled with the ability to assess regional myocardial perfusion by contrast echocardiography, the clinician will be able to institute more timely and appropriate medical and surgical therapy.

References

1. Hertzer NR: Basic data concerning associated coronary disease in peripheral vascular patients. Ann Vasc Surg 1:616–620, 1987

2. Roger VL, Ballard DJ, Hallett JJ, et al: Influence of coronary artery disease on morbidity and mortality after abdominal aortic aneurysmectomy: A population-based study, 1971–1987. J Am Coll Cardiol 14:1245–1252, 1989

3. Matsumoto M, Oka Y, Lin YT, et al: Transesophageal echocardiography: For assessing ventricular performance. N Y State J Med 79:19–21, 1979

4. Geiser EA, Wilson DC, Gibby GL: Applications of cross-correlation techniques to the quantitation of wall motion in short-axis two-dimensional echocardiographic images. J Am Soc Echocardiogr 3:266–275, 1990

5. Melton HJ, Collins SM, Skorton DJ: Automatic real-time endocardial edge detection in two-dimensional echocardiography. Ultrason Imaging 5:300–307, 1983

6. Melton HJ, Skorton DJ: Rational gain compensation for attenuation in cardiac ultrasonography. Ultrason Imaging 5:214–228, 1983

7. Melton HEJ, Collins SM, Skorton DJ: Automatic real-time endocardial edge detection in two-dimensional echocardiography. Ultrason Imaging 5:300–307, 1983

8. Skorton DJ, McNary CA, Child JS, Newton FC, Shah PM: Digital image processing of two dimensional echocardiograms: Identification of the endocardium. Am J Cardiol 48:479–486, 1981

9. Cahalan MK, Ionescu P, Melton HJ, et al: Automated real-time analysis of intraoperative transesophageal echocardiograms. Anesthesiology 78:477–485, 1993

10. Gorcsan J III, Gasior TA, Mandarino WA, et al: On-line estimation of changes in left ventricular stroke volume by transesophageal echocardiographic automated border detection in patients undergoing coronary artery bypass grafting. Am J Cardiol 72:721–727, 1993

11. Benson MJ, Cahalan MK, Hickey R, et al: Volumetric estimation of cardiac output using TEE. J Am Soc Echocardiogr 7:S47, 1994

12. Muhiudeen IA, Kuecherer HF, Lee C, Cahalan MK, Schiller NB: Intraoperative estimation of cardiac output by transesophageal pulsed Doppler echocardiography. Anesthesiology 74:9–14, 1991

13. Savino JS, Troianos CA, Aukburg S, Weiss R, Reichek N: Measurement of pulmonary blood flow with transesophageal two-dimensional and Doppler echocardiography. Anesthesiology 75:445–451, 1991

14. Katz WE, Gasior TA, Quinlan JJ, Gorcsan J III: Transgastric continuous-wave Doppler to determine cardiac output. Am J Cardiol 71:853–857, 1993

15. Gorcsan J III, Diana P, Ball BA, Hattler BG: Intraoperative determination of cardiac output by transesophageal continuous wave Doppler. Am Heart J 123:171–176, 1992

16. Darmon PL, Hillel Z, Mogtader A, Mindich B, Thys D: Cardiac output by transesophageal echocardiography using continuous-wave Doppler across the aortic valve. Anesthesiology 80:796–805, 1994

17. Nessly ML, Bashein G, Detmer PR, et al: Left ventricular ejection fraction: Single-plane and multiplanar transesophageal echocardiography versus equilibrium gated-pool scintigraphy. J Cardiothorac Vasc Anesth 5:40–45, 1991

18. Doerr HK, Quinones MA, Zoghbi WA: Accurate determination of left ventricular ejection fraction by transesophageal echocardiography with a non-volumetric method. J Am Soc Echocardiogr 6:476–481, 1993

19. Ohte N, Nakano S, Hashimoto T, et al: Continuous-wave Doppler echocardiography for evaluating left ventricular performance—clinical significance of a new systolic time interval. Jpn Circ J 55:459–464, 1991

20. Bengur AR, Snider AR, Vermilion RP, Freeland JC. Left ventricular ejection

fraction measured with Doppler color flow mapping techniques. Am J Cardiol 68:669–673, 1991

21. Ohte N, Narita H, Hashimoto T, et al: Noninvasive evaluation of left ventricular performance by the shortest distance between mitral leaflets coaptation and interventricular septum at end-systole. Clin Cardiol 15:656–659, 1992

22. Martin RW, Graham MM, Kao R, Bashein G. Measurement of left ventricular ejection fraction and volumes with three-dimensional reconstructed transesophageal ultrasound scans: Comparison to radionuclide and thermal dilution measurements. J Cardiothorac Anesth 3:260–268, 1989

23. Siu SC, Rivera JM, Guerrero JL, et al: Three-dimensional echocardiography. In vivo validation for left ventricular volume and function. Circulation 88:1715–1723, 1993

24. Pearlman AS: Measurement of left ventricular volume by three-dimensional echocardiography—present promise and potential problems. J Am Coll Cardiol 22:1538–1540, 1993

25. Sapin PM, Schroeder KD, Smith MD, DeMaria AN, King DL: Three-dimensional echocardiographic measurement of left ventricular volume in vitro: Comparison with two-dimensional echocardiography and cineventriculography. J Am Coll Cardiol 22:1530–1557, 1993

26. Handschumacher MD, Lethor JP, Siu SC, et al: A new integrated system for three-dimensional echocardiographic reconstruction: Development and validation for ventricular volume with application in human subjects. J Am Coll Cardiol 21:743–753, 1993

27. Bashein G, Sheehan FH, Nessly ML, Detmer PR, Martin RW: Three-dimensional transesophageal echocardiography for depiction of regional left-ventricular performance: Initial results and future directions. Int J Cardiol Imag 9:121–131, 1993

28. Harpole DH, Clements FM, Quill T, et al: Right and left ventricular performance during and after abdominal aortic aneruysm repair. Ann Surg 209:356–362, 1989

29. Kalman PG, Wellwood MR, Weisel RD, et al. Cardiac dysfunction during abdominal aortic operation: The limitations of pulmonary wedge pressures. J Vasc Surg 3:773–781, 1986

30. Kuecherer HF, Muhiudeen IA, Kusumoto FM, et al: Estimation of mean left atrial pressure from transesophageal pulsed Doppler echocardiography of pulmonary venous flow. Circulation 82:1127–1139, 1990

31. Kusumoto FM, Muhiudeen IA, Kuecherer HF, Cahalan MK, Schiller NB: Response of the interatrial septum to transatrial pressure gradients and its potential for predicting pulmonary capillary wedge pressure: An intraoperative study using transesophageal echocardiography in patients during mechanical ventilation. J Am Coll Cardiol 21:721–728, 1993

32. Sagawa K, Suga H, Shouas AA, Bakalar KM: End-systolic pressure/volume ratio: A new index of ventricular contractility. J Am Cardiol 40:748–753, 1977

33. Pagel PS, Kampine JP, Schmeling WT, Warltier DC: Comparison of end-systolic pressure-length relations and preload recruitable stroke work as indices of myocardial contractility in the conscious and anesthetized, chronically instrumented dog. Anesthesiology 73:278–290, 1990

34. Crottogini AJ, Willshaw P, Barra JG, et al: Inconsistency of the slope and the volume intercept of the end-systolic pressure-volume relationship as individual indexes of inotropic state in conscious dogs: Presentation of an index combining both variables. Circulation 76:1115–1126, 1987

35. Reichek N, Wilson J, St John Sutton M, et al: Noninvasive determination of left ventricular end-systolic stress: Validation of the method and initial application. Circulation 65:99–108, 1982

36. Marsh JD, Green LH, Wynne J, Cohn PF, Grossman W: Left ventricular end-systolic pressure-dimension and stress-length relations on normal human subjects. Am J Cardiol 44:1311–1317, 1979

37. Gorcsan J III, Gasior TA, Mandarino WA, et al: Assessment of the immediate effects of cardiopulmonary bypass on left ventricular performance by on-line pressure-area relations. Circulation 89:180–190, 1994

38. Feneley M, Skelton T, Kisslo K, et al: Comparison of preload recruitable stroke work, end-systolic pressure-volume and dP/dT max—end-diastolic volume relations as indexes of left ventricular contractile performance in patients undergoing routine cardiac catheterization. J Am Coll Cardiol 19:1522–1530, 1992

39. Gorcsan J III, Romand JA, Mandarino WA, Deneault LG, Pinsky MR: Assessment of left ventricular performance by on-line pressure-area relations using echocardiographic automated border detection. J Am Coll Cardiol 23:242–252, 1994

40. Nishimura R, Housmans P, Hatle L, Tajik A. Assessment of diastolic function of the heart: Background and current applications of doppler echocardiography. Part 1. Physiological and pathophysiological features. Mayo Clin Proc 64:71–81, 1989

41. Nishimura R, Abel M, Hatle L, Tajik A: Assessment of diastolic function of the heart: Background and current applications of doppler echocardiography. Part 11. Clinical studies. Mayo Clin Proc 64:181–204, 1989

42. Colan SD, Borow KM, Neumann A: Effects of loading conditions and contractile state (methoxamine and dobutamine) on left ventricular early diastolic function in normal subjects. Am J Cardiol 55:790–796, 1985

43. Choong CY, Abascal VM, Thomas JD, et al: Combined influence of ventricular loading and relaxation on the transmitral flow velocity profile in dogs measured by Doppler echocardiography. Circulation 78:672–683, 1988

44. Ishida Y, Meisner JS, Tsujioka K, et al: Left ventricular filling dynamics: Influence of left ventricular relaxation and left atrial pressure. Circulation 74:187–196, 1986

45. Harrison MR, Clifton GD, Sublett KL, DeMaria AN: Effect of heart rate on Doppler indexes of systolic function in humans. J Am Coll Cardiol 14:929–935, 1989

46. Bahler RC, Vrobel TR, Martin P. The relation of heart rate and shortening fraction to echocardiographic indexes of left ventricular relaxation in normal subjects. J Am Coll Cardiol 2:926–933, 1983

47. Stoddard MF, Pearson AC, Kern MJ, et al: Influence of alteration in preload on the pattern of left ventricular diastolic filling as assessed by Doppler echocardiography in humans. Circulation 79:1226–1236, 1989

48. Plotnick GD, Kmetzo JJ, Gottdiener JS: Effect of autonomic blockade, postural changes and isometric exercise on Doppler indexes of diastolic left ventricular function. Am J Cardiol 67:1284–1290, 1991

49. Owall A, Anderson R, Brodin LA, Samuelsson S, Juhlin DA: Left ventricular filling as assessed by pulsed Doppler echocardiography after coronary artery bypass grafting. J Cardiothorac Vasc Anesth 6:573–577, 1992

50. Stoddard MF, Pearson AC, Kern MJ, et al: Left ventricular diastolic function: Comparison of pulsed Doppler echocardiographic and hemodynamic

indexes in subjects with and without coronary artery disease. J Am Coll Cardiol 13:327–336, 1989

51. Appleton CP, Hatle LK, Popp RL: Relation of transmitral flow velocity patterns to left ventricular diastolic function: New insights from a combined hemodynamic and Doppler echocardiographic study. J Am Coll Cardiol 12:426–440, 1988

52. Marino P, Destro G, Barbieri E, Zardini P: Early left ventricular filling: An approach to its multifactorial nature using a combined hemodynamic-Doppler technique. Am Heart J 122:132–141, 1991

53. Bahl VK, Dave TH, Sundaram KR, Shrivastava S: Pulsed Doppler echocardiographic indexes of left ventricular diastolic function in normal subjects. Clin Cardiol 15:504–512, 1992

54. Benjamin EJ, Levy D, Anderson KM, et al: Determinants of Doppler indexes of left ventricular diastolic function in normal subjects (the Framingham Heart Study). Am J Cardiol 70:508–515, 1992

55. Pai RG, Shah PM: A new Doppler method for assessing left ventricular diastolic stiffness based on principles of flow wave propagation: Mathematical basis and review of the method. J Heart Valve Dis 2:167–173, 1993

56. Brun P, Tribouilloy C, Duval AM, et al: Left ventricular flow propagation during early filling is related to wall relaxation: A color M-mode Doppler analysis. J Am Coll Cardiol 20:420–432, 1992

57. Lang RM, Borow KM, Neumann A, Janzen D: Systemic vascular resistance: An unreliable index of left ventricular afterload. Circulation 74:1114–1123, 1986

58. Borow K: An integrated approach to the noninvasive assessment of left ventricular systolic and diastolic performance. In St John Sutton M, Oldershaw P (eds): Textbook of Adult and Pediatric Echocardiography and Doppler, pp. 97–153. Boston, Blackwell, 1991

59. Smith JS, Roizen MF, Cahalan MK, et al: Does anesthetic technique make a difference? Augmentation of systolic blood pressure during carotid endarterectomy: Effects of phenylephrine versus light anesthesia and of isoflurane versus halothane on the incidence of myocardial ischemia. Anesthesiology 69:846–853, 1988

60. Aronson S, Lee Bk, Wiencek JG, et al: Assessment of myocardial perfusion during CABG surgery with two-dimensional transesophageal contrast echocardiography. Anesthesiology 75:433–440, 1991

61. Tennant R, Wiggers C: The effect of coronary occlusion on myocardial contraction. Am J Physiol 112:351–361, 1935

62. Forrester JS, Wyatt HL, Da LPL, et al: Functional significance of regional ischemic contraction abnormalities. Circulation 54:64–70, 1976

63. Vatner SF: Correlation between acute reductions in myocardial blood flow and function in conscious dogs. Circ Res 47:201–207, 1980

64. Waters DD, Da Luz P, Wyatt HL, Swan HJ, Forrester JS: Early changes in regional and global left ventricular function induced by graded reductions in regional coronary perfusion. Am J Cardiol 39:537–543, 1977

65. Battler A, Froelicher VF, Gallagher KP, Kemper WS, Ross J: Dissociation between regional myocardial dysfunction and ECG changes during ischemia in the conscious dog. Circulation 62:735–744, 1980

66. Horowitz RS, Morganroth J, Parrotto C, et al: Immediate diagnosis of acute myocardial infarction by two-dimensional echocardiography. Circulation 65:323–329, 1982

67. Beaupre PN, Kremer PF, Cahalan MK, et al: Intraoperative detection of

changes in left ventricular segmental wall motion by transesophageal two-dimensional echocardiography. Am Heart J 107:1021–1023, 1984

68. Smith JS, Cahalan MK, Benefiel DJ, et al: Intraoperative detection of myocardial ischemia in high-risk patients: Electrocardiography versus two-dimensional transesophageal echocardiography. Circulation 72:1015–1021, 1985

69. Leung JM, OKelly B, Browner WS, et al: Prognostic importance of postbypass regional wall-motion abnormalities in patients undergoing coronary artery bypass graft surgery. Anesthesiology 71:16–25, 1989

70. van Daele ME, Sutherland GR, Mitchell MM, et al: Do changes in pulmonary capillary wedge pressure adequately reflect myocardial ischemia during anesthesia? A correlative preoperative hemodynamic, electrocardiographic, and transesophageal echocardiographic study. Circulation 81:865–871, 1990

71. Eisenberg MJ, London MJ, Leung JM, et al: Monitoring for myocardial ischemia during noncardiac surgery. A technology assessment of transesophageal echocardiography and 12-lead electrocardiography. The Study of Perioperative Ischemia Research Group. JAMA 268:210–216, 1992

72. Lambertz H, Kreis A, Trumper H, Hanrath P: Simultaneous transesophageal atrial pacing and transesophageal two-dimensional echocardiography: A new method of stress echocardiography. J Am Coll Cardiol 16:1143–1153, 1990

73. Hauser AM, Gangadharan V, Ramos RG, Gordon S, Timmis GC: Sequence of mechanical, electrocardiographic and clinical effects of repeated coronary artery occlusion in human beings: Echocardiographic observations during coronary angioplasty. J Am Coll Cardiol 5:193–197, 1985

74. Wohlgelernter D, Jaffe CC, Cabin HS, Yeatman LAJ, Cleman M: Silent ischemia during coronary occlusion produced by balloon inflation: Relation to regional myocardial dysfunction. J Am Coll Cardiol 10:491–498, 1987

75. London MJ, Tubau JF, Wong MG, et al: The "natural history" of segmental wall motion abnormalities in patients undergoing noncardiac surgery. Anesthesiology 73:644–655, 1990

76. Sklenar J, Jayaweera AR, Kaul S: A computer-aided approach for the quantitation of regional left ventricular function using two-dimensional echocardiography. J Am Soc Echocardiogr 5:33–40, 1992

77. Pandian NG, Skorton DJ, Collins SM, et al: Heterogeneity of left ventricular segmental wall thickening and excursion in 2-dimensional echocardiograms of normal human subjects. Am J Cardiol 51:1667–1673, 1983

78. Lehmann KG, Lee FA, McKenzie WB, et al: Onset of altered inter-ventricular septal motion during cardiac surgery. Assessment by continuous intraoperative transesophageal echocardiography. Circulation 82:1325–1334, 1990

79. Braunwald E, Kloner RA: The stunned myocardium: Prolonged, postischemic ventricular dysfunction. Circulation 66:1146–1149, 1982

80. Feinstein SB, Cheirif J, Ten CF, et al: Safety and efficacy of a new transpulmonary ultrasound contast agent: Initial multicenter clinical results. J Am Coll Cardiol 16:316–324, 1990

81. Ismail S, Johnson SH, Utsunomiya H, et al: Safety and efficacy of sonicated albumin microspheres in perfusion and vein graft patency assessments. Clin Cardiol 14(V):V29–32, 1991

82. Kaul S: Assessment of myocardial perfusion with contrast two-dimensional echocardiography. Am J Med Sci 299:113–130, 1990

83. Reisner SA, Ong LS, Fitzpatrick PG, et al: Evaluation of coronary flow re-

serve using myocardial contrast echocardiography in humans. Eur Heart J 13:389–394, 1992

84. Buffington CW, Coyle RJ: Altered load dependence of postischemic myocardium. Anesthesiology 75:464–474, 1991

85. Seeberger M, Cahalan M, Chu E, et al: Severe loading reductions may induce new segmental wall motion abnormalities in the absence of myocardial ischemia. Anesth Analg 78:S379, 1994

86. Force T, Kemper A, Perkins L, et al: Overestimation of infarct size by quantitative two-dimensional echocardiography: The role of tethering and of analytic procedures. Circulation 73:1360–1368, 1986

87. Shah PM, Kyo S, Matsumura M, Omoto R: Utility of biplane transesophageal echocardiography in left ventricular wall motion analysis. J Cardiothorac Vasc Anesth 5:316–319, 1991

88. Rouine-Rapp K, Cahalan M, Ionescu P, Muhideen I, Foster E: Detection of wall motion abnormalities: Biplane transesophageal echocardiography vs multiple transverse cross sections. Anesthesiology 77, No 3A:A481, 1992

89. Munoz E, Cohen J, Chang J, et al: Socioeconomic concerns in vascular surgery: A survey of the role of age, resource consumption, and outcome in treatment cost. J Vasc Surg 9:479–486, 1989

90. Seeberger M, Cahalan M, Chu E, et al: Sensitivity of intraoperative stress testing for detection of coronary artery disease. Anesthesiology 79:A64, 1993

91. Akosah KO, Porter TR, Simon R, et al: Ischemia-induced regional wall motion abnormality is improved after coronary angioplasty: Demonstration by dobutamine stress echocardiography. J Am Coll Cardiol 21:584–589, 1993

92. Sheikh K, Bengston J, Rankin J, et al: Intraoperative transesophageal Doppler color flow imaging used to guide patient selection and operative treatment of ischemic mitral regurgitation. Circulation 84:594–604, 1991

Arthur W. Wallace
Dennis T. Mangano

Perioperative Evaluation of the Patient with Ventricular Dysfunction

9

SIGNIFICANCE OF THE PROBLEM

Cardiovascular disease affects approximately one in four Americans (65 of 239 million),[1,2] accounting for almost 1 million deaths per year, 1.5 million myocardial infarctions, 0.6 million strokes, and 0.4 million cases of congestive heart failure (CHF). There are 2.3 to 3 million Americans with a history of CHF resulting in 37,000 deaths per year.[3] Related health care costs for cardiovascular disease exceed $109 billion per year.[3] Additionally, cardiovascular disease becomes more prevalent with age, and 25 million Americans (10%) are now 65 years or older, including 2.7 million greater than 85 years of age.[1,4] The incidence of cardiovascular disease will increase as the United States population continues to live longer.

The perioperative course of patients undergoing cardiac and noncardiac surgery is substantially compromised by the effects of cardiovascular disease. For example, the increased severity of disease in patients presenting for coronary artery bypass graft (CABG) surgery has increased the incidence of morbidity and mortality. There are approximately 50,000 cardiac perioperative deaths each year in the United States, among the more than 400,000 cardiac and 8 million noncardiac operations performed annually.[5] Ventricular dysfunction resulting in CHF contributes to perioperative cardiac morbidity and mortality.

Ventricular Function, edited by David C. Warltier. Williams & Wilkins, Baltimore © 1995.

Heart failure occurs intraoperatively in 4.8%[6] and postoperatively in 3.6%[7] of patients undergoing noncardiac surgery. In a recent study of 2400 patients undergoing CABG surgery (McSPI EPI I database), 31% had a preoperative history of CHF.

RISK FACTORS OF PERIOPERATIVE CARDIAC MORBIDITY

Clinical

Cardiac morbidity is one of the leading causes of death following anesthesia and surgery and manifests as myocardial infarction, unstable angina, CHF, serious dysrhythmia, or cardiac death. Identified clinical risk factors for perioperative cardiac morbidity and mortality include age,[8-13] previous myocardial infarction (recent <6 mo),[10,14-22] previous myocardial infarction (old),[15,20-25] angina,[8,16,22,23,25] CHF,[6,11,13,22,24] hypertension,[8,16,17,20,26-28] diabetes mellitus,[8,13,16,19,22] dysrhythmia,[11,23,24] peripheral vascular disease,[8,21,29,30] valvular heart disease,[11,31] hypercholesterolemia, cigarette smoking, previous CABG surgery,[13,21,32-41] previous percutaneous transluminal coronary angioplasty, and cardiovascular drug therapy.[13,42-48]

Numerous risk indices[7,12,13,24,29,49-54] have been defined in an effort to predict patients likely to sustain perioperative cardiac morbidity. Risk indices are variably weighted combinations of identified risk factors. Heart failure is a principle risk factor for perioperative cardiac morbidity in all risk indices.

Quantitative Indices of Ventricular Function as an Indicator of Risk

Quantitative indices of ventricular function associated with morbidity and mortality in surgical patients are limited. An ejection fraction (EF) of less than 50% was not predictive of myocardial infarction or ischemia but did predict a 4.6 (1.8 to 11.8)-fold increase in left ventricular failure.[55] Several studies suggest that a depressed preoperative EF (<0.40, as determined by radionuclear imaging or ventriculography) is prognostic of perioperative myocardial infarction, reinfarction, and ventricular dysfunction.[22,56-58] Patients with an EF of less than 40%, determined by radioisotope imaging, have a 1-year cumulative mortality of 30%. Patients with compromised left ventricular function (pulmonary capillary wedge pressure greater than 15 mm Hg) and depressed stroke work (less than 20 gm * m/m^2) have a 2-year mortality rate that exceeds

78%.[59] Left ventricular wall motion score[13] is a predictor of ventricular dysfunction. Right ventricular dysfunction, while clinically devastating, is less common and therefore less studied, resulting in fewer reported indicators of function, risk, or outcome. As new indices of ventricular function develop, their ability to predict mortality and morbidity will need to be evaluated.

LIMITATIONS OF RISK FACTORS

Studies of risk factors often do not agree as to which factors predict greatest risk. One of the only consistent predictors of adverse outcome appears to be the presence of one or more signs of severe ventricular dysfunction. Additionally, clinical studies that find a specific indicator of cardiac risk, such as severe CHF or myocardial infarction in the last 6 months, are difficult to repeat because the identification of the specific risk factor alters future surgical management and operative patient population. The population of patients studied and the presence of each identified factor is critical to the result. For example, if a group of patients all of whom have an EF above 50% are studied, the EF will not achieve statistical significance, whereas a lack of patients presenting with CHF will exclude CHF as a risk factor for poor outcome. Similarly, despite the high incidence of CHF (2 million),[60] the prognostic value of individual signs of CHF (e.g., S3, rales, pulmonary edema) is controversial. Goldman et al.[7] suggest that only two signs of CHF have predictive value—a third heart sound (S3) and jugular venous distention. A history of prior CHF was not predictive if the S3 and jugular venous distention were excluded from analysis. Finally, due to multiple criteria, indicators, and tests suggestive of CHF, clinical outcome studies often use different definitions, resulting in different incidences of perioperative cardiac morbidity associated with CHF.

CLINICAL DEFINITIONS OF VENTRICULAR DYSFUNCTION

The forms of cardiovascular disease specific to the heart include congenital heart defects, coronary artery disease, arrhythmias, valvular disease, and ventricular dysfunction. Of these, ventricular dysfunction is the major cause of death (excluding sudden death from arrhythmias). Ventricular function can be classified as systolic or diastolic as well as right or left ventricular. Systolic function is the ability of the heart to contract. Diastolic function is the ability of the heart to relax and passively fill. Loss of the contractile ability of ventricular muscle, as is common following myocardial infarction or ischemia with myocardial stunning, results in systolic dysfunction. Left ventricular hypertrophy or impaired relaxation from ischemia can result in diastolic dysfunction (see Chapter 4). Clinically, left ventricular systolic dysfunction is manifest by CHF with pulmonary edema and a poor EF. Patients who have left ventricular hypertrophy and an adequate EF but high left ventricular filling pressures or pulmonary edema with slight increases in blood volume are thought to have diastolic dysfunction. Clinically, both diastolic and systolic dysfunction result in signs of CHF, such as pulmonary edema and elevated filling pressures. The clinical distinction between the two groups depends on the adequacy of ventricular contraction.

While left ventricular failure is associated with pulmonary edema, right ventricular failure is manifest by elevated central venous pressures and hepatic engorgement. It can result from loss of right ventricular myocardium secondary to infarction, poor preservation or distention during bypass, or excessive loading in the presence of pulmonary hypertension or a pulmonary embolus. Right ventricular function is less commonly depressed and is more difficult to evaluate because of the complex geometry of the right ventricle.

These clinical definitions of ventricular function are rudimentary because adequate definition of cardiac function requires invasive measurement of pressure and volume relationships. Nevertheless, the clinical definition of CHF is critical because CHF is one of the most frequently noted and strongest indicators of perioperative cardiac morbidity.

MEASURES OF VENTRICULAR FUNCTION

CHF as a Clinical Indicator of Ventricular Dysfunction

At the present time, CHF is defined as a clinical syndrome consisting of a constellation of symptoms and signs including pulmonary edema, cardiomegaly, S3 heart sound, jugular venous distention, low cardiac output, depressed EF, elevated pulmonary venous pressure, peripheral edema, hepatojugular reflux, and hepatic enlargement. It is an abnormality of cardiac function responsible for the inability of the heart to pump blood at a rate sufficient to supply the metabolic requirements of the patient or it can only do so with abnormally elevated filling pressures. There may be abnormalities in both systolic and diastolic cardiac function. In systolic heart failure, an impaired inotropic state leads to a reduction in stroke volume and cardiac dilation. In diastolic heart failure, impaired lusitropic function leads to an elevation of ventricular diastolic pressures at normal diastolic volumes. Failure of relaxation can have an anatomical basis as caused by a thickened, stiff ventricle secondary to hypertrophy or restrictive cardiomyopathy, or a functional basis as from myocardial ischemia. While CHF can be described by a constellation of symptoms, the only clinical signs that have been shown to be associated with poor perioperative outcome include S3, jugular venous distention,[11] and an EF of less than 40%.[22,56–58] If one chooses a more specific definition of CHF, then the incidence will be lower but the severity of associated morbidity will probably be worse. Heart failure as defined by pulmonary edema, an S3, jugular venous distention, or an EF below 0.40 is an extreme example of left ventricular dysfunction and is clearly a risk factor for perioperative morbidity and mortality. More subtle disturbances of ventricular function may also be detrimental or indicative of increased risk for perioperative morbidity.

Current Quantitative Measures

Current quantitative measures permit assessment of cardiac anatomy (echocardiography, magnetic resonance imaging (MRI), computed tomography (CT), angiography), global systolic function (e.g., EF by echocardiography, radionuclide imaging, volume conductance catheterization, MRI, CT, angiography), regional ventricular function (e.g., wall motion by echocardiography, ventriculography, radionuclear imaging, MRI, CT), and coronary blood flow (angiography, CT, contrast echocardiography). Of these techniques, some can be used clinically for preoperative assessment of left ventricular function or for continuous intraoperative monitoring of function. Others are still primarily research tools.

ASSESSMENT OF VENTRICULAR FUNCTION

Perioperative evaluation of ventricular function begins with a clinical history and physical examination and then proceeds to preoperative diagnostic assessment of ventricular function and intraoperative monitoring. Routine techniques for quantifying ventricular function preoperatively include echocardiography, angiography, and radionuclide wall motion imaging. Specialized approaches include ultrafast CT scanning and MRI. Each of these techniques is useful in diagnostic evaluation, although their effect on perioperative morbidity and mortality may not yet be established.

Clinical history and physical examination are the baseline indicators of cardiac dysfunction. A history of orthopnea, paroxysmal nocturnal dyspnea, peripheral edema, or pulmonary edema indicates possible ventricular dysfunction and CHF. Poor exercise tolerance also is associated with poor ventricular function.[61] Physical examination revealing an S3, jugular venous distention, hepatojugular reflux, rales, a laterally displaced point of maximal impulse, or a systolic heave indicates poor cardiac function. Electrocardiographic evidence of left ventricular hypertrophy may be associated with poor diastolic relaxation, indicating impaired diastolic function. Chest x-ray findings of cardiomegaly, pulmonary edema, cephalization of blood flow, curley B lines, or pleural effusions may also indicate the presence of CHF, tamponade, or fluid overload.

Once a patient has been identified as having poor cardiac function, there are several options depending on the medical situation. If the medical condition allows delay of surgery, the patient should be managed with angiotensin-converting enzyme inhibitors (ACE), vasodilators, diuretics, digoxin, and oxygen as needed.[62] Medical management of a patient with CHF is essential prior to elective surgery. If the etiology of failure requires surgery (e.g., tamponade, papillary muscle rupture, or acute coronary occlusion from angioplasty), then surgical intervention may be necessary concurrent with medical stabilization. If the medical condition does not permit delay of surgery (e.g., dissecting abdominal aortic aneurysm, trauma, or intraabdominal catastrophes), failure may be managed by invasive monitoring and rapid management with oxygen, diuretics, vasodilators, and inotropes, but mortality will exceed that for nonemergent surgery. Preoperative optimization of cardiac status improves outcome, even in patients at risk for cardiac morbidity (e.g., vascular surgery patients) who do not exhibit overt CHF.[63]

TECHNIQUES FOR THE ASSESSMENT OF CARDIAC FUNCTION

Indices of Systolic Ventricular Function

There are many numerical indices of systolic ventricular function (see Chapter 3) that have been developed over the last 150 years including: pressure-area, dP/dt_{max}, dp/dt_{max} – end-diastolic volume (EDV), end-systolic pressure volume relationship (ESPVR), and preload recruitable stroke work (PRSW). The area under the systemic arterial pressure waveform (pressure-area) was at one time thought to reflect cardiac function. However, increases in systolic blood pressure elevate this index without reflecting an increase in cardiac function but, rather, an increase in afterload. The maximum change in left ventricular pressure with respect to time (dP/dt_{max}) is relatively simple to measure and is equal to 1368 ± 554 mm Hg/second in normal ventricles at normal volumes.[64] dP/dt_{max} is directly proportional to end-diastolic volume and can vary from 200 to 2500 mm Hg/second as end-diastolic volume changes (Fig. 9–1). Therefore, DP/dt_{max} is useful only if the end-diastolic volume is known. Attempts have been made to normalize the DP/dt_{max} measurement by correcting for the systolic arterial pressure, $DP/dt_{max}/P$.[65–67] However, normalization in this manner does not fully eliminate either the preload or afterload dependency of this measure.[68] The slope of the DP/dt_{max}-EDV relationship is linear, preload-, and afterload-independent and sensitive to changes in inotropic state.[64] Clinical utility of this measure of systolic function is limited by the requirement for a measure of left ventricular volume and a change in preload during the measurement. Presently, this measure is used only in the research setting.

In 1972, Suga et al.[69] proposed the ESPVR as an index of ventricular systolic function. Unlike previous indices, the ESPVR was the result of experimental observation. After placing a balloon in a canine isolated left ventricle and connecting it to a syringe, they noted that changes in the volume of blood in the balloon were directly propor-

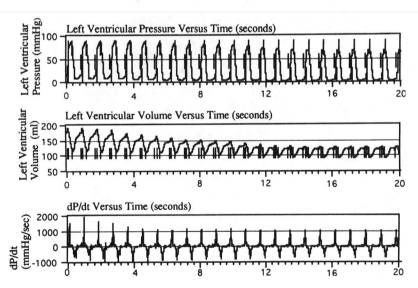

FIGURE 9-1. The *top panel* is a recording from a Millar® pressure transducer in the left ventricle of a patient undergoing CABG surgery. The *middle panel* is simultaneous recording from a volume conductance catheter also in the left ventricle. The *bottom panel* is the calculated dP/dt for the pressure signal. The pressure and volume signal were digitized at 200 Hz.

tional to changes in the developed ventricular pressure. Isovolumic ventricular contractions against an infinite afterload resulted in the development of a linear ESPVR. The slope of this relationship varied with changes in inotropic state. An identical relationship was found for ESPVR with ejecting beats, i.e., the ventricular ESPVR with infinite afterload (isovolumic contraction) was identical to that with normal afterload (ejecting beats).

The ESPVR (Fig. 9–2) reflects subtle changes in contractility that

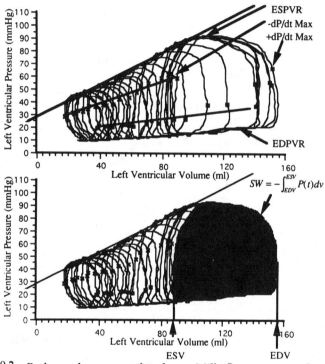

FIGURE 9-2. Both panels represent data from a Millar® pressure transducer and volume conductance catheter in the left ventricle of a patient undergoing CABG surgery. Each loop represents one cardiac cycle. The measures of global systolic ventricular contractility, ESPVR, dP/dt_{max}, dP/dt_{max} EDV, and PRSW are demonstrated in this figure. The ESPVR is derived from the linear regression of the end-systolic pressure and volume points. dP/dt_{max} occurs during isovolumic contraction. The dP/dt_{max}-EDV relationship is the linear regression of each of the dP/dt_{max} for each contraction vs the EDV for that beat. The SW is the area of an individual loop and is illustrated by the blackened loop in the *bottom panel*. The PRSW relationship is the linear regression of SW vs the EDV for that beat. The measures of global diastolic ventricular function $-dP/dt_{max}$-EDV and EDPVR are demonstrated in this figure. $-dP/dt_{max}$ occurs during isovolumic relaxation. The $-dP/dt_{max}$-EDV relationship is the linear regression of each $-dP/dt_{max}$ for each contraction vs the EDV for that beat. The EDPVR relationship is the linear regression of the end-diastolic pressure and volume points.

other indicators cannot, e.g., decreased contractility in ectopic beats or increased contractility in postextrasystolic contractions. A potential limitation of ESPVR in vivo is nonlinearity[70,71] and a nonzero or positive volume intercept.[71] However, the slope of the ESPVR relationship clearly reflects global systolic function relatively independent of preload and afterload.[69] The ESPVR relationship has been measured in humans in several studies despite the requirement for some measure of ventricular dimension.[64,72–81] Ventricular volume is the optimal dimension for global ventricular function, but ventricular area or unidirectional ventricular strain may also be used.

The stroke work (SW) performed by the ventricle can be calculated from:

$$SW = -\int_{EDV}^{ESV} P(t)dv$$

where *ESV* is end-systolic volume, *EDV* is end-diastolic volume, *P(t)* is left ventricular pressure, and *dv* is the change in volume (Fig. 9–2 *bottom panel*). The SW varies linearly with EDV. PRSW is the slope of the SW-EDV relationship. The SW-EDV relationship is more linear than the ESPVR[82] and has been suggested to be more accurate. However, linearity of a relationship is not the only important criteria for usefulness, i.e., the PRSW is less sensitive to small changes in inotropic state than the ESPVR.[64]

The use of indices of systolic ventricular function has been limited by their reliance on a measurement of ventricular dimension. Despite this limitation, these indices are used extensively in animal research. Additionally, several studies in humans[74,77] have used these indices as outcome variables, suggesting that they may soon be available for clinical use. The development of technologies that provide a ventricular dimension (acoustic quantification (AQ) echocardiography and volume conductance catheters) will increase the clinical availability of preload- and afterload-insensitive, dimensionally dependent measures of ventricular function.

Indices of Diastolic Ventricular Function

There are numerous indices of diastolic ventricular function. A few of these include $-dP/dt_{max}$, $-dP/dt_{max}$- EDV, EDPVR, and τ (Fig. 9–2, *top panel*). The maximum negative change in left ventricular pressure with respect to time ($-dP/dt_{max}$) occurs during isovolumic relaxation and, therefore, reflects an active relaxation.[83] Since $-dp/dt_{max}$ varies directly with EDV, the slope of the $-dP/dt_{max}$-EDV relationship is a preload-insensitive index of active diastolic relaxation. It can be measured at the same time as the dP/dt_{max}-EDV relationship.

The decay of left ventricular pressure over time during isovolumic relaxation can be fitted to an exponential curve, with τ as the half-life. τ reflects active diastolic relaxation without measurement of a ventricular dimension; it varies with end-diastolic volume and is therefore preload-sensitive. The end-diastolic pressure-volume relationship (EDPVR)[83] can be measured using the same techniques as those used to determine the ESPVR. EDPVR is a measure of global ventricular diastolic function and reflects passive ventricular compliance.[64,83]

Clinical investigation and measurement of ventricular diastolic function is even more limited than that for systolic function. Numerous studies have used echocardiographic measures of ventricular diastolic function as outcome variables without adequate validation. Advances in the ability to measure ventricular dimensions using AQ and volume conductance technology now make research and clinical measurement of diastolic function possible.[64,72,73,75-79,81,84,85]

In a clinical trial of 67 patients undergoing CABG surgery, volume conductance catheter measurements of systolic and diastolic indices of ventricular function were compared with EF% from catheterization and echocardiography. The patients were divided by clinical history into those with and without a history of CHF, myocardial infarction, or hypertension. Only patients with a history of CHF demonstrated differences in EF by echocardiography or catherization, and ESPVR (P<0.05). Patients with a history of infarction or hypertension did not have any differences in systolic or diastolic function indices. There were no demonstrable differences in diastolic function ($-dP/dt_{max}$-EDV or EDPVR) in any of the of the patient groups (Table 9–1).[80]

Summary of Indices of Ventricular Function

An index of ventricular contractility must be both preload- and afterload-insensitive to be meaningful at different hemodynamic states. If a measure is preload-sensitive, then it will be altered by simple volume shifts; if afterload-sensitive, it may be artifactually vulnerable to changes in systemic blood pressure. A measure of ventricular contractility must incorporate both a force and a dimension if it is to reflect an intrinsic property of the ventricle. The force is easily substituted by a measurement of pressure. The measurement of a left ventricular dimension is more difficult. Because many indices of ventricular function ignore the dimensional component (e.g., dP/dt_{max}, τ), they are influenced by changes in preload and afterload. The clinical use of preload and afterload insensitive measures of systolic and diastolic ventricular function is limited by the requirement for an easily obtainable mea-

TABLE 9–1. VOLUME CONDUCTANCE CATHETER MEASUREMENTS OF SYSTOLIC AND DIASTOLIC INDICES OF VENTRICULAR FUNCTION COMPARED WITH EF% FROM CATHETERIZATION AND ECHOCARDIOGRAPHY

Index ± SD (No. of Patients)	No CHF	History of CHF	No MI	Previous MI[a]	No HTN	History of HTN
EF% (echocardiography)	58.0 ± 9.6 (42)	43.7 ± 18.6 (6)	58.1 ± 12.7 (29)	53.6 ± 9.9 (20)	56.6 ± 11.1 (25)	55.9 ± 12.7 (24)
EF% (ventriculography)	62.4 ± 16.7 (44)	42.8 ± 5.0 (5)	61.7 ± 18.4 (28)	58.7 ± 15.2 (21)	61.4 ± 17.5 (21)	59.7 ± 16.9 (28)
LVEDP (mm Hg)	17.6 ± 5.4 (44)	17.6 ± 7.0 (5)	17.4 ± 5.6 (28)	17.9 ± 5.5 (21)	17.0 ± 6.4 (19)	18.0 ± 4.9 (30)
ESPVR (mm Hg/ml)	2.27 ± 1.98 (55)	1.30 ± 0.83 (7)	2.20 ± 2.04 (37)	2.11 ± 1.74 (25)	2.18 ± 1.64 (29)	2.15 ± 2.15 (33)
dP/dt_{max}-EDV (mm Hg/sec/ml)	15.0 ± 11.5 (55)	10.6 ± 9.1 (7)	12.5 ± 9.5 (37)	17.4 ± 13.1 (25)	15.6 ± 11.6 (29)	13.5 ± 11.1 (33)
PRSW (mm Hg)	34.1 ± 18.8 (55)	27.0 ± 20.8 (7)	29.6 ± 17.0 (37)	38.7 ± 20.8 (25)	36.3 ± 17.1 (29)	30.7 ± 20.4 (33)
$-dP/dt_{max}$-EDV (mm Hg/sec/ml)	−10.6 ± 8.1 (50)	−9.0 ± 9.2 (6)	−9.8 ± 7.7 (33)	−11.4 ± 9.0 (23)	−11.9 ± 10.3 (28)	−9.1 ± 5.2 (28)
EDPVR (mm Hg/ml)	0.071 ± 0.044 (50)	0.057 ± 0.035 (6)	0.068 ± 0.042 (33)	0.073 ± 0.044 (23)	0.074 ± 0.048	0.066 ± 0.037

[a] MI, myocardial infarction; HTN, hypertension; LVEP, left ventricular end-diastolic pressure.

surement of ventricular dimension. As techniques that provide a ventricular dimension become more reliable and easily quantifiable (AQ echocardiography), the clinical use of preload- and afterload-insensitive indices of systolic and diastolic function will be more common.

Hemodynamic Measurements

Pulmonary Artery and Central Venous Pressures

Invasive cardiac monitors should not be necessary to diagnose CHF, but invasive monitoring is often useful for the management of cardiac dysfunction. Optimal management of ventricular dysfunction requires a measure of left ventricular dimension to indicate adequacy of filling, but these measures are difficult to obtain. Pressures have been substituted as easily measured parameters of filling, but changes in atrial and ventricular compliance alter the relationship between pressure and volume. Patients with ventricular dysfunction frequently have reduced ventricular compliance complicating use of invasive monitors that rely on pressure measurement as a reflection of volume. It has been clearly demonstrated that in patients with cardiac dysfunction there is a poor correlation between pulmonary artery wedge pressure and EDV. Therefore, while the pulmonary artery catheter is very good at measuring central venous, pulmonary arterial, and pulmonary arterial wedge pressures, the wedge pressure may not be an accurate reflection of left ventricular volume in patients with ventricular dysfunction.[86]

Central venous pressure can be used as a surrogate for pulmonary artery wedge pressure in patients with EF above 0.50,[86] but in patients with ventricular dysfunction, central venous pressure neither correlates nor even indicates trends in pulmonary artery wedge pressure. Since wedge pressure does not reflect EDV in patients with ventricular dysfunction, central venous pressure is clearly not able to reflect EDV. Central venous pressure monitoring can reflect adequacy of cardiac filling in patients with normal ventricular function, but those patients rarely require more monitoring than blood pressure, heart rate, and urine output to indicate adequacy of cardiac filling.

Cardiac Output

Calculation of cardiac output by thermodilution using the pulmonary artery catheter has become a gold standard, despite its variability, because of ease of measurement. Dye dilution or Fick calculation of cardiac output is similar in accuracy. Cardiac output can be calculated with Doppler echocardiography but is operator-dependent. These technologies have allowed the measurement of cardiac output, but there are multiple etiologies for a low cardiac output state (e.g., decreased contractility, inadequate volume, reduced sympathetic tone, increases in venous capacitance from anaphylaxis or end-stage sepsis, or poor diastolic compliance). Distinguishing the etiology of reduced cardiac output states is essential to institute appropriate therapy—ventricular systolic dysfunction is only one possible diagnosis.

Acid-Base, Lactate, and Mixed Venous Saturation

The adequacy of cardiac output can be assessed by acid-base balance, lactate production, and mixed venous oxygen saturation. Abnormal laboratory results such as metabolic acidosis, lactic acidosis, and low mixed venous oxygen saturation can be the end-result of inadequate cardiac output. These tests do not identify a specific cause, merely the presence of a problem. Often, they are useful indicators of the need for further diagnostic and therapeutic efforts. Mixed venous oxygen saturation measured by either blood sampling from the pulmonary artery or by continuous reading from an oxymetric pulmonary artery catheter provides a measure of the adequacy of cardiac output relative to metabolic state.[87] Oxymetric pulmonary artery catheters are most useful in patients with ventricular dysfunction in whom continuous assessment of the adequacy of cardiac output will affect therapy.

Right Ventricular Ejection Fraction

Pulmonary artery catheters with rapid-response thermisters (50 to 90 msec) have been used to calculate right ventricular EF, stroke volume, and EDV. The rapid-response thermister provides a washout temperature trace with multiple diastolic plateaus, each plateau corresponding to successive cardiac ejections. End-diastolic plateaus also coincide with the onset of the QRS complex of the simultaneously recorded electrocardiogram. Consecutive differences between baseline and end-diastolic plateau temperature (C_1, C_2, C_3, ...) are used to calculate the mean residual fraction (K) of blood in the right ventricle according to the following equation, where n = the total number of diastolic plateaus obtained on the temperature washout curve:

$$K = \frac{\left(\dfrac{C_1}{C_2} + \dfrac{C_2}{C_3} + ... \dfrac{C_n}{C_{n-1}}\right)}{n-1}$$

Right ventricular ejection fraction (RVEF) is then calculated as $RVEF = 1 - K$, and right ventricular end-diastolic volume (RVEDV) and end-systolic volume (RVESV) are obtained from the following formulas where stroke volume ($SV = \frac{CO}{HR}$) is obtained from thermodilution cardiac output (CO) and the heart rate (HR):

$$RVEDV = \frac{\dfrac{CO}{HR}}{RVEF}$$

$$RVESV = \frac{CO}{HR} \left(\frac{1}{RVEF} - 1 \right)$$

A limitation of this technique is that the calculated values do not correlate well with simultaneously measured RVEF, RVEDV, or RVESV by echocardiography ($r^2 = 0.54$)[88] or biplane angiography ($r^2 = 0.68$).[89] Agreement is poor and with marked variability. Echocardiographic assessment of right ventricular function is superior to thermodilution measurements of RVEF and RVEDV.[90]

Electrocardiography

Electrocardiography is sensitive and specific in the diagnosis of arrhythmias, conduction disturbances, myocardial ischemia, myocardial infarction, pericarditis, and atrial or ventricular hypertrophy. Numerous studies correlate various aspects of the electrocardiogram with each cardiac abnormality. However, quantification of the severity or magnitude of abnormality by electrocardiography has remained elusive. For example, the duration, onset, offset, and area of the heart affected by myocardial ischemia can be identified by electrocardiographic analysis, but quantification of the percentage of myocardium that is ischemic is not possible. High-resolution electrocardiographic recordings demonstrate that some patients with low EF have early waves appearing at the beginning of the QRS complex. High-frequency potentials, QRS duration time, and low EF are associated with ventricular tachycardia and fibrillation. Early waves are most prominent in patients with the lowest EF, ventricular actopy, and recent myocardial infarction. Electrocardiographic abnormalities are less common in patients with normal EF and no history of ventricular tachycardia fibrillation or myocardial infarction.[91] However, this relationship does not indicate that the EF can be estimated by the electrocardiogram. It simply demonstrates that patients with poor EF are more likely to have electrocardiographic abnormalities. Efforts to correlate the ratio of the peak waveform amplitude of different electrocardiogram elements (R/T) to the EF or other measures of contractility have not yet produced a reliable clinical index. The electrocardiogram remains critical to the identification and diagnosis of cardiac abnormalities but cannot be used as quantitative index of ventricular function.

Echocardiography

Cardiac echocardiography can be performed either from the transthoracic or transesophageal approach. Cardiologists initially use transthoracic imaging because of simplicity, patient comfort, and lack of need for sedation. However, image quality is inferior to that achieved with the transesophageal approach because of difficulty in imaging through anatomical structures, such as ribs and lung. Additionally, continuous cardiac monitoring using the transthoracic approach is challenging, because it is difficult to stabilize the externally applied probe. Anesthesiologists commonly use transesophageal imaging for intraoperative monitoring because patients are already unconscious; this approach permits surgical access to the patient's chest and abdomen, and probe stabilization is simplified. Preoperatively, transthoracic echocardiography is the more common technique, while intraoperatively, transesophageal imaging is more common. Although the two techniques use different planes of orientation, the information obtained and analysis are similar. Both approaches are valuable to perioperative assessment, but intraoperative two-dimensional transesophageal echocardiography (TEE) monitoring is the anesthesiologist's preference and will be emphasized (see Chapter 8).

TEE allows continuous and serial measurement and monitoring of cardiac anatomy and function, including cardiac chambers, wall motion, valves, pericardium, and connecting vasculature. Because of the proximity of the esophagus to the heart, ultrasound passes through only the esophagus and pericardium before reaching the heart, resulting in less image distortion from structures with poor acoustic transmission (ribs and lung). TEE can be used to monitor cardiac function during all types of surgery except oral, esophageal, and gastric procedures. Complications are rare but include esophageal perforation, vocal cord paralysis, hemodynamic compromise due to pressure on the atrium, tracheal extubation, dental damage, and sore throat. TEE can be used to describe function and anatomy in congenital heart disease, atrial septal defects, ventricular septal defects, valvular stenosis, valvular regurgitation, aortic dissection, aortic calcification, and cardiac tamponade.

TEE Monitoring of Myocardial Ischemia

Wall motion abnormalities develop within 5 to 10 seconds after a reduction in myocardial blood flow (Tennant and Wiggers, 1935). Changes in wall motion progress from normal contraction to hypokinesia, akinesia, and then dyskinesia indicating myocardial ischemia. Changes in wall motion precede electrocardiographic or metabolic changes indicative of ischemia.[92] Thus, TEE often detects myocardial ischemia prior to ECG or pulmonary artery catheter pressure measurement.[92-94] However, changes in regional wall motion do correlate with ST segment elevation[94] indicative of myocardial ischemia and infarction.[95] Dobutamine stress testing for diagnosis of coronary artery disease relies on echocardiographic detection of changes in regional wall motion.[96]

Regional wall motion and thickening abnormalities are difficult to quantify. First, the ventricle twists when it contracts and may cause sections of the myocardium in the imaging plane during early systole to move out of the imaging plane in late systole. Thus, the region imaged is different throughout the cardiac cycle. Second, the endocardial border often cannot be completely identified. Enhancement of the endocardial blood border with echogenic contrast media has been attempted,[97] but no proven, reliable, FDA-approved, echogenic contrast media is available for venous injection with pulmonary transit sufficient to enhance the left ventricular cavity or arterial injection without risk of infarction from cerebral embolization. Wall thickening measurements require visualization of both the endocardial and epicardial borders. The epicardial border is even more difficult to visualize throughout the entire circumference of the cross-section than the endocardial border, preventing quantification of wall thickening. However, qualitative grading of wall motion and thickening abnormalities can be used to predict cardiac morbidity.[95]

Echocardiographic Measurement of Global Systolic Function

Echocardiography also can be used to measure global ventricular function. The commonly measured echocardiographic indices of ventricular systolic function are end-diastolic area (EDA), end-systolic area (ESA), fractional area change (FAC), regional wall motion abnormalities (RWMA), regional thickening, and EF. Experimental indices of left ventricular contractility include LV end-systolic wall stress[98] or the LV end-systolic pressure-area relationship[99] (Figs. 9–3 and 9–4). Quantification of these parameters is difficult. First, the fractional area change, which is defined as $FAC = \frac{EDA - ESA}{EDA}$, varies with the ventricular imaging plane (Fig. 9–5 to 9–7, all from same patient). Measured at the base or apex, the valve of

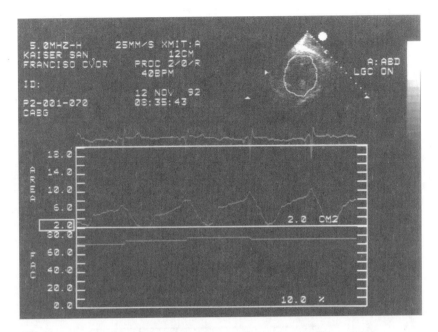

FIGURE 9-3. In the *upper right* there is an acoustic quantification (AQ)-enhanced short-axis view of the left ventricle of a patient undergoing CABG surgery. AQ is able to detect tissue-blood, and tissue-air interfaces, highlight them in real time, and then track the interface providing a real-time ventricular area measurement without hand measurement. The *solid line* defines the area of interest for area calculations. The left ventricular short-axis area as well as fractional area change (FAC) are plotted in real time on the lower two panels. The ECG is also provided for timing. AQ-derived dimensional measurements can be used in the calculation of indices of ventricular function.

FAC is less than at the level of the papillary muscles. If a section of myocardium with a wall motion abnormality is included, the FAC will be lower than at a level with no wall motion abnormality. FAC measured in one plane and at one level, provides only a limited representation of the ventricle. TEE measurement of FAC in the long-axis view often does not include the apex because it is difficult to visualize except with omniplane TEE. Although more complex measures of ventricular systolic function such as LV end-systolic wall stress or the LV end-systolic pressure-area relationship can be derived from TEE measures,[79,99,100] their absolute magnitude may be poorly reproducible. These parameters can be improved if normalized or corrected for stroke volume calculated from cardiac output and heart rate, and they may then become clinically useful.

Automatic detection of endocardial and epicardial borders from

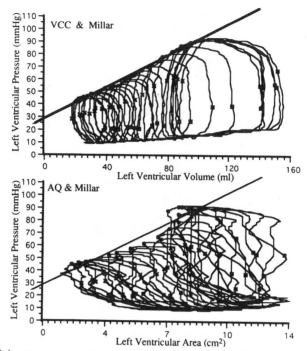

FIGURE 9-4. The *top panel* represents data from a Millar® pressure transducer and volume conductance catheter in the left ventricle of a patient undergoing CABG surgery. Each loop represents one cardiac cycle. The *bottom panel* is simultaneously acquired data using AQ echocardiography to measure the left ventricular short-axis area at the midpapillary level. The measures of global systolic ventricular function end-systolic pressure-area (ESPAR), $-dP/dt_{max}$-end-diastolic area, and preload recruitable stroke work area, as well as measures of global diastolic ventricular function end-diastolic pressure-area relationship, $-dP/dt_{max}$-end diastolic pressure-area relationship can be derived from a left ventricular pressure and AQ-derived measure of left ventricular area.

the echocardiographic images is limited by the quality of available image and computer processors. Hewlett Packard recently released a system that is able to identify the boundary between tissue and fluid, using a technique called acoustic quantification (AQ). This technique easily tracks the endocardial border and provides accurate on-line measurements of FAC[101] that correlate with off-line measurements obtained from echocardiographic images,[101] CT scans,[102] and nuclear angiography.[103] However, AQ images only one plane and thus does not give a full representation of the ventricle. AQ also attempts to estimate cardiac volume from a single long-axis view. Calculations are derived from a single imaging plane and do not measure true ventricular volume, limiting the utility of indices of cardiac function that rely on true

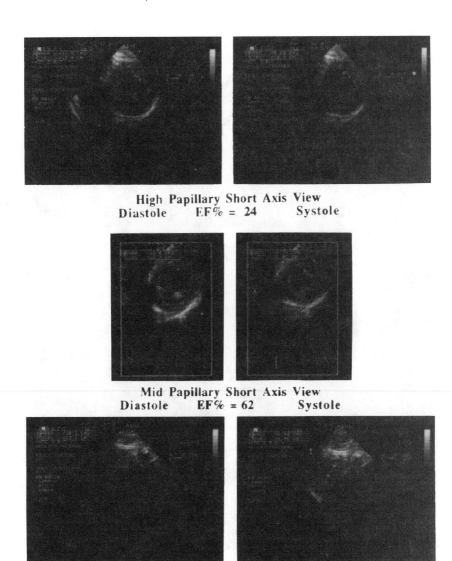

High Papillary Short Axis View
Diastole   EF% = 24   Systole

Mid Papillary Short Axis View
Diastole   EF% = 62   Systole

Low Papillary Short Axis View
Diastole   EF% = 39%   Systole

FIGURE 9-5. Manual calculations of end-diastolic and end-systolic areas with EF% calculations from three short-axis echo images are demonstrated in the same patient. This method requires hand tracing of the endocardial border after identification of the end-diastolic and end-systolic images. Papillary muscles are included in the ventricular volume. The *top panel* is slightly above the midpapillary level, the *middle panel* is at the midpapillary level, and the *bottom panel* is slightly below the midpapillary level. The level imaged affects the ejection fraction.

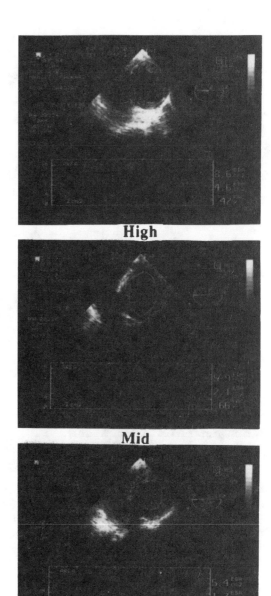

High

Mid

Low

FIGURE 9-6. Automatic border detection by AQ with calculation of EF% at three short-axis echo planes is shown in the same patient. This method automatically identifies the tissue-blood interface and therefore the endocardial border. Papillary muscles are excluded from the ventricular volume as tissue. The *top panel* is slightly above the midpapillary level, the *middle panel* is at the midpapillary level, and the *bottom panel* is slightly below the midpapillary level. The level imaged affects the ejection fraction.

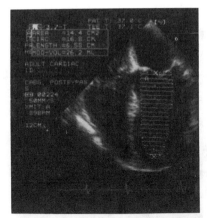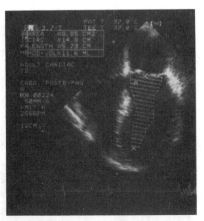

Four Chamber View
Diastole   EF% = 56   Systole

FIGURE 9-7. Manual calculation of end-diastolic and end-systolic area with EF% calculation from a four-chamber echo image. This method requires hand tracing of the endocardial border after identification of the end-diastolic and end-systolic images.

volume measurement.[79] Nonetheless, AQ is a significant advance over manual endocardial border detection, and once measures of systolic function accounting for AQ limitations are developed, this technique will provide noninvasive measures of global cardiac function.

Echocardiographic Measurement of Diastolic Function

Echocardiography has also been used to measure left ventricular diastolic function. Volumetric filling rates have been calculated from M-mode echocardiography[104] and pulsed Doppler echocardiography.[104-107] Echocardiographic measurement of left ventricle diastolic function is derived from the velocity of blood flow across the top of the mitral valve leaflets or at the level of the mitral valve annulus during diastole, when the annulus has a constant cross-sectional area (Fig. 9–8). Velocity of blood flow across the annulus is therefore related to volumetric flow. Higher peak velocity during early passive filling than during late filling produced by atrial contraction is thought to characterize normal diastolic function. Similar or reduced velocities during early vs late filling defines impaired diastolic function typical of a stiff or noncompliant ventricle.

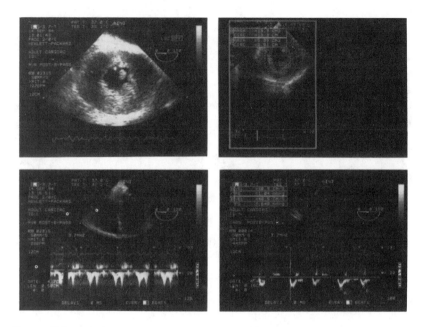

FIGURE 9-8. Two examples of the transmitral valve flow velocity vs time by Doppler. The leftmost velocity profile is the early (E) wave labeled (A), and the rightmost is the atrial (A) wave labeled (B). The ratio of early to atrial velocities may give a qualitative assessment of diastolic function. The *upper left panel* is a short-axis view of a patient with left ventricular hypertrophy. The *lower left panel* is the transmitral velocity profile from this patient demonstrating decreased early diastolic flow velocity. The *upper right panel* is a short-axis view of a patient with a normal ventricle. The *lower right panel* demonstrates normal transmitral flow velocities.

Another index of diastolic function is the time from closure of the aortic valve (determined by phonocardiography) to the onset of mitral flow (Doppler echocardiography) and is defined as the isovolumic relaxation time (IVRT). The early to late filling velocities and IVRT have been used to quantify the effects of drugs on diastolic function.[108,109] This analysis is truly qualitative in nature because the transmitral flow velocity is dependent on multiple factors. The velocity of blood flow across the mitral valve depends on the instantaneous pressure gradient across the valve and the resistance to flow. If the pressure gradient across the valve changes for any reason, velocity also changes. Although a change in diastolic compliance will alter the gradient, a simple elevation in diastolic pressure will slow filling velocity. Increased EDV also slows filling. Myocardial ischemia slows active diastolic relaxation and may or may not affect the diastolic pressure-volume relationship.[110] The IVRT depends on the pressure gradient across the valve, not the diastolic compliance. Flow may begin at higher left ventricular pressures during myocardial ischemia, thereby shortening the time from closure of the aortic valve to the onset of mitral flow, but leaving the EDPVR unchanged.[110] Thus, a simple measurement of velocity of filling is not alone sufficient to reflect changes in diastolic compliance.

Echocardiographic measurement of left ventricular diastolic function has been used to identify and define mechanisms, establish etiology, quantify severity, follow serial changes, and assess prognosis of a variety of disorders,[111–118] without establishing the sensitivity or specificity of the technique for these applications. Despite this limitation, the measurement of volumetric filling rates presently is the most commonly used test of diastolic function, and Doppler echocardiography is a convenient, noninvasive test for two primary etiologies of left ventricular diastolic dysfunction: impaired myocardial relaxation and restricted filling due to ventricular stiffness. Variations in ventricular loading may obscure the diagnosis of diastolic dysfunction in individual patients and prevent quantification.

TEE with AQ

TEE with AQ can measure a ventricular dimension. If pressure within the left ventricle is simultaneously measured, then the left ventricular end diastolic pressure area relationship may be obtained. Calculations derived from area must account for nonuniformity of ventricular contraction. The end-diastolic pressure-area relationship should be insensitive to changes in loading conditions and may more accurately reflect passive diastolic function. Indices of ventricular function derived from TEE will need to be validated by comparison with other techniques to establish accuracy, reproducibility, and validity.

Echocardiography is a relatively noninvasive, safe, real-time, continuous measure of cardiac anatomy and function. However, it requires a substantial investment of time and financial resources to learn the technique and acquire the equipment. Clearly, echocardiography can be used to define anatomy, determine valve competency and gradients, detect myocardial ischemia, estimate volume status, calculate cardiac output, measure EF, and obtain transmitral filling velocities. Although its measurements are primarily qualitative, in some cases, echocardiography can be used to quantify systolic and diastolic function.

Cardiac Catheterization, Ventriculography, and Angiography

Cardiac catheterization is one of the most useful and indispensable techniques for complete evaluation of the heart and to date is considered the gold standard for defining cardiac anatomy and physiology. Catheterization allows the measurement of pressure, flow, volume, oxygen saturation, and electrical potential (electrophysiology). With iodinated contrast medium, it also visualizes chamber, valvular, and coronary anatomy. Other techniques can complement some aspects of cardiac catheterization. For example, color Doppler echocardiography can be used to identify stenotic or regurgitant flow and calculate valvular gradients, while cardiac catheterization provides direct measurement of the pressure gradient across a valve and visualization of the flow with contrast. Similarly, evaluation of congenital anomalies is possible with echocardiography, but catheterization allows a more complete and precise evaluation. Presently, cardiac catheterization with angiography is the only technique with sufficient resolution to provide the anatomical detail necessary for coronary revascularization. Cardiac catheterization also allows electrophysiological mapping and ablation. It can also be used therapeutically for angioplasty, septoplasty, valvuloplasty, and closure of atrial and ventriculoseptal defects.

Uses of catheterization in evaluation of cardiac function are multiple. After definition of the anatomy of the chambers, valves, and coronary arteries, ventriculography can be completed to estimate EF and determine the presence and severity of wall motion abnormalities. Biplane ventriculography can clearly define wall motion abnormalities. Experimentally, radioopaque beads have been placed in the myocardium to determine local dimensional changes, permitting the calculation of regional cardiac function.[119–127] Although ventriculography is excellent for evaluation of cardiac function, serial measurements for monitoring are limited by risk of iodinated contrast-induced renal toxicity and radiation exposure.

Volume Conductance

Cardiac catheterization led not only to the common use of pulmonary artery catheters, which have become a standard for cardiac output measurements and central venous, pulmonary artery, and wedge pressures, but also to the development of volume conductance catheters. A volume conductance catheter is a standard electrophysiology recording catheter that has a number of electrodes at equal spacing along the distal end. Catheters with 12 electrodes are commonly used in humans. An alternating electric field is produced between the first and last electrode. The conductivity between the remaining pairs of electrodes is then measured, and total conductivity is related to the volume of conductive material around the catheter. Time-varying conductivity is defined by $G_i(t)$:

$G_i(t)$ for $i = 1 - 5$ where $G_i(t)$ represents the conductance of a single pair of electrodes. The sum of the time-varying conductances is defined by $G(t)$:

$$G(t) = \sum_{i=1}^{5} G_i(t)$$ where $G(t)$ represents the sum of the conductances from the five pairs of electrodes. The total volume is given by $V(t)$:

$$V(t) = \left(\frac{1}{\alpha} \frac{L^2}{\sigma}\right)[G(t) - G^p]$$ where α is defined as a slope constant relating conductance to volume, L is the interelectrode distance, σ is the conductivity of blood, and G^p is the parallel conductance. Parallel conductance is conductance of current through nonblood structures, i.e., myocardium and lung, and is constant throughout the cardiac cycle.[128] It is subtracted from the total conductance to derive the conductance of blood.

The volume conductance catheter allows continuous measurement of left ventricular volume.[129] This volume measurement can be used in the calculations of indices of global ventricular contractility such as ESPVR, dP/dt_{max}-EDV, and PRSW. Volume conductance catheter measurements of ventricular contractility have also been used in several clinical trials.[64,72–79,81]

Changes in volume can be measured accurately using the volume conductance catheter, but absolute volume is difficult to obtain.[130] This technique is used most often to measure left ventricular volume, but also can be used to quantify right ventricular and right atrial volume.[131–133] Advantages of the volume conductance catheter are that it is a continuous, repeatable, nontoxic (no use of iodinated contrast, x-rays, radioactivity) technique that provides a measure of volume and not just area (echocardiography). Its greatest limitation is the requirement for an invasive catheter.

NUCLEAR TECHNIQUES

Scintigraphy

There are numerous types of nuclear cardiac imaging, the choice of radioisotope depending on the goal of the test. One of the earliest descriptions of the use of nuclear imaging was published in 1927 when radioactive radon was injected intravenously, and circulation time was measured with a Wilson cloud chamber.[134] Prinzmetal and Corday first described nuclear imaging of the heart in 1949. The scintillation camera, also known as the Anger or gamma camera, detects single gamma rays from an injected radiopharmaceutical, and reports their detected location. The camera consists of a collimator that absorbs scattered gamma rays and passes parallel, unscattered ones through a series of holes in a lead plate. The gamma rays are then absorbed by a sodium iodide crystal that converts the energy in the gamma ray to a photon that can be amplified by a photo multiplier tube next to the crystal. The photons detected by the photomultiplier tube are converted to an electrical signal indicating the detection of one gamma ray in a certain location.

Collimators differ by providing either greater sensitivity or image resolution. Collimators that are more sensitive, pass more gamma rays, thereby decreasing resolution; those with better resolution reject gamma rays, reducing sensitivity. Time-dependent studies, such as exercise thallium-201 and gated blood pool imaging, use general purpose collimators with moderate sensitivity and resolution. High-resolution collimators are used for studies of anatomy at rest, where sensitivity is not of primary importance. High-sensitivity collimators are used in first-pass radionuclide angiography when photon count may be limited.

A second type of camera, the multicrystal scintillation camera, uses signal processing of photomultiplier row and column tubes to provide spatial identification of scintillation events. This design provides imaging with high count rates (e.g., 500,000 events/sec and is therefore useful for dynamic studies, such as first-pass radionuclide angiography. A third type of detector, the single-probe scintillation detector, allows measurement of EF, cardiac output, and pulmonary transit time. The advantages of this unit are that it is small and portable. The most common crystal is sodium iodide; however, cadmium telluride crystals have been used to obtain serial measurements over prolonged periods.

After injection of a radiopharmaceutical, such as technetium-99m, passage through the right heart, pulmonary circulation, and the left heart can be recorded by measuring count rates during the systolic and diastolic cycles. The radiopharmaceutical may also be used to label albumin or red blood cells and the study gated to the electrocardiogram following equilibration. End-systolic and end-diastolic counts, EF, cardiac output, and pulmonary transit time may be measured from the time activity curves.

Acute Myocardial Infarction

Acute myocardial infarction can be diagnosed by technetium-99m pyrophosphate scintigraphy (hot-spot imaging) and thallium-201 perfusion scintigraphy (cold-spot imaging). Infarct avid myocardial scintigraphy (hot-spot imaging) relies on the selective affinity of the infarcted segment of the myocardium for technetium-99m pyrophosphate. Once taken up, the increase in activity of the infarcted area can be detected by a gamma camera. Normal tissue or areas of old scarring do not have an affinity for pyrophosphate and are not visualized. The uptake in acute myocardial infarction depends on the regional blood flow, the concentration of calcium in the myocardium, the reversibility of the myocardial injury, and the time of infarction. The earliest detectable images are obtained at 12 to 16 hours following the event, but maximum abnormality occurs between 48 and 72 hours. The intensity of the image returns to normal after 5 to 7 days.

Uptake of radioactive potassium and rubidium by normal myocardium produces an image with perfusion scintigraphy (cold-spot imaging). Defects in the normal pattern, known as cold spots, represent areas of decreased blood flow, possibly associated with ischemia or myocardial infarction. Because of the high-photon energies associated with radioactive potassium and rubidium, thallium-201 was developed and is currently the radiopharmaceutical of choice for myocardial perfusion scintigraphy. Thallium is a potassium analog extracted by normal myocardium and distributed in proportion to regional myocardial blood flow within minutes of an intravenous injection. The image appears as a donut of normal myocardium with a central hole which represents the ventricular cavity. Despite normal flows, a false-positive perfusion defect will be apparent in the apex in 20% of normal patients. Additionally, the specificity of thallium imaging for myocardial infarction is greater within 6 hours of the event but less useful after 24 hours.

Myocardial Stress Perfusion Imaging

Myocardial stress perfusion imaging using thallium-201 provides information regarding the extent, localization, reversibility, and stress response of the coronary circulation, permitting a quantitative assessment of the functional significance of coronary artery disease (Fig. 9–9). In the absence of myocardial infarction, coronary blood flow, even distal to ar-

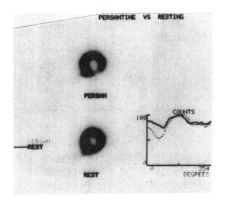

FIGURE 9-9. Reversible perfusion defect in a short-axis persantine thallium-201 scan. The rest phase is a complete donut. The persantine infusion images have a bite out of the donut at 5 o'clock indicating an area of inadequate perfusion.

teries with a 75% stenosis, is homogeneous in the resting state. Only in the presence of a severe coronary stenosis (i.e., greater than 90%) can perfusion defects be detected on resting thallium images. Thallium injected during metabolic stress will demonstrate the heterogeneity of coronary blood flow caused by coronary artery disease. Imaging is performed within 5 to 10 minutes after injection of thallium-201, during maximal exercise or infusion of a coronary vasodilator such as dipyridamole. Perfusion defects will be detectable for approximately 30 to 60 minutes, with redistribution over the next 2 to 3 hours. Repeat imaging is performed 3 to 4 hours after the initial injection. The initial perfusion defects will either persist or disappear. Those that persist indicate areas of infarction, and those that disappear are classified as areas with transient myocardial ischemia. It has been suggested that dipyridamole thallium scintigraphy be used for cardiac risk stratification of all patients undergoing vascular surgery procedures, but two clinical trials have found it not to be predictive of adverse cardiac events.[55,135,136]

Radionuclear Evaluation of Cardiac Mechanics

First-pass radionuclear angiography and gated blood pool imaging are the primary techniques used to evaluate cardiac mechanics (Fig. 9–10). Both provide information about ventricular function, including EF, end-systolic and end-diastolic volume, cardiac output, pulmonary transit time, and intracardiac shunt. First-pass radionuclear angiography allows a temporal separation of the right and left sides of the heart. With this technique, a bolus of a radiopharmaceutical, usually technetium-99m, is injected into a peripheral vein, and radioactive emissions are counted as this bolus passes through the central circulation. The entire sequence is measured for 10 to 15 seconds and allows acute assessment of cardiac performance, particularly in unstable patients. Repeat assessments can be made at multiple time intervals but require additional injections of the radiopharmaceutical.

The scintillation counters used with this technique are usually multicrystal digital cameras that allow rapid acquisition and measurement of high radioisotope count rates. With each cardiac cycle, the measured activities at end-diastole and end-systole are proportional to the respective ventricular volumes. The maximal count rates during a cardiac cycle correspond to end-diastole, and the minimal count rates correspond to end-systole. Left ventricular EF can be computed by the difference between the end-diastolic and end-systolic count, subtracted from the background count. Typically, EF is computed over 3 to 5 cycles and averaged. This first-pass EF technique correlates well with contrast angiography ($r = 0.94$ to 0.97).[137–139]

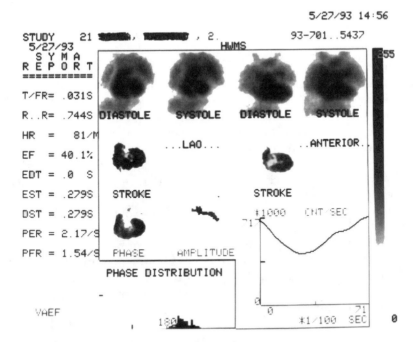

FIGURE 9-10. Gated blood pool nuclear imaging ventriculogram with calculation of EF. The cardiac cycle is divided into 10-msec intervals and a plot of the counts/10-msec is produced. The ratio of end-diastolic-end-systolic to end-diastolic corrected for background count rate gives a measure of the EF.

Right ventricular EF has been measured using similar methodology. This technique is particularly useful since the geometry of the right ventricle is variable and complex, making other techniques using geometric calculations less precise. Right ventricular EF has been shown to have a normal value of 0.55, with a lower limit of 0.45 by the first-pass technique.[140] The first-pass technique can also be used for calculation of EDV,[141] left ventricular ejection phase indices such as ejection rate,[138] and peak diastolic filling rate.[142] These indices are difficult to validate and at the present time, only relative changes seem to be clinically useful.

Gated blood pool imaging is the second radionuclide imaging technique for assessment of ventricular function.Radionuclides such as technetium-99m-labeled human serum albumin or technetium-99m-labeled red blood cells are used to differentiate the intravascular space after equilibration. The gamma camera accumulates activity over the region of interest and identifies end-systole and end-diastole by gating to the R-wave of the electrocardiogram. Data from 300 to 500 cardiac cycles are averaged to produce count rates of 300,000 over the 2- to 10-minute imaging time. Image resolution is high because of the high number of counts. Background activity is measured (by selecting a noncardiac area, i.e., lung) and subtracted from the measured cardiac volumes to produce a relative ventricular volume. Global EF can be obtained from the difference in end-systolic and end-diastolic count rates.

Regional EF and wall motion may be measured using a series of geometric models and processing algorithms.[143–145] Absolute determinations are difficult to validate, but relative changes in these indices of regional function provide useful information. Advantages of gated blood pool imaging over first-pass imaging include higher count rates, resulting in greater resolution, and the ability to obtain serial measurements without repeat injections.

Radionuclear imaging provides unique information regarding detection of myocardial infarction, quantification of myocardial perfusion abnormalities, and calculation of ventricular performance and wall motion indices. These techniques can be used to quantify myocardial perfusion and ventricular function.

CT Scanning

Computed tomography with iodinated contrast delineates the cardiac chambers and quantifies area, calculates volume, and identifies congenital lesions (e.g., transposition of the great vessels, tetrology of Fallot, aortic stenosis, and coarctation.[146]) or acquired lesions (e.g., dissection,[147,148] areas of decreased perfusion, and infarction.[149–151]). CT scans can identify coronary artery calcification which may suggest the presence of coronary artery disease[152,153] and can be used to determine saphenous graft patency.[154] Multiple images gated to the electrocardiogram can be used to quantify wall motion, wall thickness, end-systolic and end-diastolic volume, and EF.[155]

Ultrafast CT scans which steer an electron beam across multiple fixed tungsten targets and have complete rings of fixed x-ray detectors can scan the entire heart in 50 msec and produce multiple complete reconstructions of the heart throughout the cardiac cycle. The short scan time reduces some motion artifact and enables high-quality imaging of dynamic processes in rapidly moving organs. However, the rapid scan time will not eliminate cardiac motion artifacts until the scan time is less than 19 msec.[156] Quantification of volumes, perfusion, and wall motion is possible.[150,151,153,157–162] Because the resolution of CT scanning is not sufficient to determine detailed intracoronary anatomy, it cannot substitute for x-ray contrast angiography.

CT scanning is a rapid, quantifiable, noninvasive imaging technique for evaluation of cardiac anatomy and function. The dose of radiation is substantially less than that with angiography.

MRI Scanning

MRI scanning permits noninvasive imaging of cardiac anatomy and function. The patient is placed in a high magnetic field. The primary magnetic field aligns atomic nuclei having a net spin and a magnetic moment due to an uneven number of nucleons (protons + neutrons). With adjustments in primary magnetic field strength and tuning of the stimulation frequency, imaging of atomic nuclei with magnetic moments, including ^1H, ^{13}C, ^{19}F, ^{23}Na, and ^{31}P, can be performed. Each nuclei processes at a specific frequency (Larmor frequency) in a given magnetic field. The approximate Larmor procession frequencies (f_L) of biomedically significant nuclei in a magnetic field of 1.0 Tesla (10,000 Gauss) are provided below[163] (Table 9–2).

^1H nuclei are the most frequently imaged because they are abundant and thus yield a greater signal. Three gradient magnetic fields change the local magnetic field for specific locations in the patient. Each gradient magnetic field has a zero point. The zero point for all three gradient fields is the point imaged. The zero point of the three fields is moved in the volume of interest to obtain a complete image. A radiofrequency transmitted at the Larmor frequency causes the nuclei to misalign, momentarily, with the magnetic field. When the nuclei realign with the field, they emit a radiofrequency signal at the Larmor frequency, which is detected by an antenna. The magnitude of the detected signal is proportional to the number of nuclei in the area of interest. The three gradient magnetic fields are altered to sample each location in the imaging plane. Imaging planes are then moved to sample a new cross-section. Timing of signal acquisition and processing can be manipulated, thereby varying the imaging technique.

TABLE 9–2. LARMOR PROCESSION FREQUENCIES (f_L) OF
BIOMEDICALLY SIGNIFICANT NUCLEI

Nucleus	f_L (mHz/T)
^1H	42.58
^{13}C	10.70
^{19}F	40.05
^{23}Na	11.26
^{31}P	17.32

MRI scanning can provide excellent anatomical detail of fixed structures (Figs. 9–11 to 9–13). The imaging time can be prolonged, depending on the technique chosen. At the present time, prolonged sampling with electrocardiographic gating is required for cardiac imaging. MRI can clearly define cardiac chambers, detect atrial septal defect (ASD) and ventricular septal defect (VSD), measure the EF of the right and left ventricles,[164] detect blood flow, and quantify oxyhemoglobin saturation. Because there is no ionizing radiation dose, data can be acquired over a prolonged time and at multiple levels, allowing serial calculation of volumes and wall motion.

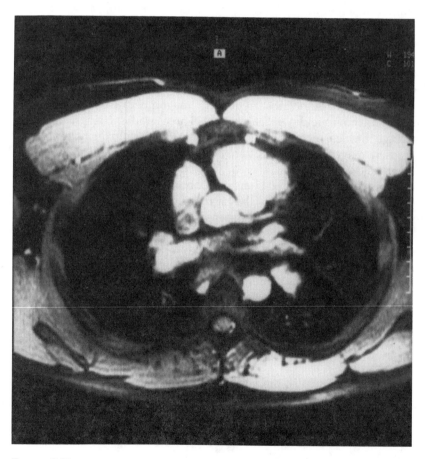

FIGURE 9-11. Example of transverse plane MRI image of the heart. Anatomical description of left and right atrium, aorta, pulmonary artery, and coronary arteries is possible. With special techniques calculation of blood flow in the pulmonary and coronary arteries is possible.

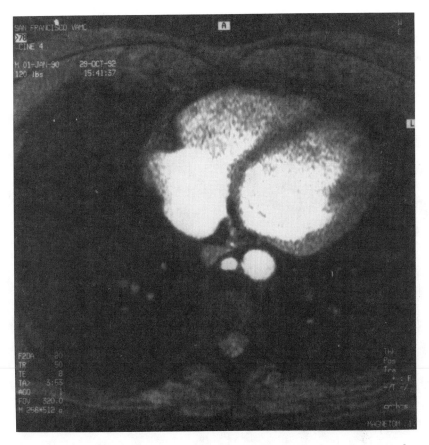

FIGURE 9-12. Example of transverse plane MRI image of the heart. Anatomical description of left and right ventricle, aorta, and intraventricular septum is possible. With gating of the image by the ECG calculation of EF% and identification of wall motion abnormalities is possible. Ventricular septal defects have been identified with MRI. With special techniques, calculation of aortic flow and distensibility can also be made.

Stress MRI

Stress MRI scanning has been used to detect coronary artery disease.[165] Comparison of MRI stress scanning with dobutamine-stress thallium-201 scintigraphy in 21 patients demonstrated close correspondence for the two techniques in detection of perfusion defects. The MRI scan can also provide a measure of aortic flow and of the velocity of ventricular wall motion. Ischemia can be detected by MRI evidence

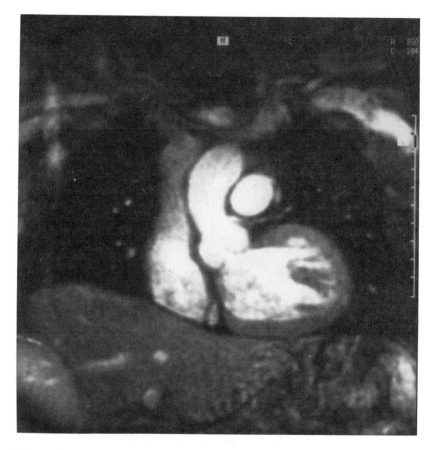

FIGURE 9-13. Example of frontal plane MRI image of the heart. Anatomical description of vena cava, right atrium, left ventricle with papillary muscles, aortic valve, aortic arch, and coronary arteries is possible. With gating of the image calculation of EF%, identification of wall motion abnormalities is possible. With special techniques calculation of flow can also be made.

of either wall motion abnormalities or failure to increase peak aortic flow during infusion of dobutamine.[165]

There are limitations to the MRI technology. Current scanners are long, narrow tubes into which patients must be placed for imaging. Some patients feel claustrophobic and require sedation. Because the area around the patient is very limited, MRI scanning is not currently useful intraoperatively. Additionally, patients with ferromagnetic implants (e.g., cerebral aneurysm clips, pacemakers) should not be placed in MRI scanners, and equipment used near an MRI scanner must be non-ferromagnetic to avoid damage to the scanner or severe injury to the patient. MRI scanners rely on superconducting magnets cooled by liquid helium to provide the large currents necessary to produce the large magnetic fields. Ingestion of a ferromagnetic object into the scanner may damage the container for the liquid helium cooling the superconducting magnet. Leakage of helium will rapidly neutralize the superconductivity of the magnetic coils. The resulting current can produce heat that will boil the remaining liquid helium and cause a large volume of gaseous helium to be released. This may cause suffocation and possible barotrauma if not adequately vented from the environment. A related limitation of MRI technology is the induction of electrical currents in loops of wire placed in the scanner, such as those contained in a pacemaker or pulmonary artery catheter. The time-varying magnetic field produces a current in wires that may burn the patient. Additionally, many electronic and mechanical devices do not function near the scanner due to either current induction or mechanical interference.

MRI scanning is presently used for cardiac imaging of both structure (hydrogen) and function (phosphorous) nuclei. MRI also can provide information on the chemical environment of each nuclei based on changes in the Larmor frequency. Despite its limitations, MRI has become an effective clinical and research tool. Although not currently used for intraoperative monitoring, MRI scanning often requires the clinical service of anesthesiologists to provide sedation and monitoring.

Impedance Cardiography

Blood is a conductor, and as it moves through the body, it alters local conductance. Time-varying changes in conductivity are described by a change in the impedance of an object. For example, the movement of blood during each heart beat alters thoracic impedance. Measurement of the thoracic impedance can detect changes in cardiac blood volume during each beat. Impedance is measured by passing a high-frequency alternating current across the thorax and measuring the resulting changes in voltage. The amplitude and phase of the resulting voltage at each frequency gives the impedance spectrum. Thoracic impedance changes with the cardiac cycle and can be used to calculate stroke volume and cardiac output. There is some correlation between measurements of stroke volume derived from thoracic impedance and thermodilution measurements.[166–173] but precise, reproducible quantification of stroke volume with impedance cardiography has remained elusive.

Several indices have been developed for use with impedance cardiography (Fig. 9–14). Preejection period (PEP) is defined as the time

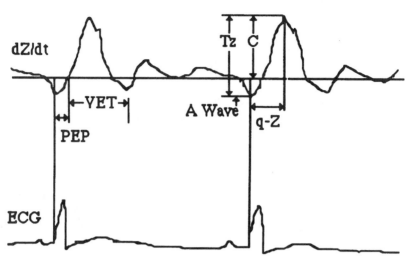

FIGURE 9-14. Example of first derivative with respect to time (*dZ/dt*) of the thoracic impedance waveform and ECG is shown to demonstrate the following features: systolic time intervals (*PEP* and *VET*). C-wave (maximum acceleration of blood during ventricular systole), A-*wave* (caused by atrial systole), T*z* (the sum of C- and A-wave magnitudes), and *q-Z* (the interval from the start of electrical ventricular systole to the point of maximum acceleration of blood during systole).

from the onset of electrical systole indicated by the electrocardiogram (as defined by the Q or R-wave) to the onset of changes in electrical impedance caused by ejection of blood from the ventricle. The ventricular ejection time (VET) is the time for the ejection of blood from the left ventricle defined by changes in electrical impedance. The ratio of PEP to VET is increased in hearts with reduced ventricular function. However, the correlation ($r = -0.90$) between the PEP to VET and EF measured by radionuclear techniques is negative.[174–176] That is, the PEP to VET ratio correlated poorly with radionuclear findings in patients with EF below 40%.[177]

The Heather index[178] is derived from the ratio of the magnitude of the impedance signal (C) divided by the time to peak of the maximum wave (q-Z). This index C/(q-Z) is lower in patients with New York Heart Association (NYHA) grade III to IV functional capacity than in patients who are NYHA grade I or II ($P = 0.001$).[178] Patients with reduced cardiac function have a reduction in the Heather index.[178–180]

Other ratios derived from the impedance waveforms include the C/T_z,[181,182] but the correlation of this index with radionuclear measurement of EF is poor.[183,184] The O-wave, a small, upward deflection in the first derivative with respect to the time of the impedance waveform, is enlarged in patients with CHF.[180,185] Indices of poor ventricular function have also been developed. In one study, the combination of historical cardiac risk factors with bioimpedance cardiodynamic measurements to stratify patients for operative risk proved predictive of cardiac death and potentially lethal cardiac complications.[186] However, none of these indices has been sufficiently reliable to be adopted for routine clinical use.

CONCLUSIONS

Prevention of deterioration of cardiac function is critical to perioperative survival. The preoperative evaluation of cardiac function can help to identify those patients at greatest risk for perioperative cardiac morbidity and mortality. The history and physical examination with specific attention to a recent myocardial infarction, presence of unstable angina, angina at rest, and CHF remain the key elements in perioperative evaluations of cardiac function. Echocardiographic or nuclear medicine evaluation of EF and wall motion analysis can predict perioperative survival. Coronary angiography and thallium radionuclide imaging can determine the presence of areas at risk for myocardial ischemia and the need for either coronary artery bypass surgery or angioplasty. The overall surgical mortality needs to be considered when making recommendations for preoperative cardiac procedures. Preoperative cardiac intervention is sensible only if the perioperative morbidity and mortality for the planned operation without surgical correction of the cardiac problem is greater than the combined mortality of a preoperative cardiac intervention plus that for the planned operation. The morbidity and mortality of angioplasty and coronary artery bypass graft surgery is substantial, and there remains a significant mortality for further surgeries despite coronary revascularization. Any strategy for the reduction of cardiac morbidity and mortality that relies on interventions that have risk must calculate the combined risk of all the procedures, not just the reduced risk to the planned procedure. Perioperative evaluation of cardiac function is critical to the prevention of cardiac morbidity and mortality.

Acknowledgments: We would like to thank Winifred Von Ehrenburg for her editorial assistance in the preparation of this chapter.

Bibliography

1. Frye R, Higgins M, Beller G, et al: Major demographic and epidemiologic trends affecting adult cardiology. J Am Coll Cardiol 12:840–846, 1988

2. Goldman L, Caldera D: Risks of general anesthesia and elective operation in the hypertensive patient. Anesthesiology 50:285–292, 1979
3. American Heart Association: 1992 Heart and Stroke Facts, p. 35, 1992
4. US Department of Commerce, Bureau of the Census. CPR: Current Population Reports, p. 23. Washington DC, US Department of Commerce, 1988
5. Mangano DT. Perioperative cardiac morbidity. Anesthesiology 72:153–84, 1990
6. Rao T, Jacobs K, El-Etr A. Reinfarction following anesthesia in patients with myocardial infarction. Anesthesiology 59:499–505, 1983
7. Goldman L, Caldera D. Nussbaum S, et al. Multifactorial index of cardiac risk in noncardiac surgical procedures. N Engl J Med 297:846–850, 1977
8. Driscoll A, Hobika J, Etsten B, et al. Clinically unrecognized myocardial infarction following surgery. N Engl J Med 264:633–639, 1961
9. Dack S. Symposium on cardiovascular-pulmonary problems before and after surgery: Postoperative problems. Am J Cardiol 12:423–430, 1963
10. Arkins R, Smessaert A, Hicks R. Mortality and morbidity in surgical patients with coronary artery disease. JAMA 190:485–488, 1964
11. Goldman L, Caldera DL, Nussbaum SR, et al. Multifactorial index of cardiac risk in noncardiac surgical procedures. N Engl J Med 297:845–850, 1977
12. Carliner NH, Fisher ML, Plotnick GD, et al. Routine preoperative exercise testing in patients undergoing major noncardiac surgery. Am J Cardiol 56:51–58, 1985
13. Foster E, Davis D, Carpenter J, et al. Risk of noncardiac operation in patients with defined coronary disease: The Coronary Artery Surgery Study (CASS) Registry Experience. Ann Thorac Surg 41:42–50, 1986
14. Knapp R, Topkins M, Artusio JJ: The cerebravascular accident and coronary occlusion in anesthesia. JAMA 182:332–334, 1962
15. Topkins M, Artusio J: Myocardial infarction and surgery: A five year study. Anesth Analg 43:716–720, 1964
16. Tarhan S. Moffitt E, Taylor W, et al: Myocardial infarction after general anesthesia. JAMA 220:1451–1454, 1972
17. Steen P, Tinker J, Tarhan S. Myocardial infarction after anesthesia and surgery. JAMA 239:2566–2570, 1978
18. Eerola M, Eerola E, Kaukinen S, et al. Risk factors in surgical patients with verified preoperative myocardial infarction. Acta Anaesthesiol Scand 24: 219–223, 1980
19. Hertzer N. Myocardial ischemia. Surgery 97–101, 1983
20. von Knorring J. Postoperative myocardial infarction: A prospective study in a risk group of surgical patients. Surgery 90:55–60, 1981
21. Schoeppel SL, Wilkinson C, Waters J, et al. Effects of myocardial infarction on perioperative cardiac complications. Anesth Analg 62:493–498, 1983
22. Larsen S. Olesen K, Jacobsen E, et al. Prediction of cardiac risk in non-cardiac surgery. Eur Heart J 8:179–185, 1987
23. Sapala JA, Ponka JL, Duvernoy WF. Operative and nonoperative risks in the cardiac patient. J Am Geriatr Soc 23:529–534, 1975
24. Cooperman M, Pflug B, Martin EJ, et al. Cardiovascular risk factors in patients with peripheral vascular disease. Surgery 84:505–509, 1978
25. Jamieson W, Janusz M, Miyagishima R, et al. Influence of ischemic heart disease on early and late mortality after surgery for peripheral occlusive vascular disease. Circulation 66:I92–I97, 1982
26. Mauney MJ, Ebert P, Sabiston DJ. Postoperative myocardial infarction: A study of predisposing factors, diagnosis and mortality in a high risk group of surgical patients. Ann Surg 1972:497–503, 1970

27. Prys-Roberts C, Meloche R, Foex P: Studies of anesthesia in relation to hypertension. I. Cardiovascular responses to treated and untreated patients. Br J Anaesth 43:122–137, 1971
28. Schneider AJ: Assessment of risk factors and surgical outcome. Surg Clin North Am 63:1113–1126, 1983
29. Jeffrey CC, Kunsman J, Cullen DJ, et al: A prospective evaluation of cardiac risk index. Anesthesiology 58:462–464, 1983
30. Boucher C. Brewster D, Darling R, et al. Determination of cardiac risk by dipyridamole thallium imaging before peripheral vascular surgery. N Engl J Med 312:389–394, 1985
31. Skinner J, Pearce M. Surgical risk in the cardiac patient. J Chron Dis 17:57–72, 1964
32. Scher K, Tice D. Operative risk in patients with previous coronary artery bypass. Arch Surg 111:807–809, 1976
33. McCollum C, Garcia-Rinaldi R, Graham J, et al. Myocardial revacularization prior to subsequent major surgery in patients with coronary artery disease. Surgery 81:302–304, 1977
34. Mahar L, Steen P, Tinker J. Peroperative myocardial infarction in patients with coronary artery disease with and without aorta-coronary bypass grafts. J Thorac Cardiovasc Surg 76:533–537, 1978
35. Crawford ES, Morris G Jr, Howell JF, et al. Operative risk in patients with previous coronary artery bypass. Ann Thorac Surg 26:215–221, 1978
36. Read R, Murphy M, Hultgren J, et al. Survival of men treated for chronic stable angina pectoris. A cooperative randomized study. J Thorac Cardiovasc Surg 75:1–16, 1978
37. Kimbris D, Segal B. Coronary disease progression in patients with and without saphenous vein bypass surgery. Am Heart J 102:811–818, 1981
38. Wells P, Kaplan J. Optimal management of patients with ischemic heart disease for noncardiac surgery by complementary anesthesiologist and cardiologist interactions. Am Heart J 102:1029–1037, 1981
39. Diehl J, Cali R, Hertzer N, et al: Complications of abdominal aortic reconstruction: An analysis of perioperative risk factors in 557 patients. Ann Surg 197:49–56, 1983
40. Hertzer NR, Beven EG, Young JR, et al: Coronary artery disease in peripheral vascular patients. A classification of 1000 coronary angiograms and results of surgical management. Ann Surg 199:223–233, 1984
41. Reul G Jr, Cooley DA, Duncan JM, et al. The effect of coronary bypass on the outcome of peripheral vascular operations in 1093 patients. J Vasc Surg 3:788–798, 1986
42. Miller R, Olson H, Amsterdam E, et al. Propranolol-withdrawal rebound phenomenon. Exacerbation of coronary events after abrupt cessation of anti-anginal therapy. N Engl J Med 293:416–418, 1975
43. Bruce D, Croley T, Lee J. Preoperative clonidine withdrawal syndrome. Anesthesiology 51:90–92, 1979
44. Foex P, Beta-blockade in anaesthesia. J Clin Hosp Pharm 8:1983–190, 1983.
45. Engelman R, Hadji-Rousou, I, Breyer R, et al. Rebound vasopasm after coronary revascularization in association with calcium antagonist withdrawal. Ann Thorac Surg 37:469–472, 1984
46. Cucchiara R, Benefiel D, Matteo R, et al. Evaluation of esmolol in controlling increases in heart rate and blood pressure during endotracheal intubation in patients undergoing carotid endarterectomy. Anesthesiology 65:528–531, 1986
47. Magnusson J, Thulin T, Werner O, et al. Haemodynamic effects of pre-

treatment with metroprolol in hypertensive patients undergoing surgery. Br J Anaesth 58:251–260, 1986

48. Stone JG, Foex P, Sear JW, et al. Myocardial ischemia in untreated hypertensive patients: Effect of a single small oral dose of a beta-adrenergic blocking agent. Anesthesiology 68:495, 1988

49. Vacanti C, VanHouten R, Hill R. A statistical analysis of the relationship of physical status to postoperative mortality in 68,388 cases. Anesth Analg 49:565–566, 1970

50. Djokovic J, Hedley-Whyte J: Prediction of outcome of surgery and anesthesia in patients over 80. JAMA 242:2301–2306, 1979

51. Zeldin RA: Assessing cardiac risk in patients who undergo noncardiac surgical procedures. Can J Surg 27:402–404, 1984

52. Detsky AS, Abrams HB, Forbath N, et al: The risk of anesthesia. Anesthesiology 33:130, 1970

53. Lewin I, Lerner A, Green S, et al. Physical class and physiological status in the prediction of operative mortality in the aged sick. Ann Surg 174:217–231, 1971

54. Gerson MC, Hurst JM, Hertzberg VS, et al. Cardiac prognosis in noncardiac geriatric surgery. Ann Intern Med 103:832–837, 1985

55. Baron JF, Mundler O, Bertrand M, et al. Dipyridamole-thallium scintigraphy and gated radionuclide angiography to assess cardiac risk before abdominal aortic surgery [see comments]. N Engl J Med 330:663–669, 1994

56. Mangano D. Biventricular function after myocardial revascularization in humans. Deterioration and recovery patterns during the first 24 hours. Anesthesiology 62:571–577, 1985

57. Pasternack PF, Imparato AM, Bear G, et al. The value of radionuclide angiography as a predictor of perioperative myocardial infarction in patients undergoing abdominal aortic aneurysm resection. J Vasc Surg 1:320–325, 1984

58. Pasternack PF, Imparato AM, Riles TS, et al. The value of the radionuclide angiogram in the prediction of perioperative myocardial infarction in patients undergoing lower extremity revascularization procedures. Circulation 72:II13–II17, 1985

59. Moraski R, Russel RJ, Smith M, et al. Left ventricular function in patients with and without myocardial infarction and one, two, or three vessel coronary artery disease. Am J Cardiol 35:1–10, 1975

60. National Center for Health Statistics, United States, pp. 10–17, 66, 67, 100, 101 Washington, DC, US Government Printing Office, 1988

61. Lewis BS, Emmott SN, Smyllie J, et al: Left ventricular systolic and diastolic function, and exercise capacity six to eight weeks after acute myocardial infarction. The DEFIANT Study Group. Doppler Flow and Echocardiography in Functional Cardiac Insufficiency: Assessment of Nisoldipine Therapy. Am J Cardiol 72:149–153, 1993

62. Young JB: Angiotensin-converting enzyme inhibitors in heart failure: New strategies justified by recent clinical trials. Int J Cardiol 43:151–163, 1994

63. Berlauk JF, Abrams, JH, Gilmour IJ, et al. Preoperative optimization of cardiovascular hemodynamics improves outcome in peripheral vascular surgery. Ann Surg 214:289–299, 1991

64. Wallace A, Lam HW, Nose PS, et al. Changes in systolic and diastolic ventricular function with cold cardioplegic arrest in man. J Card Surg 9:497–502, 1994

65. Fry DL, Griggs DM, Greenfield JCJ. Myocardial mechanics: Tension-velocity-length relationships of heart muscle. Circ Res 14:73–85, 1964

66. Ross JJ, Covell JW, Sonnenblick EH, et al. Contractile state of the heart char-

acterized by force-velocity relations in variably afterloaded and isovolumic beats. Circ Res 17:163–169, 1966

67. Covell JW, Ross JJ, Sonnenblick EH, et al. Comparison of force-velocity relation and the ventricular function curve as measures of the contractile state of the intact heart. Circ Res 19:364–372, 1966

68. Parmley WW. Mechanics of ventricular muscle. In Levine HJ, Gausch WH (eds): The Ventricle: Basic and Clinical Aspects, pp. 41–64. Boston, Martinus Nijhoff, 1985

69. Suga H, Sagawa K, Shoukas AA. Load independence of the instantaneous pressure-volume ratio of the canine left ventricle and effects of epinephrine and heart rate on the ratio. Circ Res 32:314–322, 1973

70. Burkhoff D, Sugiura S, Yue DT, et al. Contractility-dependent curvilinearity of end-systolic pressure-volume relations. Am J Physiol 252:H1218–H1227, 1987

71. Kass DA, Beyar R, Lankford E, et al: Influence of contractile state on curvilinearity of in situ end-systolic pressure-volume relations. Circulation 79:167–178, 1989

72. Liu CP, Ting CT, Yang TM, et al: Reduced left ventricular compliance in human mitral stenosis. Role of reversible internal constraint. Circulation 85:1447–1456, 1992

73. Takaoka H, Takeuchi M, Odake M, et al: Assessment of myocardial oxygen consumption (Vo2) and systolic pressure-volume area (PVA) in human hearts. Eur Heart J 13:85–90, 1992

74. Takaoka H, Takeuchi M, Odake M, et al. Comparison of the effects on arterial-ventricular coupling between phosphodiesterase inhibitor and dobutamine in the diseased human heart. J Am Coll Cardiol 22:598–606, 1993

75. Takaoka H, Takeuchi M, Odake M, et al. Comparison of hemodynamic determinants for myocardial oxygen consumption under different contractile states in human ventricle. Circulation 87:59–69, 1993

76. Takeuchi M, Takaoka H, Odake M, et al. Assessment of left ventricular function using a conductance catheter in the human heart. Jpn Circ J 56:730–734, 1992

77. Cho PW, Levin HR, Curtis WE, et al. Pressure-volume analysis of changes in cardiac function in chronic cardiomyoplasy. Ann Thorac Surg 56:38–45, 1993

78. Odake M, Takeuchi M, Takaoka H, et al. Determination of left ventricular volume using a conductance catheter in the diseased human heart. Eur Heart J 13:22–27, 1992

79. Wallace A, Bellows W, Moores W, et al. Left ventricular pressure-dimension relationship derived from invasive and non-invasive methods in man. Anesth Analg 78:s462, 1994

80. Wallace AW, Lam HW, Mangano DT, et al. Linearity, load dependence, hysteresis, and clinical associations of systolic and diastolic indices of left ventricular function in man. Card Surg in press, 1995

81. Liu CP, Ting CT, Lawrence W, et al. Diminished contractile response to increased heart rate in intact human left ventricular hypertrophy. Systolic versus diastolic determinants. Circulation 88:1893–1906, 1993

82. Takeuchi M, Odake M, Takaoka H, et al: Comparison between preload recruitable stroke work and the end-systolic pressure-volume relationship in man. Eur Heart J 13:80–84, 1992

83. Shintani H, Glantz SA: Influence of filling on left ventricular diastolic pressure-volume curve during pacing ischemia in dogs. Am J Physiol 266: H1373–H1385, 1994

84. Gorosan J, Gaslor TA, Deneault LG, et al: Transesophageal echocardiographic automated border detection for intraoperative evaluation of left ventricular pressure-area relationships. J Am Coll Cardiol 19:55A, 1992
85. Gorosan J, Deneault LG, Pinsky MR. Echocardiographic automated border detection for on-line determination of left ventricular function during acute alterations in preload. J Am Coll Cardiol 19:262A, 1992
86. Mangano DT. Monitoring pulmonary arterial pressure in coronary-artery disease. Anesthesiology 53:364–370, 1980
87. Dorman BH, Spinale FG, Kratz JM, et al. Use of a combined right ventricular ejection fraction-oximetry catheter system for coronary bypass surgery. Crit Care Med 20:1650–1656, 1992
88. Jardin F, Gueret P, Dubourg O, et al. Right ventricular volumes by thermodilution in the adult respiratory distress syndrome: A comparative study using two-dimensional echocardiography as a reference method. Chest 88:34–39, 1985.
89. Urban P, Scheidegger D, Gabathuler J, et al. Thermodilution determination of right ventricular volume and ejection fraction: A comparison with biplane angiography. Crit Care Med 15:652–655, 1987
90. Jardin F, Brun-Ney D, Hardy A, et al. Combined thermodilution and two-dimensional echocardiographic evaluation of right ventricular function during respiratory support with PEEP. Chest 99:162–168, 1991
91. Walczak F, Kepski R, Hoffman M. Early and late potentials in postinfarction patients. Clin Cardiol 15:898–902, 1992
92. Battler A, Froelicher VF, Gallagher KP, et al: Dissociation between regional myocardial dysfunction and ECG changes during ischemia in the conscious dog. Circulation 62:735–744, 1980
93. Roizen MF, Beaupre PN, Alpert RA, et al: Monitoring with two-dimensional transesophageal echocardiography. J Vasc Surg 1:300–305, 1984
94. London MJ, Tubau JF, Wong MG, et al: The "natural history" of segmental wall motion abnormalities detected by intraoperative transesophageal echocardiography: A clinically blinded, prospective approach. Anesthesiology 69:A7, 1988
95. Leung JM, O'Kelly B, Browner WS, et al. Prognostic importance of postbypass regional wall-motion abnormalities in patients undergoing coronary artery bypass graft surgery. SPI Research Group. Anesthesiology 71:16–25, 1989
96. Davila-Roman VG, Barzilai B, Wareing TH, et al. Intraoperative ultrasonographic evaluation of the ascending aorta in 100 consecutive patients undergoing cardiac surgery. Circulation 84:III47–III53, 1991
97. Crouse LJ, Cheirif J, Hanly DE, et al. Opacification and border delineation improvement in patients with suboptimal endocardial border definition in routine echocardiography: Results of the phase III Albunex Multicenter Trial. J Am Coll Cardiol 22:1494–1500, 1993
98. O'Kelly BF, Tubau JF, Knight AA, et al. Measurement of left ventricular contractility using transeophageal echocardiography in patients undergoing coronary artery bypass grafting. The Study of Perioperative Ischemia (SPI) Research Group. Am Heart J 122:1041–1049, 1991
99. Gorcsan J III, Gasior TA, Mandarino WA, et al. Assessment of the immediate effects of cardiopulmonary bypass on left ventricular performance by on-line pressure-area relations. Circulation 89:180–190, 1994
100. Gorcsan J III, Romand JA, Mandarino WA, et al. Assessment of left ventricular performance by on-line pressure-area relations using echocardiographic automated border detection. J Am Coll Cardiol 23:242–252, 1994

101. Cahalan MK, Ionescu P, Melton H Jr, et al: Automated real-time analysis of intraoperative transesophageal echocardiograms. Anesthesiology 78: 477–485, 1993

102. Marcus RH, Bednarz J, Coulden R, et al: Ultrasonic backscatter system for automated on-line endocardial boundary detection: Evaluation by ultrafast computed tomography. J Am Coll Cardiol 22:839–847, 1993

103. Gorcsan JIII, Lazar JM, Schulman DS, et al: Comparison of left ventricular function by echocardiographic automated border detection and by radionuclide ejection fraction. Am J Cardiol 72:810–815, 1993

104. Bahler RC, Vrobel TR, Martin P. The relation of heart rate and shortening fraction to echocardiographic indexes of left ventricular relaxation in normal subjects. J Am Coll Cardiol 2:926–933, 1983

105. Rokey R, Kuo LC, Zoghbi WA, et al. Determination of parameters of left ventricular diastolic filling with pulsed Doppler echocardiography: Comparison with cineangiography. Circulation 71:543–550, 1985

106. Friedman BJ, Drinkovic N, Miles H, et al. Assessment of left ventricular diastolic function: Comparison of Doppler echocardiography and gated blood pool scintigraphy (published erratum appears in J Am Coll Cardiol 9(5):1199, 1987). J Am Coll Cardiol 8:1348–1354, 1986

107. Spirito P, Maron BJ, Bonow RO. Noninvasive assessment of left ventricular diastolic function: Comparative analysis of Doppler echocardiographic and radionuclide angiographic techniques. J Am Coll Cardiol 7:518–526, 1986

108. Iwase M, Sotobata I, Takagi S, et al. Effects of diltiazem on left ventricular diastolic behavior in patients with hypertrophic cardiomyopathy: Evaluation with exercise pulsed Doppler echocardiography. J Am Coll Cardiol 9:1099–1105, 1987

109. Myreng Y, Myhre E. Effects of verapamil on left ventricular relaxation and filling dynamics in coronary artery disease: A study by pulsed Doppler echocardiography (see comments). Am Heart J 117:870–875, 1989

110. Shintani H, Glantz SA: Influence of filling on left ventricular diastolic pressure-volume curve during pacing ischemia in dogs. Am J Physiol 266:H1373–H1385, 1994

111. Klein AL, Hatle LK, Burstow DJ, et al: Doppler characterization of left ventricular diastolic function in cardiac amyloidosis. J Am Coll Cardiol 13:1017–1026, 1989

112. Pearson AC, Labovitz AJ, Mrosek D, et al: Assessment of diastolic function in normal and hypertrophied hearts: Comparison of Doppler echocardiography and M-mode echocardiography. Am Heart J 113:1417–1425, 1987

113. Wind BE, Snider AR, Buda AJ, et al. Pulsed Doppler assessment of left ventricular diastolic filling in coronary artery disease before and immediately after coronary angioplasty. Am J Cardiol 59:1041–1046, 1987

114. Takenaka K, Dabestani A, Gardin JM, et al. Pulsed Doppler echocardiographic study of left ventricular filling in dilated cardiomyopathy. Am J Cardiol 58:143–147, 1986

115. Takenaka K, Dabestani A, Gardin JM, et al. Left ventricular filling in hypertrophic cardiomyopathy: A pulsed Doppler echocardiographic study. J Am Coll Cardiol 7:1263–1271, 1986

116. Bryg RJ, Pearson AC, Williams GA, et al. Left ventricular systolic and diastolic flow abnormalities determined by Doppler echocardiography in obstructive hypertrophic cardiomyopathy. Am J Cardiol 59:925–931, 1987.

117. Appleton CP, Hatle LK, Popp RL. Demonstration of restrictive ventricu-

lar physiology by Doppler echocardiography (see comments). J Am Coll Cardiol 11:757–768, 1988

118. Appleton CP, Hatle LK, Popp RL. Cardiac tamponade and pericardial effusion: Respiratory variation in transvalvular flow velocities studied by Doppler echocardiography. J Am Coll Cardiol 11:1020–1030, 1988

119. Doss JK, Hillis LD, Curry G, et al. A new model for the assessment of regional ventricular wall motion. Radiology 143:763–770, 1982

120. Douglas AS, Rodriquez EK, O'Dell W, et al. Unique strain history during ejection in canine left ventricle. Am J Physiol 260:H1596–H1611, 1991

121. Liu YH, Bahn RC, Ritman EL: Dynamic intramyocardial blood volume: Evaluation with a radiological opaque marker method. Am J Physiol 263:H963–H967, 1992

122. Lipscomb K: Cardiac dimensional analysis by use of biplane cineradiography: Description and validation of method. Cathet Cardiovasc Diagn 6:451–464, 1980

123. Leshin SJ, Horwitz LD, Mitchell JH: Dimensional analysis of the left ventricle: Effects of acute aortic regurgitation. Am J Physiol 228:536–542, 1975.

124. Omens JH, Covell JW. Transmural distribution of myocardial tissue growth induced by volume-overload hypertrophy in the dog. Circulation 84:1235–1245, 1991

125. Rodriquez EK, Hunter WC, Royce MJ, et al. A method to reconstruct myocardial sarcomere lengths and orientations at transmural sites in beating canine hearts. Am J Physiol 263:H293–H306, 1992

126. Waldman LK, Fung YC, Covell JW. Transmural myocardial deformation in the canine left ventricle. Normal in vivo three-dimensional finite strains. Circ Res 57:152–163, 1985

127. Tsakiris AG, Mair DD, Seki S, et al. Motion of the tricuspid valve annulus in anesthetized intact dogs. Circ Res 36:43–48, 1975

128. Lankford EB, Kass DA, Maughan WL, et al. Does volume catheter parallel conductance vary during a cardiac cycle: Am J Physiol 258:H1933–H1942, 1990

129. Baan J, Van Der Velde ET, Steendijk P, et al. Calibration and application of the conductance catheter for ventricular volume measurement. Automedica 11:357–365, 1989

130. Burkhoff D. The conductance method of left ventricular volume estimation. Methodologic limitations put into perspective. Circulation 81:703–706, 1990

131. Woodard JC, Bertram CD, Gow BS. Right ventricular volumetry by catheter measurement of conductance. Pace Pacing Clin Electrophysiol 10:862–870, 1987

132. Woodard JC, Bertram CD, Gow BS. Detecting right ventricular volume changes using the conductance catheter. Pace Pacing Clin Electrophysiol 15:2283–2294, 1992

133. Carlson DE, Brunner MJ, Gann DS. Carotid baroreceptor control of right atrial mechanics in dogs. Am J Physiol 261:H1903–H1912, 1991

134. Blumgart HC, Weiss S: Studies on the velocity of blood flow. VII. The pulmonary circulation time in normal resting individuals. J Clin Invest 4:399, 1927

135. Mangano DT, Massie BM, Browner WS: the dipyridamole-thallium test [letter; comment]. Circulation 84:1879–1880, 1991

136. Mangano DT, London MJ, Tubau JF, et al: Dipyridamole thallium-201 scintigraphy as a preoperative screening test. A reexamination of its pre-

dictive potential. Study of Perioperative Ischemia Research Group [see comments]. Circulation 84:493–502, 1991
137. Jengo JA, Mena J, Blaufuss A, et al. Evaluation of left ventricular function (ejection fraction and segmental wall motion) by a single pass radioisotope angiography. Circulation 57:326, 1978
138. Marshall RC, Berger HJ, Costin JC, et al. Assessment of cardiac performance with quantitative radionuclide angiocardiography: Sequential left ventricular ejection fraction, normalized left ventricular ejection rate and regional wall motion. Circulation 56:820, 1977
139. Schelbert HR, Verba JW, Johnson AD, et al. Non traumatic determination of left ventricular ejection fraction by radionuclide angiography. Circulation 51:902, 1975
140. Berger HJ, Matthay RA, Loke J, et al. Assessment of cardiac performance with quantitative radionuclide angiocardiography. Right ventricular ejection fraction with reference to findings in chronic obstructive pulmonary disease. Am J Cardiol 41:897, 1978
141. Sandler H, Dodge HT. The use of single plane angiocardiograms for the calculation of left ventricular volume in man. Am Heart J 75:325, 1968
142. Polak JF, Kemper AJ, Bianco JA, et al. A sensitive index of myocardial dysfunction in patients with coronary artery disease. J Nucl Med 23:471, 1982.
143. Papapietro SE, Yester MV, Logic JR, et al. Method for quantitative analysis of regional left ventricular function with first pass and gated blood pool scintigraphy. Am J Cardiol 47:618, 1981
144. Ratib O, Henze E, Schon H, et al. Phase analysis of radionuclide ventriculograms for the detection of coronary artery disease. Am Heart J 104:1, 1982
145. Vos PH, Vossepoel AM, Pauwels EKJ: Quantitative assessment of wall motion in multiple-gated studies using temporal fourier analysis. J Nucl Med 24:388, 1983
146. Vogel M, Buhlemeyer K. [Diagnosis of congenital heart defects today. Part 2: Aortic stenosis, aortic isthmus stenosis, tetralogy of Fallot, transposition of great vessels]. Fortschr Med 110:319–321, 1992
147. Roudaut RP, Marcaggi XL, Deville C, et al. Value of transesophageal echocardiography combined with computed tomography for assessing repaired type A aortic dissection. Am J Cardiol 70:1468–1476, 1992
148. George G, Erbel R, Gerber T, et al. [Intravascular ultrasound in patients with suspected aortic dissection: Comparison with transesophageal echocardiography]. Z Kardiol 81:37–43, 1992
149. Skioldebrand CG, Lipton MJ, Redington RW, et al. Myocardial infarction in dogs, demonstrated by non-enhanced computed tomography. Acta Radiol [Diagn] 22:1–8, 1981
150. Hamada S. Naito H, Takamiya M. Evaluation of myocardium in ischemic heart disease by ultrafast computed tomography. Jpn Circ J 56:627–631, 1992
151. Naito H, Saito H, Ohta M, et al. Significance of ultrafast computed tomography in cardiac imaging: Usefulness in assessment of myocardial characteristics and cardiac function. Jpn Circ J 54:322–327, 1990
152. Khan A, Mond DJ, Kallman CE, et al. Computed tomography of normal and calcified coronary arteries. J Thorac Imaging 9:1–7, 1994
153. Kaufman RB, Sheedy P II, Breen JF, et al. Detection of heart calcification with electron beam CT: Interobserver and intraobserver reliability for scoring quantification. Radiology 190:347–352, 1994

154. Muhlberger V, zur Nedden D, Knapp E, et al. [Evaluation of coronary artery graft patency by computed tomography. Comparison with coronary arteriography (author's transl)]. Z Kardiol 70:377–379, 1981

155. Senda Y, Tohkai H, Kimura M, et al: ECG-gated cardiac scan and echocardiographic assessments of left ventricular hypertrophy: Reversal by 6-month treatment with diltiazem. J Cardiovasc Pharmacol 16:298–304, 1990

156. Ritchie CJ, Godwin JD, Crawford CR, et al: Minimum scan speeds for suppression of motion artifacts in CT. Radiology 185:37–42, 1992

157. Flicker S, Naidech HJ, Altin RS, et al: Ultrafast computed tomography techniques in cardiac disease. J Thorac Imaging 4:42–49, 1989

158. Mathru M, Wolfkiel CJ, Jelnin V, et al. Measurement of right ventricular volume in human explanted hearts using ultrafast cine computed tomography. Chest 105:585–588, 1994

159. Rich S, Chomka EV, Stagl R, et al. Determination of left ventricular ejection fraction using ultrafast computed tomography. Am Heart J 112:392–396, 1986

160. MacMillan RM, Rees MR, Maranhao V, et al. Rapid acquisition computed tomographic assessment of left ventricular regional wall motion using a new long axis view. Angiology 37:372–377, 1986

161. Feiring AJ, Rumberger JA, Reiter SJ, et al. Determination of left ventricular mass in dogs with rapid-acquisition cardiac computed tomographic scanning. Circulation 72:1355–1364, 1985

162. Lipton MJ, Farmer DW, Killebrew EJ, et al. Regional myocardial dysfunction: Evaluation of patients with prior myocardial infarction with fast CT. Radiology 157:735–740, 1985

163. Partain CL, Jones JP. Physics of magnetic resonance. In Taveras J, Ferrucci J, (eds): Radiology: Diagnosis—Imaging—Intervention, vol. 1, pp. 1–14. Philadelphia, JB Lippincott, 1991

164. Zhang Y, Imai K, Araki Y, et al. Assessment of ejection fraction of the right and left ventricles in patients with acute myocardial infarction by magnetic resonance imaging. Jpn Circ J 57:512–520, 1993

165. Pennell DJ, Underwood SR. The cardiovascular effects of dobutamine assessed by magnetic resonance imaging. Postgrad Med J 67:S1–S9, 1991.

166. Secher NJ, Thomsen A, Arnsbo P: Measurement of rapid changes in cardiac stroke volume. An evaluation of the impedance cardiography method. Acta Anaesthesiol Scand 21:353–358, 1977

167. Goldstein DS, Cannon RO, Zimlichman R, et al: Clinical evaluation of impedance cardiography. Clin Physiol 6:235–251, 1986

168. Donovan KD, Dobb GJ, Woods WPD, et al: Comparison of transthoracic electrical impedance and thermodilution methods for measuring cardiac output. Crit Care Med 14:1038–1044, 1986

169. Judy WV, Powner DJ, Parr K, et al. Comparison of electrical impedance and thermal dilution measured cardiac output in the critical care setting. Crit Care Med 13:305, 1985

170. Appel PL, Kram HB, Mackabee J, et al. Comparison of measurements of cardiac output by bioimpedance and thermodilution in severely ill surgical patients. Crit Care Med 14:933–935, 1986

171. Spinale FG, Reines HD, Crawford FA. Comparison of bioimpedance and thermodilution methods for determining cardiac output. Experimental and clinical studies. Ann Thorac Surg 45:421–425, 1988

172. Saladin V, Zussa C, Risica G, et al. Comparison of cardiac output estimation by thoracic electrical bioimpedance, thermodilution, and fick methods. Crit Care Med 16:1157–1158, 1988

173. Castor G, Molter G, Helms J, et al. Determination of cardiac output during positive end-expiratory pressure—noninvasive electrical bioimpedance compared with standard thermodilution. Crit Care Med 18:544–546, 1990

174. Garrad CL, Weissler AM, Dodge HT. The relationship of alterations in systolic time intervals to ejection fraction in patients with cardiac disease. Circulation 52:455–462, 1970

175. Capan LM, Bernstein DP, Patel KP, et al. Measurement of ejection fraction by bioimpedance method. Crit Care Med 15:402, 1987

176. Hanna L, Lopez-Majano V, Ward J, et al: Non-invasive ejection fraction monitoring: A comparison of the impedance method to the radionuclide cardiography. Anaesthesia 69:A308, 1988

177. Appel PL, Bernstein DP, Patel KP, et al: Evaluation of a continuous, on line, real time non invasive cardiac output and ejection fraction measurement by electrical bioimpedance in critically ill patients. Crit Care Med 15:364, 1987

178. Heather LW: A comparison of cardiac output values by the impedance cardiograph and dye dilution techniques in cardiac patients. Natl Aeronaut Space Admin CR.10 N70–10015:247–258, 1969

179. Richards NT, McBrien DJ. Changes in the impedance cardiogram occurring with change in posture in patients with heart disease. Int J Cardiol 20:365–372, 1988

180. Hubbard WN, Fish DR, McBrien DJ. The use of impedance cardiography in heart failure. Int J Cardiol 12:71–79, 1986

181. Judy WV, Hall JJ, Elliot WC. Left ventricular ejection fraction measured by the impedance cardiographic method. Fed Proc 42:1006, 1983

182. Judy WV, Demeter RJ, Toth PD. Fluid challenge assessment by bioelectric impedance. Crit Care Med 14:379, 1986

183. Fuller HD, Turpie F, Raskob G, et al. Validity of ejection fraction determination by impedance cardiography. Clin Invest Med 14(suppl A):A22, 1991

184. Miles DS, Gotshall RW, Quinones JD, et al. Impedance cardiography fails to measure accurately left ventricular ejection fraction. Crit Care Med 18:221–228, 1990

185. Gabriel S, Oro L. The effect of posture on the first derivative thoracic impedance cardiogram in patients with myocardial infarction. Acta Med Scand 198:219–221, 1975

186. Jivegard L, Haljamae H, Holm J, et al. Cardiac risk screening of peripheral arterial surgical patients by the use of combined simple clinical and non-invasive cardiodynamic parameters. Eur J Vasc Surg 7:180–187, 1993

Index

Page numbers followed by t or f indicate tables or figures, respectively.